Endometrial Ablation

For Churchill Livingstone

Publisher: Peter Richardson
Project Editor: Lucy Gardner
Editorial Co-ordination: Editorial Resources Unit
   Copy Editor: Rich Cutler
   Indexer: John R. Sampson
Production Controller: Neil Dickson
Design: Design Resources Unit
Sales Promotion Executive: Kathy Crawford

Endometrial Ablation

Edited by

B. Victor Lewis MD FRCS (Edin) FRCOG
Consultant Obstetrician/Gynaecologist, Watford General Hospital, Watford, UK

Adam L. Magos BSc MD MRCOG
Consultant Obstetrician and Gynaecologist, University Department of Obstetrics and Gynaecology, Royal Free Hospital, London, UK

Foreword by
Milton Goldrath MD
Department of Obstetrics & Gynecology, Sinai Hospital of Detroit, Detroit, Michigan, USA

CHURCHILL LIVINGSTONE
EDINBURGH LONDON MADRID MELBOURNE NEW YORK AND TOKYO 1993

CHURCHILL LIVINGSTONE
Medical Division of Longman Group UK Limited

Distributed in the United States of America by Churchill
Livingstone Inc., 650 Avenue of the Americas, New York,
N. Y. 10011, and by associated companies, branches and
representatives throughout the world.

First published 1993

ISBN 0-443-04587-9

British Library Cataloguing in Publication Data
A catalogue record for this book is available from the British
Library.

Library of Congress Cataloging in Publication Data
Endometrial ablation/edited by B. Victor Lewis, Adam L.
Magos; foreword by Milton Goldrath.
     p.   cm.
   Includes index.
   ISBN 0-443-04587-9
   1. Endometrium--Endoscopic surgery. I. Lewis, B.
Victor. II. Magos, Adam L.
   [DNLM: 1. Endometrium--surgery. WP 400 E554]
RG104.7.E53 1992
618. 1'45--dc20
DNLM/DLC
for Library of Congress   92–21014
                     CIP

The
publisher's
policy is to use
**paper manufactured
from sustainable forests**

Printed in Hong Kong
NPC/01

Foreword

When I was asked to write the foreword for the volume *Endometrial Ablation*, I looked upon it with great humility mixed with considerable pride. The development of endometrial ablation and its continued application have occupied a large portion of my professional career and I am particularly pleased that the procedure has gained so much popularity that a volume devoted to it has become necessary.

Since Asherman in 1948 first described the syndrome which bears his name, gynaecologists have used numerous methods to attempt to duplicate the clinical picture. Endometrial ablation was first consistently performed using the Nd:YAG laser in 1979. It was felt that the procedure would achieve acceptance in a relatively short period of time, and indeed, in many parts of the world this has been so.

Interest in endometrial ablation led to rapid proliferation of hysteroscopy as a diagnostic procedure. This resulted in more accurate preoperative evaluations of patients with bleeding disorders and more appropriate selection of patients for ablative techniques or other hysteroscopic surgery. This is very well described in the volume.

Subsequent to the development of endometrial ablation utilizing the Nd:YAG laser, other methods have been used successfully to destroy the endometrium. These are very well described in this volume. With time I am confident additional methods will be developed. Hysteroscopic use of the urologic resectoscope was first performed by Neuwirth in 1976 for the removal of submucous leiomyomas. Following the development of endometrial ablative techniques, this was extended to endometrial resection and other hysteroscopic methods for treatment of leiomyomata of the uterus. Proliferation of these techniques has been geometric.

Of more importance is the increasing incidence of complications as more and more gynaecologists perform endometrial ablation and other hysteroscopic operations. These complications are very adequately described in this volume and point out that increased training and skill are necessary in performing hysteroscopic procedures. There can be no progress without some complications. However, physicians must be aware of the possibility and be alert to prevention and treatment.

I look forward to the further development of this very interesting approach to the management of uterine bleeding disorders and I'm sure the future will bring additional procedures which will be much less skill-dependent and which hopefully will result in fewer complications.

1993   M. G.

Preface

This book seeks to review the rapidly expanding subject of endometrial ablation. There has been enormous worldwide interest in a simple surgical alternative to abdominal or vaginal hysterectomy. It is a relatively short time since Goldrath first described laser ablation and De Cherney described electroresection for functional bleeding. In the last 5 years, there has been an exponential growth of interest in the subject, and, in the United States and Europe, numerous training courses and clinical meetings are being held. This is important because high technology is involved and, as the use of video cameras is needed, surgeons must retrain to master new surgical skills. National and International Laparoscopic and Hysteroscopic Societies have been formed by enthusiastic practitioners, which are responsible for organizing meetings and training courses, and a new Journal— *Gynaecological Endoscopy*—will publish data on this exciting and expanding field.

The main aim of this book is to review critically the different technologies available for ablation of the endometrium, with recognized experts from the United States and Europe as contributors. The object is to provide a balanced view of current clinical opinion, bearing in mind the short time during which these operations have been performed. Wherever possible, comparative results from the literature are given, together with the medium- and short-term complication rates. It must be remembered however that the complication rates are those described by experts, and may be higher with inexperienced surgeons. Dr Gordon rightly emphasizes that, in the early phase of the learning curve, diagnostic hysteroscopy must first be performed until familiarity with the appearance of the normal endometrium during different phases of the menstrual cycle is understood.

Long-term complication rates are not yet available. The experience of individual surgeons is relatively small, but it is hoped that national surveys will soon be started to provide a database from which the complications can be calculated. Ablation should be considered in women in whom hysterectomy is the only alternative procedure because of heavy bleeding which limits social activity and causes anaemia. Endometrial ablation should not be performed in women with minor menstrual disturbance, or without careful patient selection and detailed clinical and hysteroscopic examination to exclude unexpected pathology such as pelvic inflammatory disease and endometriosis. Endometrial ablation should only be performed at present in women with severe functional bleeding, or submucous myomas, although it may be helpful in dysmenorrhoea due to adenomyosis.

Because long-term follow-up studies are not available there is minimal information about the annual recurrence rates of menorrhagia, and there is no information available on women who have had endometrial ablation and subsequently present for hysterectomy. However, if patients are carefully selected, an annual recurrence rate of 5 or 10% is acceptable, particularly when the ablation is performed in perimenopausal women.

There are considerable practical difficulties in performing randomized controlled trials between drug treatment, endometrial ablation and hysterectomy. The main problem is that of obtaining sufficient numbers of cooperative women, and of persuading women to agree to randomization. Many patients will choose an ablation procedure in preference to a hysterectomy when they know they can be treated as out-patients, or with a minimal hospital stay. In spite of these problems, three randomized trials are currently being evaluated in the United Kingdom, and it is probable that further trials will soon be published in the international literature, and thus the definitive role of endometrial ablation will become apparent.

Watford and   B. V. L.
London, 1993   A. L. M.

Contributors

Stephen G. Bown MD FRCP
ICRF Professor of Laser Medicine and Surgery and Director of the National Medical Laser Centre, University College London, The Rayne Institute, London, UK

J. A. Mark Broadbent BSc MB BS MRCOG
Research Fellow, Minimally Invasive Therapy Unit, University Department of Obstetrics and Gynaecology, The Royal Free Hospital, London, UK

Julie Crow BSc MB BS FRCPath
Senior Lecturer, Department of Histopathology, Royal Free Hospital School of Medicine, London, UK

Alan H. De Cherney MD
Phaneuf Professor and Chairman, Department of Obstetrics and Gynecology, Tufts University School of Medicine, Boston, Massachusetts, USA

Jonathan A. Davis FRCOG
Consultant Gynaecologist, Department of Gynaecology, Stobhill Hospital, Glasgow, UK

Sjoerd de Blok MD PhD
Consultant Obstetrician and Gynaecologist, Onze Lieve Vrouwe Gasthuis, Amsterdam; Lecturer/Secretary, Hysteroscopic Training Centre, Spaarne Hospital, The Netherlands

Maurizio Colafranceschi MD
Associated Professor of Pathology, Institute of Pathology, University of Florence, Italy

C. J. Richard Elliott MB BS FRCAnaes DA
Consultant, Departments of Anaesthesia, Queen Elizabeth II, Welwyn Garden City and St. Albans City Hospital (Retired); Locum Consultant, Department of Anaesthesia, Royal Free Hospital, London, UK (Retired)

A. Gallinat MD
Center of Gynaecological Endoscopy, Hamburg, Germany

Ray Garry MD FRCOG
Medical Director, Women's Endoscopic Laser Foundation; Consultant Gynaecologist, South Cleveland Hospital, Middlesbrough, UK

Alan G. Gordon MB FRCS FRCOG
Consultant Gynaecologist, Princess Royal Hospital, Hull, UK

N. C. W. Hill MD MRCOG
Lecturer/Honorary Senior Registrar, University Department of Obstetrics and Gynaecology, The Royal Free Hospital and Medical School, London, UK

Michelle D. Judd MRCOG
Research Registrar in Gynaecology, National Medical Laser Centre, University College London, The Rayne Institute, London, UK

Annette I. La Morte MD
Postdoctoral Associate, Department of Obstetrics and Gynaecology, Yale University School of Medicine, New Haven, Connecticut, USA

B. Victor Lewis MD FRCS(Edin) FRCOG
Consultant Obstetrician and Gynaecologist, Watford General Hospital, Watford, UK

Franklin D. Loffer MD
Director, Gynecological Endoscopy, Maricopa Medical Center, Phoenix, Arizona, USA

R. P. Leuken MD
Centre of Gynaecological endoscopy,
Hamburg, Germany

Russell Macdonald MB FRCS MRCOG
Senior Registrar in Obstetrics and Gynaecology,
Hillingdon Hospital and Queen Charlotte's and
Chelsea Hospitals, London, UK

Adam L. Magos MD MRCOG
Consultant Obstetrician and Gynaecologist,
University Department of Obstetrics and
Gynaecology, Royal Free Hospital, London, UK

Klim McPherson MA PhD
Professor of Public Health Epidemiology, Unit
of Health Promotion Sciences, Department of
Public Health and Policy, London School of
Hygiene and Tropical Diseases, London, UK

Colin D. Miller MB ChB FRCAnaes
Consultant Anaesthetist, Stobhill General
Hospital, Glasgow, UK

V. J. Page MB ChB FRCAnaes
Senior Registrar, Department of
Anaesthesia, Royal Postgraduate
Medical School, Hammersmith Hospital,
London, UK

Jeffrey H. Phipps BSc MRCOG
Consultant Gynaecologist, The George Eliot
Centre for Minimally Invasive Surgery,
Nuneaton, UK

Terry Smith BSc MSc PhD
Senior Scientist, Section of Medical Physics,
Clinical Research Centre, Harrow, UK

C. J. G. Sutton MB BChir FRCOG
Consultant Gynaecologist, Royal Surrey County
Hospital, Guildford, UK

Thierry G. Vancaillie MD
Director, Center for Gynecological Endosurgery,
San Antonio, Texas, USA

Kees Wamsteker MD PhD
Director, Hysteroscopy Training Centre (HTC-
NL); Senior Staff Gynaecologist, Department of
Obstetrics and Gynaecology, Spaarne Hospital,
Haarlem, The Netherlands

Contents

1. History of operative hysteroscopy

A. LaMorte   A. H. De Cherney

Over the past two decades, operative hysteroscopy has become a widely implemented technology. Its roots, however, date back to almost two centuries ago when Bozzini in 1805 suggested that a device called a light conductor be used to study the interior of the uterus for a variety of conditions (Bauer 1966). He examined the nasal passage, the vagina and the rectum. The device consisted of a tubular speculum through which candlelight was directed by a concave mirror. The results were unsatisfactory.

In 1865, Desormeaux introduced the first endoscope that actually permitted inspection of internal organs. The instrument consisted of a straight tube with a kerosene lamp or candle used as a light source. He intended the instrument to be used for examination of the bladder and urethra.

Historically, advances in hysteroscopy paralleled developments in cystoscopy. The former tended to lag behind, however, due to problems with uterine distention and adequate visualization.

Credit for the first hysteroscopy is often given to Pantaleoni. In 1869 he used a device similar to the one developed by Desormeaux to view the interior of the uterus in a 60-year-old woman with therapy-resistant bleeding. A polypoid growth was observed and cauterized with silver nitrate.

A cystoscope closer to modern-day design was introduced by Nitze (1879). His cystoscope had optical lenses built into the instrument and the illuminator was inserted with the examination device directly into the urinary bladder. These improvements helped to achieve a wider field of vision and more intense illumination within the bladder.

Bumm was one of the first to extensively study hysteroscopy and its use in gynaecology: using a modified urethroscope he reported the results of a series of intrauterine endoscopic examinations to the Vienna Congress in 1895. By direct inspection he was able to diagnose such conditions as endometritis, carcinomas and other tumours in the corpus. In addition, he called attention to the difficulties met with when bleeding obscured the view. A headlamp with an incandescent light reflector served as an illuminator.

Modern hysteroscopy began in the early 1900s when David performed hysteroscopy using a cystoscope with an internal light and lens system. In his report (David 1908) he fully described the technique, indications, contraindications, dangers and uses of the hysteroscope; 25 cases without complication were presented. His instrument consisted of a sheath into which fitted the cystoscope closed at the far end by a glass crystal and containing near it an incandescent lamp. A magnifying lens was attached at the ocular or near end. David suggested that, by enclosing the lamp, compromise of the visual field by bleeding was avoided. By varying the size of the sheath in accordance with anatomical variations, anaesthesia was not necessary.

Heineberg published an account of his hysteroscopic method 6 years later (Heineberg 1914). He described an internally illuminated endoscopic tube with a water-irrigating system surrounding the inner opening. The purpose of the water was to wash away obscuring blood. The number of examinations performed with the instrument was 20, most with satisfactory results. The need for a hysteroscopic method was strongly emphasized and illustrated by two cases which had been erroneously diagnosed after examination by conventional means.

In 1925, Rubin published a hallmark paper in which he compared the use of hysteroscopy to that of cystoscopy. Conceptually, both procedures resembled each other. Hysteroscopy, however, had failed to become widely used and accepted to the degree cystoscopy had. Rubin regarded the small slit-like uterine cavity and propensity for bleeding from the endometrium as obstacles to the development of hysteroscopy. Techniques intended to overcome these obstacles were detailed in his paper. Adequate uterine distention was achieved with carbon dioxide gas or dry air by insufflating the uterus with the carbon dioxide tank or a rubber bulb or syringe.

Rubin considered the cystourethroscope as devised by McCarthy to be the best adapted for the purpose of hysteroscopy. The outer sheath with the obturator in place had a well-rounded tip for easy insertion and resulted in less trauma to the endometrium.

In his publication, Rubin included 26 hysteroscopic cases in which he detailed points of technical interest or described interesting findings. He described using a wider sheath that allowed use of an operating instrument such as scissors or fulguration wire. A method of amputating objects by sucking or pressing them into an oval window and rotating an outer sheath over this window to sever the base of the object was reported. The advantages of hysteroscopy and contraindications to the procedure were also included.

Rubin experimented with water irrigation and found that positive pressure was necessary to dislodge clots or cleanse the instrument tip. Negative pressure was felt to be gentler, however, and was therefore preferred. The inability of negative-pressure irrigation to remove coagulated blood or have a haemostatic effect caused Rubin to abandon water use.

Seymour (1925) reported using suction for removing blood during hysteroscopy. His hysteroscope resembled a bronchoscope. Along the length were arranged three channels. In one channel there was a replaceable tubular light. Continuous suction was maintained through the other two channels. Since the field of vision was limited, the examination had to be done in stages.

In 1927, von Mikulicz-Radecki & Freund presented an account of their experiences with hysteroscopy. They used a water rinsing system to keep the objective lens clean. Saline was admitted through an inlet tube and discharged through an outlet tube. It was considered purposeless to try to keep the uterine cavity dilated by means of a liquid because the liquid would mix with the blood and prevent adequate visualization. Attempts were made at catheterization of the fallopian tubes and biopsies were made under direct visualization.

Gauss (1928) achieved adequate intrauterine visualization by means of an optical instrument into which a flow of liquid was directed from a height of 50 cm. The outflowing liquid was drained into a receptacle. Gauss wrote enthusiastically about his experiences and remarked that hysteroscopy would find wide application.

Schroeder (1934), a student of Gauss', continued his work and improved on the right-angle lens by making the optic system forward-viewing. He attempted one of the first hysteroscopic sterilizations using electrocoagulation. His two cases both failed.

Norment continued attempts at improving visualization during hysteroscopy. He published a summary of his experiences and detailed his hysteroscopic technique (Norment et al 1957). The development of his instrument encompassed a period of 18 years. Initially, an inflatable rubber bag over the objective lens was used to keep the uterus dilated. The rubber bag was transparent and allowed examination of the uterine cavity in some cases, but in others it became wrinkled and rendered direct inspection impossible. After a few years he abandoned this method and used a piece of transparent plastic. Blood and secretions were removed using a water rinsing system. Based upon his results, Norment pointed out the superiority of hysteroscopy over hysterography.

The use of a water-filled balloon to distend the uterine cavity and prevent bleeding was reported by Silander (1962) 5 years later. Others found this method unsatisfactory because the balloon compressed the endometrium and therefore modified its appearance.

The development of glass fibre optics during the late 1950s and early 1960s helped to advance hysteroscopy and the field of endoscopy in general. In 1963, Mohri and co-workers introduced a hysterofibrescope which they used to observe intrauterine phenomena late in pregnancy (Mohri et al 1986). Although the fibreoptic hysteroscope may be useful for specific procedures, the major contribution of fibreoptics technology to operative hysteroscopy to date has been in providing a convenient, flexible light source.

During the 1970s, various methods were introduced to improve uterine distention. Edstrom & Fernstrom (1970) used 32% dextran 70 and found it superior to previously described methods. Due to high viscosity it was not miscible with blood. This property allowed continued examination with good visibility in the presence of a modest amount of bleeding and made it useful in both diagnostic and operative hysteroscopy. Allergic reactions and rare pulmonary oedema were reported with intrauterine instillation of 32% dextran 70 (Maddi et al 1969, Leake et al 1987), but limiting the amount of medium instilled has helped to prevent these complications. Levine & Neuwirth (1972) used 30% dextran successfully. Lindemann (1973) used carbon dioxide gas and a hysteroscope adaptor that fitted over the cervix which he developed to prevent escape of the gas. Early use of insufflation equipment in the uterus with high flow rates designed for laparoscopy resulted in cardiac arrhythmias and arrest (Porto 1974). Insufflators especially designed for hysteroscopy have made use of this medium safe. A disadvantage of carbon dioxide in operative hysteroscopy is the presence of air bubbles that mix with blood and obscure the field. 5% dextrose and saline were found to be safe distention media and easy to deliver. Their low viscosity makes them miscible with blood and therefore not good media for operative hysteroscopy where bleeding may occur. Saline also has excellent conductance and cannot be used if an electric current is involved in a hysteroscopic procedure.

With improvements in uterine distention methods 20 years ago, operative hysteroscopy in its modern form began to develop. Edstrom (1974) was one of the first to describe a number of intra-uterine surgical procedures during hysteroscopy. He addressed removal of intra-uterine devices using the hysteroscope and suggested use of strong, firmly attached forceps

for this procedure. Siegler & Kemmann (1976) reported hysteroscopic removal of misplaced or embedded intrauterine devices using a grasping forceps through the operating channel. Valle et al (1977) used hysteroscopy as a primary method to locate and remove intrauterine devices with missing filaments.

The use of hysteroscopy offered an improvement over previously described methods in the diagnosis and treatment of intrauterine adhesions. Levine & Neuwirth (1973) used hysteroscopy and laparoscopy to evaluate ten patients with hysterographic diagnosis of Asherman's syndrome. In four of these patients, synechiae were dissected under direct vision through the hysteroscope using miniature scissors or an electrocautery probe. This report served to focus attention on important advantages gained with the use of the hysteroscope in patients with Asherman's syndrome. The procedure was felt to show promise because it was more accurate than blind curettage or dissection and safer than laparotomy. Laparoscopy was pointed out as being essential in this procedure to serve as a safety precaution to avoid uterine perforation. An alternative technique was reported by Edstrom (1974), who described a series of nine patients who had intrauterine synechiae either simply ruptured by the endoscope or excised at the base and top with the biopsy forceps. March et al (1978) published a series of 66 patients who underwent hysteroscopic lysis of adhesions using miniature scissors. Short-term results were excellent with 98% incidence of resumption of normal menses in women with secondary amenorrhoea and hypomenorrhoea. Of those studied postlysis of adhesions, 94% had a normal uterine cavity. Sugimoto (1978) reported hysteroscopic adhesiolysis by using the outer sleeve of the hysteroscope to break the adhesion under visual control. In both March's and Sugimoto's series the pregnancy rate among those who wished to conceive surpassed that achieved with earlier therapeutic modalities, such as repeat curettage or hysterotomy (March & Israel 1981).

In addition to lysing intrauterine adhesions, hysteroscopy also was employed to develop new techniques of myomectomy. One of the first references to hysteroscopic myomectomy was by

Norment in 1957. He described a resecting loop for the resection of wide based polyps and submucosal fibroids. An analogy to transurethral prostatic resection was made. Norment specified tumours to be removed with a cutting current and the base fulgurated later. No specific cases were reported.

In 1976, Neuwirth & Amin reported five cases of transcervical removal of submucosal fibroids in which hysteroscopic guidance was used. All of the cases involved pedunculated fibroids; the pedicles were cut with scissors or twisted off using ovum forceps. Diathermic cutting and morcellation were used with a cutting loop in two cases. A 'new' hysteroscopic technique for removal of sessile submucosal fibroids was described 2 years later (Neuwirth 1978). Neuwirth used a modified urological resectoscope that was adapted to the higher pressures necessary in 32% dextran 70 hysteroscopy. A cutting loop that moved to and fro beyond the telescope was used. Four patients were treated in this manner. De Cherney & Polan (1983) removed both pedunculated and sessile myomas less than 3 cm in diameter using an unmodified urological resectoscope. There were no immediate or later complications.

During the past three decades, hysteroscopic methods for female sterilization have been developed but none has found widespread use. Between 1953 and 1969, Ishikawa designed electrodes capable of coagulating the fallopian tubes under the control of hysteroscopy or fluoroscopy (Hayashi 1972). Results were poor, with pregnancy rates ranging from 5 to 83%. Quinones Guerror et al (1973) and Richart et al (1973) published reports on clinical trials using hysteroscopically directed electrodes to fulgurate the uterine tubal openings. Initial results were encouraging, but subsequent reports of high failure rates and significant complications led to the abandonment of this technique (Richart 1974, Cibils 1975, March & Israel 1975).

In contrast to previously employed coagulation methods, Lindemann and Mohr (1976) used hysteroscopy to inject a chemical used for tubal occlusion, methyl 2-cyanoacrylate (MCA), into the oviducts of 150 women. Several other agents have been utilized in attempts at achieving permanent tubal occlusion, but none has found widespread clinical use.

Investigators have also attempted to provide reversible tubal occlusion via the hysteroscope. In 1979, Reed & Erb described preliminary formed-in-place silicone rubber plugs which were placed hysteroscopically. An update of their experience 2 years later (Reed et al 1981) showed an overall success rate for bilateral occlusion of 71.5% (239 women). After improvements in the delivery device they raised their bilateral occlusion rate to 92.3% (25 patients). The authors found that proper case selection was important and estimated that approximately 10% of patients would not be considered good candidates for the procedure due to anatomical reasons.

Hysteroscopic excision of uterine septa has been reported to result in a high rate of reproductive success without the associated risks of more traditional therapies. Edstrom (1974) described resection of uterine septa in two cases using the hysteroscopic approach. Rigid, firmly attached forceps were used and the septum resected in piecemeal fashion. Chervenak & Neuwirth (1981) described a new approach to the symptomatic uterine septum, utilizing hysteroscopic resection under laparoscopic control. Two cases were reported. Very fine scissors were used to resect the septa. Bleeding was controlled by focal cautery using a coagulating current. Daly et al (1982) reported 14 patients with uterine septa who underwent hysteroscopic septal divisions. Small scissors were used to incise the septa. Laparoscopy was used to monitor the depth of resection. A year later, Daly et al (1983) reported a series of 25 patients in which the anatomical outcome after hysteroscopic septal division was as good or better than after Jones or Tompkins metroplasties. De Cherney & Polan (1983) reported 11 patients with intrauterine septa less than 1 cm at the broadest point that were resected using an unmodified urological cystoscope. Nine patients carried a fetus to term during the 5–25 month follow-up. March (1987) incised 91 septa using flexible scissors under hysteroscopic guidance. Most septa were 3–5 cm in depth and width. Two were 8 cm wide. A history of recurrent abortion was reported in 79 patients. Their gestational outcome post-therapy markedly improved.

The treatment of intractable uterine bleeding has recently been approached by use of the hysteroscope. Goldrath et al (1981) first reported on 22 patients who had excessive and disabling uterine bleeding and were treated with hysteroscopic endometrial ablation using neodymium: yttrium aluminium garnet (Nd:YAG) laser photovaporization. Successful results were obtained for 21 patients, with the longest period of observation being 23 months. The one failure occurred in an anticoagulated patient with an artificial mitral valve. The Nd:YAG was chosen over other lasers because of its greater energy output, degree of tissue damage, and greater portability, which facilitated its use in the operating room. De Cherney & Polan (1983) used an unmodified urological resectoscope to cauterize the entire endometrial surface in patients with intractable uterine bleeding unresponsive to hormonal therapy. Results up to 18 months were good. In 1987 De Cherney et al reported a series of 21 patients who had undergone hysteroscopic endometrial ablation using the resectoscope; 18 of the patients had blood dyscrasias or were poor anaesthetic risks. The follow-up period ranged from 6 months to 5 years. The technique was noted to be efficient and beneficial.

The role of lasers in operative hysteroscopy continues to be explored. The carbon dioxide laser is absorbed by liquid distention media and, if gas distention is used, the plume is difficult to evacuate without losing the pneumometra. The Nd:YAG laser has properties that are particularly well suited for endometrial ablation, such as deep coagulation, ability to pass through fluids, and a fibre delivery system. Following Goldrath's favourable report, its successful use has been further documented (Goldfarb 1990). The argon and potassium titanyl phosphate 532 (KTP-532) lasers have less depth of penetration than the Nd:YAG laser, but their properties include a fibre delivery system and ability to pass through fluid. Both can be used in the uterus. Diamond et al (1987) used the KTP-532 laser to lyse intrauterine adhesions and partially treat extensive intracavitary uterine fibroids. The laser was easy to use but required sophisticated equipment, including specialized electrical wiring in the operating room. The relative usefulness of laser as opposed to non-laser operative techniques remains to be established.

THE FUTURE OF HYSTEROSCOPY

Hysteroscopy has an exciting future as it becomes a continually more important modality in treating uterine bleeding disorders. Better technology, including optics and dispensing media, will make removal of larger and multiple myomas more accessible. In addition, ablation of the endometrium will become a safer and more efficient procedure, yielding greater numbers of patients with amenorrhoea.

The work-up of a patient with irregular bleeding will not be complete without a hysteroscopic examination to rule out an anatomical lesion. This will include the postmenopausal woman as well.

Advancing technology, especially with better audiovisual equipment, will allow much more elaborate operations with the hysteroscope.

The use of office hysteroscopy under sedation will also increase in importance and perhaps become part of routine gynaecologic examination.

REFERENCES

Bauer K 1966 Cited in: Zystoskopische Diagnostik. Schattauer Verlag, Stuttgart
Bumm E 1895 Zur aetiologie der endometritis. Verhandlungen Deutschen Gesellschaft für Gynakologie 6: 524
Chervenak F A, Neuwirth R S 1981 Hysteroscopic resection of the uterine septum. American Journal of Obstetrics and Gynecology 141(3): 351–353
Cibils L A 1975 Permanent sterilization by hysteroscopic cauterization. American Journal of Obstetrics and Gynecology 121: 513–520
Daly D C, Tohan N, Walters C A, Riddick D H 1982 Hysteroscopic resection of uterine septa. Surgical Forum 33: 637–639
Daly D C, Walters C A, Soto-Albors C E, Riddick D H 1983 Hysteroscopic metroplasty: surgical technique and obstetric outcome. Fertility and Sterility 39(5): 623–628
David C 1908 Lendoscopie uterine (hysteroscopie) applications au diagnostic et au traitement des affections intrauterines. In: Jaques G (ed) Thèse de Paris. Paris, 132
De Cherney A, Polan M L 1983 Hysteroscopic management of intrauterine lesions and intractable uterine bleeding. Obstetrics and Gynecology 61(3): 392–397

De Cherney A H, Diamond M P, Lavy G, Polan M L 1987 Endometrial ablation for intractable uterine bleeding: hysteroscopic resection. Obstetrics and Gynecology 70: 668–670

Desormeaux A-J 1865 De l'endoscope et de ses applications au diagnostic et au traitement des affections de l'urethra et de la vessie. Baillière, Paris

Diamond M P, Boyers S P, Lavy G, Shapiro B S, Grunfeld L, De Cherney A H 1987 Endoscopic use of the potassium-titanyl-phosphate 532 laser in gynecologic surgery. Colposcopy and Gynecologic Laser Surgery 3(4): 213–216

Edstrom K, Fernstrom I 1970 The diagnostic possibilities of a modified hysteroscopic technique. Acta Obstetrica et Gynecologica Scandinavica 49: 327–330

Edstrom KGB 1974 Intrauterine surgical procedures during hysteroscopy. Endoscopy 6: 175–181

Gauss C J 1928 Hysteroskopie. Archiv für Gynakologie 133: 18

Goldfarb H A 1990 A review of 35 endometrial ablations using the Nd:YAG laser for recurrent menometrorrhagia. Obstetrics and Gynecology 76: 833–835

Goldrath M H, Fuller T A, Segal S 1981 Laser photovaporization of endometrium for the treatment of menorrhagia. American Journal of Obstetrics and Gynecology 140(1): 14–19

Hayashi M 1972 Tubal sterilization by cornual coagulation under hysteroscopy. In: Richart R M, Praeger D J (eds) Human sterilization. Charles C Thomas, Springfield, pp 334–338

Heineberg A 1914 Uterine endoscopy; an aid to precision in the diagnosis of intra-uterine disease, a preliminary report, with the presentation of a new uteroscope. Surgery, Gynecology and Obstetrics 18: 513–515

Leake J L, Murphy A A, Zacur E N 1987 Noncardiogenic pulmonary edema: a complication of operative hysteroscopy. Fertility and Sterility 48: 497–499

Levine R U, Neuwirth R S 1972 Evaluation of a method of hysteroscopy with the use of 30% dextran. American Journal of Obstetrics and Gynecology 113: 696

Levine R U, Neuwirth R S 1973 Simultaneous laparoscopy and hysteroscopy for intrauterine adhesions. Obstetrics and Gynecology 42(3): 441–445

Lindemann H J 1973 Historical aspects of hysteroscopy. Fertility and Sterility 24(3): 230–243

Lindemann H J, Mohr J 1976 Review of clinical experience with hysteroscopic sterilization. In: Sciarra J J, Droegemueller W, Speidel J J (eds) Advances in female sterilization technizues. Harper and Row, Hagerstown, p 153–161

Maddi V I, Wyso E M, Zinner E N 1969 Dextran anaphylaxis. Angiology 20: 243

March C M, Israel R 1975 A critical appraisal of hysteroscopic tubal fulguration for sterilization. Contraception 11: 261–269

March C M, Israel R 1981 Gestational outcome following hysteroscopic lysis of adhesions. Fertility and Sterility 36(4): 455–459

March C M, Israel R 1987 Hysteroscopic management of recurrent abortion caused by septate uterus. American Journal of Obstetrics and Gynecology 156: 834–842

March C M, Israel R, March A D 1978 Hysteroscopic management of intrauterine adhesions. American Journal of Obstetrics and Gynecology 130(6): 653–657

Mohri T, Mohri C, Yamadori F 1986 The original production of the glassfibre hysteroscope and a study on the intrauterine observation of the human fetus, things attached to the fetus and inner side of the uterus wall in late pregnancy and the beginning of delivery by means of hysteroscopy and its recording on the film. Journal of the Japanese Obstetrics and Gynecology Society 15(2): 87–95

Neuwirth R S 1978 A new technique for and additional experience with hysteroscopic resection of submucous fibroids. American Journal of Obstetrics and Gynecology 131(1): 91–94

Neuwirth R S, Amin H K 1976 Excision of submucus fibroids with hysteroscopic control. American Journal of Obstetrics and Gynecology 126(1): 95–99

Nitze M 1879 Uber eine neues Behandlungsmethode der Hohlen des menschlichen Korpers. Medical Press, Wien, p 851–858

Norment W B, Sikes H, Berry F, Bird I 1957 Hysteroscopy. Surgical Clinics of North America 37: 1377–1386

Pantaleoni D C 1869 On endoscopic examination of the cavity of the womb. Medical Press Circular 8: 26–27

Porto R 1974 Hysteroscopie. Encyclopedie medico-chirurgicale. Searle/Laboratories Clin-Comar-Byla, Paris

Quinones Guerror R, Ramos R A, Duran A A 1973 Tubal electrocauterization under hysteroscopic control. Contraception 7: 195–201

Reed T P, Erb R A 1979 Hysteroscopic oviductal blocking with formed-in-place silicone rubber plugs. Journal of Reproductive Medicine 23(2): 69–72

Reed T P, Erb R A, DeMaeyer J 1981 Tubal occlusion with silicone rubber. Update, 1980. Journal of Reproductive Medicine 26(10): 534–537

Richart R M 1974 Complications of hysteroscopic sterilization. Contraception 10: 230

Richart R M, Neuwirth R S, Israngkun C, Phaosavasdi S 1973 Female sterilization by electrocoagulation of tubal ostia using hysteroscopy. American Journal of Obstetrics and Gynecology 117: 801–804

Rubin I C 1925 Uterine endoscopy, endometroscopy with the aid of uterine insufflation. American Journal of Obstetrics and Gynecology 10(3): 313–327

Schroeder C 1934 Uber den Ausbau und die Leistungen der Hysteroskopie. Archiv für Gynakologie 156: 407

Seymour H J 1925 Endoscopy of the uterus: with a description of hysteroscopy. British Medical Journal 2: 1220

Siegler A M, Kemmann E 1976 Location and removal of misplaced or embedded intrauterine devices by hystero-scopy. Journal or Reproductive Medicine 16(3): 139–144

Silander T 1962 Hysteroscopy through a transparent rubber balloon. Surgery, Gynecology and Obstetrics 114: 125–127

Sugimoto O 1978 Diagnostic and therapeutic hysteroscopy for traumatic intrauterine adhesions. American Journal of Obstetrics and Gynecology 131(5): 539–547

Valle R F, Sciarra F F, Freeman D W 1977 Hysteroscopic removal of intrauterine devices with missing filaments. Obstetrics and Gynecology 49(1): 55–60

Von Midulicz-Radecki F, Freund A 1927 Ein neues Hysteroskop und sein praktische Anwendung in der Gynakologie. Zeitschrift für Geburtshilfe und Gynakologie

2. Safety and training

A. Gordon

INTRODUCTION

Diagnostic hysteroscopy has been widely practised as an out-patient procedure both in Europe and North America for the past 20 years, and during the past decade its use has spread to other countries. The history of the technique has been discussed in Chapter 1 but it is the modern developments, including the use of improved distension media such as carbon dioxide (Lindemann 1972) and dextran 70 (Edstrom & Fernstrom 1970), fibreoptic light cables with safe proximal illumination (Fourestiere 1943) and the designing of a complex lens system allowing variable magnification (Hamou 1980), which have allowed hysteroscopy to provide a safe and accurate means of diagnosing pathological lesions within the uterine cavity. Four different but complementary techniques are in use:

1. **Panoramic hysteroscopy.** This is the most widely used technique in which the distended uterine cavity is examined through a telescope, allowing the diagnosis of intrauterine pathology such as polyps, fibroids, synechiae or defects of the müllerian ducts. Accessory instruments allow operative procedures to be performed.

2. **Microhysteroscopy and microcolpohysteroscopy.** These are performed using a telescope which has been modified by the introduction of a system of magnifying lenses, allowing both panoramic and microscopic vision. The fine structure of the endometrial vasculature can be seen at a magnification of $\times 20$ with the optic 1 cm from the surface. Detailed study of the superficial cellular layer of the cervical canal and uterine cavity can be made at magnifications of $\times 80$ and $\times 150$ in the contact mode, allowing diagnosis of cellular atypia to be made.

3. **Contact hysteroscopy.** Contact hysteroscopy utilizes a hysteroscope with no separate light source and there is no uterine distension. Illumination of the cavity is from the ambient light in the examination room transmitted through a chamber in the proximal end of the instrument. Interpretation of the findings is more difficult than with panoramic hysteroscopy and it has no application for intrauterine surgery so its use will not be discussed further.

4. **Flexible hysteroscopy.** Flexible hysteroscopy is favoured by some gynaecologists. The advantages are that the telescope can be directed to all parts of the uterus and a more extensive examination may be possible. The hysteroscope incorporates a separate channel through which a laser fibre and other instruments can be passed, allowing operative procedures to be performed. The disadvantage of the flexible hysteroscope is that the definition is not as good as that of the rod lens system in the rigid hysteroscope.

Although diagnostic hysteroscopy is usually a simple procedure, the learner may find it difficult initially and may even decide that the technique is not worth learning. Attempts at inserting the hysteroscope by an inexperienced surgeon may cause traumatic bleeding from the cervix or endometrium and failure to maintain adequate uterine distension will interfere with vision. Complications may result from incorrect usage of the instruments, failure to maintain adequate uterine distension or from anaesthetic agents, but should be rare in expert hands.

The instrumentation for modern diagnostic hysteroscopy has been available for the past decade. The only major advance in this time has been the development of high-resolution chip cameras which allow diagnostic hysteroscopy and operative hysteroscopy to be performed using a video screen instead of viewing through the lens. This has increased the ease of hysteroscopic surgery, improved the ability to train surgeons, and allows the operator to work in comfort.

INDICATIONS FOR DIAGNOSTIC HYSTEROSCOPY

The surgeon must become proficient in diagnostic techniques before considering undertaking operative hysteroscopy. Only by doing so will he learn to recognize all the landmarks, appreciate the importance of adequate uterine distension and develop skill in the use of instruments within the uterine cavity. The surgical skills required for hysteroscopic surgery are quite different from those required for laparotomy or even laparoscopic surgery. He must also learn to accommodate to the two-dimensional image and then to operate from the video screen.

The wide range of indications for diagnostic hysteroscopy gives ample opportunity for the gynaecologist to acquire skills in hysteroscopy. The indications are:

1. Abnormal uterine bleeding
2. Infertility
3. Misplaced intrauterine contraceptive devices (IUCDs)
4. Endometrial carcinoma
5. Investigation of uterine scars
6. Investigation of cervical intraepithelial neoplasia.

Abnormal uterine bleeding

Disorders of uterine bleeding are the commonest indications for diagnostic hysteroscopy. About 33% of all gynaecological consultations are for disorders of menstruation and this figure rises to 69% when only perimenopausal women are considered (Mencaglia & Perino 1986). Out-patient or office hysteroscopy should replace dilatation and curettage, which usually requires general anaesthesia and hospitalization and is a blind technique which may fail to identify focal lesions such as polyps, fibroids and localized areas of endometrial carcinoma in 25% of cases (Word et al 1958, Grimes 1982). It is essential to perform preliminary diagnostic hysteroscopy to define the pathology in all cases of disordered uterine bleeding where endometrial ablation or resection may be considered. Difficulties and failures may result from operating on a uterus more than 13 cm in length or because a uterine fibroid was missed at the preliminary assessment or because endometrial atypia or even carcinoma has not been diagnosed.

Infertility

The traditional methods of investigating the uterine cavity in infertility have been hysterosalpingography and endometrial biopsy. Hysteroscopy provides much more specific information about pathology such as submucous fibroids, polyps or synechiae, and on the normality of the tubal ostia, and also allows accurate assessment of the cavity in cases of recurrent abortion. In comparison with hysteroscopy, hysterosalpingography produces dubious or erroneous results in up to 40% of cases (Taylor & Cumming 1979) and thus, if the findings at hysterosalpingography are unclear, the value of hysteroscopy becomes even more apparent (Seigler 1977). Again, diagnostic hysteroscopy is an essential prerequisite to operative hysteroscopy in cases of infertility or repeated pregnancy loss to establish the precise pathology and allow specific treatment.

Misplaced IUCDs

Intrauterine foreign bodies and misplaced IUCDs constitute the third main indication for hysteroscopy, which allows accurate localization of the IUCD and its removal under direct vision.

Carcinoma of the endometrium

Endometrial carcinoma or atypical hyperplasia may be detected at an early stage by out-patient microhysteroscopy. Focal areas of carcinoma can also be recognized as irregular excrescences which are friable, necrotic or haemorrhagic with an irregular vascular pattern. Visually directed endometrial biopsy is always necessary to confirm the diagnosis. Focal or generalized premalignant or malignant changes constitute a contra-indication to hysteroscopic endometrial resection or ablation, so, again, preliminary diagnostic hysteroscopy is imperative.

Previous uterine scars

Investigation of a uterine scar following myomec-tomy or caesarean section is sometimes necessary to advise on future pregnancies, although the risk of uterine rupture is small. The degree of fibrosis and the depth of any defect can be readily assessed by hysteroscopy.

Cervical intraepithelial neoplasia

Microcolpohysteroscopy is a necessary adjunct to colposcopy when the transformation zone is within the cervical canal and should form part of normal colposcopic examination in these cases. Occult cervical carcinoma is, however, a contra-indication to hysteroscopy because of the risk of disseminating malignant cells.

TRAINING IN DIAGNOSTIC HYSTEROSCOPY

Any practising gynaecologist should have ade-quate opportunity in his daily work to perform diagnostic hysteroscopy and practise its use until he is ready to proceed to operative hysteroscopy. First, however, the gynaecologist should learn hysteroscopy correctly under supervision.

Initially, especially if early attempts have been made without supervision or training, hystero-scopy may seem difficult and it is common in the early part of the learning curve not to obtain a clear view of the cavity. Unless the trainee is aware of the pitfalls he may commence with enthusiasm and confidence only to be disillusioned by his failure and abandon the technique altogether. It should be remembered that the cervical canal must be negotiated gently, atraumatically and under direct vision to enter the uterine cavity

without bleeding. The cavity itself is a small cleft in a thick muscle which must be distended before a panoramic view can be obtained.

It is important not to be in a hurry. Time spent in familiarizing oneself with the instrument and its assembly, learning the extent and, particularly, the direction of the field of vision when an oblique lens is used and on the choice and pro-perties of the distension medium will be amply repaid. It is always advantageous to visit an expert who will take time to teach and demon-strate the way to avoid or deal with problems. Most workshops on hysteroscopy are directed at the clinician who already has some degree of skill and may not cater for the novice who wishes to acquire the basic skills which are vital before per-forming even the most simple surgical procedures.

The first attempts at hysteroscopy must be under general anaesthesia during a theatre list in which there is time to practise on a suitable patient. The most favourable patient is the parous woman of child-bearing age with a normal-sized uterus of less than 8 cm in length. Out-patient hysteroscopy should not be attempted until at least 25 successful procedures have been per-formed under general anaesthesia.

While most hysteroscopists in Europe favour carbon dioxide as the distension medium for diagnostic hysteroscopy, it may present problems for the beginner. Bleeding provoked by the hysteroscope negotiating the cervical canal usually prevents further examination and bubbles produced by the cervical mucus may also make visualization difficult. The learner will often find it easier to use a fluid medium such as 32% dextran 70 in 10% dextrose (Hyskon) until he has gained confidence before progressing to carbon dioxide hysteroscopy.

The main advantages of Hyskon are that it has excellent optical properties, does not mix with blood and is viscous, so little fluid escapes along the fallopian tubes or leaks back through the cervix. This makes its use preferable to dextrose or saline in the early stages of training. However, the high viscosity may cause blockage of the stopcocks of the hysteroscope if they are not cleaned very carefully, and spill on the operator's eyelids may cause the lids to stick together which, while embarrassing for the surgeon, is amusing for his staff! Hyskon also inhibits blood coagulation, may cause interstitial pulmonary oedema and, in about 1:10 000 cases, intravasation may lead to a serious or even fatal anaphylactic reaction.

The technique of insertion of the hysteroscope must be modified if Hyskon is used. After inserting the telescope about 1 cm into the cervical canal, 5 ml of Hyskon should be injected to distend the lumen of the canal and allow further progress to be made under direct vision. If on entering the uterine cavity there is bleeding sufficient to impair vision, the telescope should be advanced to the fundus or into one of the uterine cornua and then slowly withdrawn while continuing to inject Hyskon. The injected medium will first flow towards the fundus and then back towards the cervix, carrying with it blood and clots, thus rinsing the cavity and producing a clear field of vision.

Once experience has been gained with a fluid medium, the learner can progress to carbon dioxide hysteroscopy. A number of problems may be encountered initially, and much frustation and waste of time may be avoided by awareness of them:

1. Leaks in the distension system
2. Gas bubbles
3. Angle of the hysteroscope lens
4. Negotiation of the cervical canal.

Leaks in the distension system

The commonest difficulty is failure to obtain clear vision, which may be due to leaks in the tubing system. It is important to check the tightness of the system. As soon as the hysteroscope is in contact with the external cervical os, the pressure in the system should rise to 10–30 mmHg with a flow rate of 20–30 ml/min. Audible backleak from the cervix confirms the free flow of gas and the absence of a block in the hysteroscope sheath.

Bubbles of carbon dioxide

When using carbon dioxide as the distension medium, bubbles of cervical mucus frequently obscure vision in diagnostic hysteroscopy. These may be minimized by cleaning the cervix carefully and gently with a moist swab to remove excess mucus without causing bleeding. If the mucus is still copious or viscous it may be precipitated with 3% acetic acid solution. Alternatively, the outer half of the cervical canal may be negotiated under direct vision but without the gas flowing, the hysteroflator being switched on just before the telescope passes through the internal os. When the uterine cavity has been reached, back and forth movements of the telescope should be avoided. If it is withdrawn through the internal os, mucus may be deposited on the lens, further obscuring vision and producing more bubbles.

The oblique hysteroscope

Most hysteroscopies are performed using a 30° telescope. The beginner may initially find it difficult to orient his view, especially during insertion of the instrument. If the cervical os is seen in the middle of the visual field, the telescope is actually angled towards the posterior wall of the cervical canal and progress will be difficult and traumatic bleeding likely (Fig. 2.1). The image of the cervical canal should always be kept to the lower third of the visual field at 6 o'clock on the video screen (Fig. 2.2). The reverse is true if the uterus is retroverted (Figs 2.3 and 2.4).

Anteverted uterus

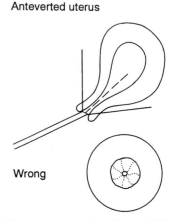

Wrong

Fig. 2.1   The *wrong* way to introduce a 30° hysteroscope into the cervical canal of an anteverted uterus. There is risk of posterior wall perforation if the image of canal is kept centrally. (Redrawn with permission from Hill et al (1992).)

Anteverted uterus

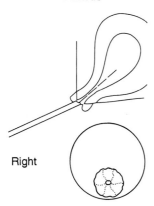

Fig. 2.2 The *right* way to introduce a 30° hysteroscope into the cervical canal of an anteverted uterus. The image of the canal is kept at 6 o'clock in the eyepiece. (Redrawn with permission from Hill et al (1992).)

Retroverted uterus

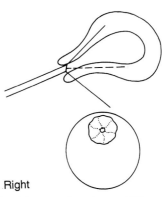

Fig. 2.4 The *right* way to introduce a 30° hysteroscope into the cervical canal of a retroverted uterus. The image of the canal is kept at 12 o'clock in the eyepiece. (Redrawn with permission from Hill et al (1992).)

Retroverted uterus

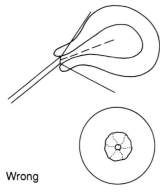

Fig. 2.3 The *wrong* way to introduce a 30° hysteroscope into the cervical canal of a retroverted uterus. There is risk of anterior wall perforation if the image of the canal is kept centrally. (Redrawn with permission from Hill et al (1992).)

Negotiating the cervical canal

The cervical canal is rarely straight and so its curvature and the folds in its wall must be negotiated by altering the angle of the hysteroscope to enable smooth progress to be made. It must be remembered that movement of the tip of the telescope by a few millimetres requires the eyepiece to be moved several centimetres. Failure to appreciate this fact may lead to insufficient movements of the tip of the hysteroscope and failure to make progress through the cervical canal. On the other hand, slight rotation of the eyepiece produces quite significant alterations in the visual field because of the deviation produced by the viewing angle. Familiarity with these physical characteristics of the hysteroscope is essential to a successful examination. It is common to encounter resistance to progress as the internal os is approached. One must never use force to overcome this resistance as it may lead to perforation of the cervix or uterus and will usually produce bleeding which then obscures vision, and the examination has to be abandoned. When resistance is encountered, the telescope should be withdrawn a few millimetres to allow the carbon dioxide to form a small space in front of the lens. If necessary, the optic should be rotated to allow detailed examination of the anatomy of the canal but usually the lumen will be evident. If not, the position of the carbon dioxide bubbles will indicate the direction. Difficulty at the internal os may be overcome by rotating the hysteroscope optic 180° so that its blunt tip reaches the cervical os first.

Attention to detail, avoiding trauma, patience and practice will be rewarded by a rapid increase in expertise and the ability to visualize the uterine cavity in nearly every case. Only when this degree of skill has been attained should the hysteroscopist progress from diagnostic to operative procedures.

CONTRAINDICATIONS TO HYSTEROSCOPY

Although diagnostic hysteroscopy is a safe procedure in expert hands, there are well-defined contraindications to its use:

1. Infection
2. Cardiorespiratory disease
3. Metabolic acidosis
4. Pregnancy
5. Uterine bleeding
6. Occult cervical malignancy.

Infection

Vaginitis and cervicitis constitute absolute contraindications to hysteroscopy because of the danger of causing an ascending infection which may lead to salpingitis or peritonitis. Investigations should be delayed until the infection has been cured. For the same reason, hysteroscopy should be avoided in suspected pelvic inflammatory disease. The only exception to this rule is infection in the presence of a 'lost' IUCD where hysteroscopy may be necessary to locate and remove it, but the operation should be performed under antibiotic cover.

Cardiorespiratory disease

In severe cardiorespiratory disease, the use of carbon dioxide as the distension medium may cause pulmonary embolism. The risk has probably been under-reported because of the high solubility of carbon dioxide and the difficulty in confirming the diagnosis.

Metabolic acidosis

Metabolic acidosis should always be corrected before any surgical procedure, including hysteroscopy, is performed.

Pregnancy

Pregnancy is generally considered a contraindication to hysteroscopy but it may be necessary to perform hysteroscopy to remove an IUCD or to diagnose retained products of conception where there has been persistent postabortal bleeding, although ultrasound has replaced endoscopy in many cases. The myometrium in the gravid uterus is much more distensible than in the non-pregnant organ, which has a strong, resistant muscular wall. Uterine distension with gas can cause the uterus to distend like a balloon, resulting in a depot of carbon dioxide accumulating, which may lead to separation of the placenta and retroplacental bleeding. The accumulated gas may then flow into the ruptured uterine veins, causing a massive pulmonary embolus. It is important, therefore, that hysteroscopy in pregnancy is only performed by an expert surgeon who is aware of these possibilities and that the gas flow is restricted to 20 ml/min with an intrauterine pressure of less than 50 mmHg. It is also important to remember that the optic nerve may be damaged by the hysteroscope light after the 10th week of pregnancy although there does not appear to be any danger before this stage (Lindemann, unpublished observation).

Uterine bleeding

Scanty or moderate uterine bleeding does not prevent adequate observation of the uterine cavity but heavy bleeding will prevent a clear view regardless of the distension medium. Heavy bleeding should usually be suppressed to allow full evaluation of the endometrium and prevent intravasation of the distension medium. Despite this there have been reports of hysteroscopy being performed in persistent heavy bleeding and the bleeding areas of the endometrium coagulated (Haeri 1990).

Cervical carcinoma

Hysteroscopy should not be performed in the presence of occult cervical carcinoma because of the danger of disseminating malignant cells. However, microcolpohysteroscopy is necessary as an adjunct to colposcopy when the transformation zone is within the cervical canal or when the ectocervix appears normal in a patient with an abnormal cervical smear.

COMPLICATIONS OF HYSTEROSCOPY

Diagnostic hysteroscopy is a safe procedure when performed correctly by a trained surgeon. As with any invasive technique, there may be complications. Lindemann (1986) carried out a postal survey of the experience of European hysteroscopists and found the incidence of serious complications such as cardiorespiratory accidents, anaesthetic reactions, allergies and uterine perforation was 0.012%. In addition, there were a number of minor complications but no deaths were recorded. It must be remembered that all the surgeons involved in this survey were expert hysteroscopists and that, in 1986, few were performing operative hysteroscopy, which carries a much higher risk of serious complications.

Cervical trauma

The most important complication of diagnostic hysteroscopy is trauma caused by the instruments. It is unusual to dilate the cervix except in the postmenopausal woman or, less commonly, in the nulliparous patient. It is preferable to utilize the passive dilation produced by the carbon dioxide to permit atraumatic introduction of the hysteroscope. If the cervix has to be dilated then there may be laceration by the cervical tenaculum and the dilators frequently produce bleeding from vessels in the cervical canal. This may sometimes be avoided by the use of prostaglandin pessaries 1–2 hours prior to examination.

Uterine perforation

Uterine perforation is unlikely to occur if the hysteroscope is passed under continuous direct vision. Perforation in diagnostic hysteroscopy does not usually produce side-effects and can be treated conservatively. However, perforation when scissors, an electric current or a laser are being used always demands laparotomy to exclude bowel damage and must never be treated conservatively.

Distension medium

The distension medium may also produce complications. Gas embolism with carbon dioxide is unlikely in diagnostic hysteroscopy because the procedure should be fairly brief and the volume of gas used should not exceed 200–400 ml. Embolism is probably underdiagnosed because carbon dioxide is so soluble in tissue fluids and is absorbed before the occurrence of embolism can be proved. Fluid overload, which is a major theoretical problem in operative hysteroscopy, should also be rare in diagnostic procedures because, again, the duration should be short, the volume of fluid used should be small and the uterine vessels should not be ruptured to permit intravasation of fluid.

The trainee hysteroscopist should be aware of all these complications and be able to recognize any variation from normal. Unless the trainee has had experience in diagnostic hysteroscopy, he may not be aware of the pitfalls in operative procedures, thus increasing the risk to the patient if unfavourable circumstances develop.

OPERATIVE HYSTEROSCOPY

Introducing instruments to perform therapeutic procedure is a logical extension of diagnostic hysteroscopy. The exciting prospect of performing hysteroscopic surgery has resulted in a sudden and rapid increase in the popularity of hysteroscopy with the consequent danger of surgeons being tempted to perform difficult surgery in an unaccustomed environment before they have achieved competence in diagnostic techniques.

The earliest operations were performed by passing fine scissors or forceps alongside the hysteroscope to biopsy lesions under direct vision or to remove polyps or small submucous fibroids. Later, the hysteroscope was adapted to allow insertion of instruments through an operating channel, directed by a bridge on the sheath of the hysteroscope. More recently the urological resectoscope has been used for intrauterine surgery and hysteroscopes with channels for the insertion of neodymium:yttrium aluminium garnet (Nd:YAG) laser fibres for destruction of the endometrium or submucous fibroids have been developed.

Hysteroscopic surgery has distinct advantages over hysterectomy and other conventional uterine operations. In general the patient will require a shorter stay in hospital and recovery will be quicker. It is unusual for a patient to remain in hospital more than 24 hours after hysteroscopic surgery and she should be fit to resume normal activity within a few days, significantly reducing the cost of the operation. The woman who has had endometrial ablation rather than hysterectomy may feel better as she will avoid the psychological trauma that removal of the uterus may produce. Many women have a wish to retain their menses as evidence of their femininity and resent the loss of their menstrual periods in the late 30s or early 40s, which, they may equate with the menopause. In addition, conservative hysteroscopic surgery for submucous fibroids or a uterine septum does not scar the uterus for a subsequent pregnancy.

Changes in attitude

The majority of gynaecologists have been trained in abdominal or vaginal surgery and, possibly later in their careers, have developed an interest in laparoscopy and hysteroscopy. When commencing operative endoscopy the surgeon must appreciate that the instruments are different from those used in conventional surgery and it may frequently be difficult for a senior surgeon to adapt to these techniques and to accept that new skills must be acquired. Indeed, the more experienced the surgeon is in the old operations, the more difficult it maybe for him to change to new ones and the learning curve may therefore be significantly longer than for a younger surgeon.

The surgeon must learn to operate in a new environment and accommodate to the two-dimensional image offered by the telescope and then learn to operate from the video screen. This latter technique should be adopted as soon as possible in the training period as in many cases it is difficult to work without it. In addition to learning to use the new instruments, he must appreciate their capabilities, their risks and their limitations. Initially the staff in the operating room must accept that operations may take longer although, with experience, hysteroscopic surgery will take approximately the same or even less time than conventional surgery. Most experienced surgeons should be able to complete endometrial resection or ablation in an average of 20–40 min. The nursing staff must also learn to use the new instruments in order to function as a team. This will be helped by the use of video cameras so that they can see the operation and, when necessary, assist.

Training programmes

Before undertaking operative hysteroscopy, the surgeon must have extensive experience in diagnostic hysteroscopy. He must be able at all times to obtain a clear view of the uterine cavity and know to stop the operation if vision is compromised. Tragedies have resulted from inexperienced hysteroscopic surgeons failing to appreciate this and continuing to use a high-frequency current or laser when the uterine distension system has failed, resulting in perforation of the uterus and damage to organs such as major vessels, the ureter and bowel. There can be no fixed rule for the number of diagnostic hysteroscopies which one should perform before proceeding to operative hysteroscopy as everybody's learning curve is different and, in recent years, the teaching of endoscopy has improved to such an extent that any arbitrary number is meaningless. Nevertheless, the need for expertise in diagnostic hysteroscopy before attempting any operative procedure cannot be overemphasized.

Having achieved expertise in diagnostic hysteroscopy, the surgeon will wish to extend his experience and commence hysteroscopic surgery. Initially he may obtain an overview of the possibilities by attending conferences where hysteroscopy is discussed or, better, where live operations are relayed to the auditorium from the operating room. Video recordings make excellent teaching aids but they can be criticized because editing can make the operation look both easier and better than it really is. Few surgeons will produce a recorded video containing the failures of their techniques as well as the successes.

Conferences are organized in many countries in Europe and North America, either sponsored by institutions or by the instrument manufacturers, to whom much credit must be given for their interest in education and promoting safety in these techniques. National and international societies are now developing in many countries which seek to educate by means of endoscopy courses and to monitor the success of the procedures and the incidence of complications. Their meetings also provide a forum for discussion and allow the surgeon who wishes to learn operative hysteroscopy to listen and watch the expert at work.

Workshop format

Workshops should last 1–2 days and include lectures and discussion on the theory and practice of hysteroscopy. The groups should be small enough to allow all the participants to contribute and to have the opportunity of 'hands on' training. Six surgeons is probably the ideal number and in order to obtain the maximum benefit they should already have some preliminary experience in diagnostic hysteroscopy and have attended at least one larger conference. Longer attachment to a training unit is desirable but not always possible because of financial constraints and the time involved. There may be inefficient use of time if the trainer has limited access to the operating room and so a week at a centre may only allow attendance at two or three operating sessions.

Initial training can commence on inert models which consist of a plastic case with a replaceable wax lining resembling the uterine cavity which can be excised by the resectoscope loop without using electricity. Biological tissue can be provided by an excised bovine uterus which is larger than the human organ but provides a readily available substitute on which to practice the use of the instruments. Alternatively an excised human uterus can be used in vitro to gain experience before commencing hysteroscopic surgery. Some surgeons use the laparoscope as a safety measure to avoid perforation of the uterus until they are competent to operate without these precautions.

In organizing a workshop, practical experience should be offered in diagnostic hysteroscopy initially under general anaesthesia and then in an out-patient setting prior to operative hysteroscopy. Each trainee can perform part of the operation, treating a segment of the uterine cavity with the resectoscope or laser under supervision using the video screen.

When a surgeon has gained experience in diagnostic hysteroscopy and has attended courses, conferences or workshops where he will have learnt the scope, risks and complications of operative hysteroscopy, he will then benefit by attending a colleague's operating session and learning on a one-to-one basis. He can then be allowed to perform more operations under supervision than are possible at a workshop and his surgical skills will probably increase faster and with greater safety than if he were to work unsupervised. Alternatively, the trainer may go to the trainee's hospital, which has the advantage that all the operating room staff have the opportunity to learn. Difficult or complex operations should be under supervision, especially those involving junior surgeons.

CLASSIFICATION OF HYSTEROSCOPIC OPERATIONS

Hysteroscopic surgery has been classified into minor, intermediate and advanced operations. This classification has merit in that it gives some indication of the progression which surgeons in training should undertake. They should commence with simple procedures before attempting complicated ones and should recognize the degree of difficulty of each operation.

Minor hysteroscopic surgery

Suggested types of operations which any competent surgeon with experience in diagnostic hysteroscopy should be able to perform are:

1. Hysteroscopically directed endometrial biopsy
2. Removal of small polyps
3. Removal of non-embedded IUCDs
4. Division of simple adhesions.

Initially orientation may be difficult but, with practice, these operations should be possible within a few weeks of training.

Endometrial biopsy

Endometrial biopsy under direct vision allows accurate sampling of suspicious areas of endometrium and is the simplest type of procedure.

Removal of small polyps

This can be done either with hysteroscopic forceps or scissors or, better, with the resectoscope and gives the opportunity to practice electrosurgery.

Removal of non-embedded IUCDs

Before any attempt is made to remove an IUCD, pregnancy must be excluded and the presence of the coil in the uterus should be confirmed by an ultrasound scan. Hysteroscopic visualization of the device permits accurate identification of its position and allows the string to be grasped and the coil removed.

Division of simple adhesions

Fine adhesions may be broken down with the tip of the hysteroscope but firmer ones are best divided with scissors or an electric knife.

Intermediate hysteroscopic surgery

1. Cannulation of the tubal ostia
2. Tubal sterilization.

Cannulation of the tubal ostia

This is a controversial procedure whose aim is to cure proximal tubal obstruction caused by a fine membrane. It is doubtful if it is ever necessary and it is possible that tubal mucosal damage could be caused by the passage of the catheter. Pathological obstruction by polyps or salpingitis isthmica nodosa would not respond to such measures. Transcervical gamete intrafallopian transfer via the hysteroscope has been attempted but the success rate is low and it has been superceded by ultrasound-guided techniques.

Tubal sterilization

Attempts have been made for many years to find a simple out-patient hysteroscopic sterilization procedure. The insertion of silastic plugs now offers a technique which is simple, safe and effective. This demands reasonable skill in intra-

uterine manipulation but appears to have merit as a relatively non-invasive procedure.

Advanced hysteroscopic surgery

When expertise in diagnostic and minor surgery has been achieved and the surgeon is familiar with intrauterine manipulation and his instruments, he can then proceed to advanced hysteroscopic surgery, commencing with simple, small submucous myomas and progressing to more complex procedures, as listed below:

1. Myomectomy
2. Removal of large polyps
3. Endometrial resection or ablation
4. Resection of uterine septa
5. Removal of IUCD in pregnancy
6. Extensive adhesiolysis.

Myomectomy

Fibroids which are less than 3 cm in diameter and more than 75% submucous are ideal cases for the initial use of the resectoscope or Nd:YAG laser. With more experience the surgeon may progress to larger fibroids up to 5 cm in diameter and with a greater intramural component, but these should not be attempted until considerable expertise has been gained or uterine perforation is possible (see Ch. 13).

Removal of large polyps

Large polyps can be difficult to remove as they may fill the uterine cavity and, because they are vascular, they may bleed if traumatized. The pedicle may be transected with scissors but, increasingly, laser or electrosurgery is being used to remove them under direct vision. The cavity should always be inspected on completion to ensure that removal has been complete.

Endometrial resection or ablation

Endometrial resection or ablation will soon be the preferred surgical method of treating menorrhagia and should replace up to 60% of hysterectomies. When the surgeon has mastered all the previous techniques, he should be ready to advance to using the resectoscope or laser. Using either technique the full thickness of the endometrium is removed or destroyed, together with about 1 mm of myometrium. If the myometrium is resected too deeply there may be excessive bleeding or uterine perforation, which is more likely when operating near the cornua where the myometrium may be only 0.5 cm thick. Accuracy and the ability to judge exactly the depth of the incisions are therefore essential in performing hysteroscopic surgery (see Chs 8–11).

Division of uterine septa

Uterine septa may be resected with scissors, an electric knife or a laser. The exact configuration of the uterine body must be determined by preliminary laparoscopy and the operation performed under laparoscopic or ultrasound control to ensure that an adequate thickness of uterine fundus remains.

Removal of an IUCD in pregnancy

Removal of a misplaced IUCD in pregnancy presents additional hazards which the surgeon must remember. The importance of introducing the distension medium slowly and at low pressure and of passing the telescope under direct vision to prevent perforation of the uterus or pregnancy sac cannot be overemphasized.

Division of extensive synechiae

Division of extensive synechiae is one of the most difficult and dangerous hysteroscopic operations. If the normal anatomy of the cavity has been lost and it is impossible to see the tubal ostia, perforation with the instruments is always possible.

This is the only condition where coincidental laparoscopy is essential.

SUMMARY

Provided that progress is made systematically, that the surgeon never attempts to perform too difficult operations and that all the safety protocols are adhered to, hysteroscopic surgery should be within the capabilities of most gynaecologists. Failure to appreciate the risks and failure to undergo continuous training in the learning period will inevitably lead to complications which should otherwise be avoidable.

Hysteroscopic surgery offers many advantages over conventional surgery and, like many other methods of minimally invasive surgery, appears to be the surgery of the future. Endoscopic surgery will not supplant open surgery but will become another essential part of practice which the patient will expect and, indeed, demand. There will be problems. Training programmes must be established to try to prevent complications. There must be continuous education and research into the value and results of new techniques and instruments both for laser surgery and electrosurgery.

It is possible that in the future new biophysical approaches may render laser surgery and electrosurgery obsolete. Safer forms of physical energy and new forms of hormone therapy are all undergoing trials with promising preliminary results. Whichever technique eventually proves to be the most effective and safe, the benefits to patients of these new methods of uterine surgery and the need for gynaecologists to undergo training in them are such that 'old dogs must learn new tricks... or perish'.

REFERENCES

Bozzini P 1807. Der Lichleiter oder Beschveibung Einer Lingachen Vonichtung und ihrer Anwendung zur Erleuchtung inerer Hohlen und Zuischeraumt des lebenden animalischen korpts. Landes-Industrie-Comptoi, Weimar. Cited in: Bauer K 1966 Zystoskopische Diagnostic. Schattauer Verlag

Edstrom K, Fernstrom I 1970 The diagnostic possibilities of a modified hysteroscopic technique. Acta Obstetrica et Gynecologica Scandanivica 49: 327

Grimes D A Diagnostic dilatation and curettage: a reappraisal. Obstetrics and Gynaecology 3: 1–6

Fourestiere M, Gladu A, Vulmiere J 1947 La peritoneoscopie. Presse Medicale 5: 46–47

Haeri A D 1990 Uterine haemorrhage controlled by hysteroscopic electrocoagulation. Case report presented to the British Society for Gynaecological Endoscopy Annual Scientific Meeting, Hull

Hamou J E 1980 Hysteroscopie et microhysteroscopie arte un instrument nouveau: lt microhysteroscope. Endoscopia Ginecologica 2: 131

Hill NCW, Broadbent J A M, Magos A L, Bauman R, Lockwood G M 1992 Local anaesthesia and cervical dilatation for outpatient diagnostic hysteroscopy. Journal of Obstetrics and Gynaecology 12 (in press).

Lindemann H J 1972 The use of CO_2 in the uterine cavity for hysteroscopy. International Journal of Fertility 17: 221

Lindemann H-J 1979 CO_2 Hysteroscopies today. Endoscopy 11: 94

Lindemann H-J 1986 Complications of hysteroscopy. Presented to the European Society of Hysteroscopy, Antwerp

Mencaglia L, Perino A 1986 Diagnostic hysteroscopy today. Acta Europ. Fertil. 17: 431–439

Siegler A M 1977 Hysterography and hysteroscopy in the infertile patient. Journal of Reproductive Medicine 18: 143–148

Taylor P J, Cumming C D 1979 Hysteroscopy in 100 infertile patients. Fertility and Sterility 31: 301–304

Word G, Gravlee L C, Wideman G L 1958 The fallacy of simple uterine curettage. Obstetrics and Gynecology 12: 642

3. Patient selection for endometrial ablation

V. Lewis

Choosing the correct patient for endometrial ablation is critical. If patients with minimal symptoms are selected the results will be biased and if unsuitable patients are chosen the operation will fail. Careful attention to the clinical history and physical signs should result in a simple operative procedure, minimal hospital stay and a successful long-term outcome (Rutherford et at 1991).

AGE

Most women with functional bleeding or submucous myomas will be over 40 years of age and this is the group which should be considered above all for elective ablation (see Table 3.1). Younger women should probably be treated by alternative measures such as cyclical steroid therapy, at least initially, because of three factors. First, functional bleeding is often a temporary hormonal imbalance which may resolve spontaneously; secondly, future fertility may be a major consideration; and finally the recurrence rate seems to increase with time (Derman et al 1991). Younger women should be considered for surgery if they do not respond to drugs or develop unacceptable side-effects, if they have been sterilized or if they suffer from very severe menstrual dysfunction which interferes significantly with home life and work. In young girls, ablation may be the only alternative to hysterectomy, especially if there is an underlying blood dyscrasia.

Women close to the menopause must be carefully selected because they may be able to avoid any surgical intervention. Therefore, all perimenopausal women should have luteinizing hormone/follicle-stimulating hormone (LH/FSH) and oestrogen levels measured because this might indicate whether expectant treatment is appropriate.

Postmenopausal women taking hormone replacement therapy with regular withdrawal bleeds represent a special case. In most instances the cyclical withdrawal bleed is small in amount and acceptable, but ablation can be considered if bleeding is heavy. Of course, other causes of postmenopausal bleeding must be excluded, especially endometrial hyperplasia or malignancy.

PARITY

Most patients being considered as candidates for ablation will have had children. The nulliparous patient is a special case because the cervix is closed and usually long and rigid. The os needs to be dilated to at least Hegar size 10 in order to insert the resectoscope, although this is usually easy. The cervix can be softened prior to dilation by inserting a prostaglandin pessary about 2 hours before surgery commences.

FITNESS FOR SURGERY

An endometrial ablation may take almost as long to perform as a hysterectomy but may be preferable in an unfit patient (DeCherney & Polan 1983, Lockwood et al 1990, Baggish &

Table 3.1 Age in selecting patients for endometrial ablation

Age (years)	
50+	If cyclical bleeding on hormone replacement therapy
40–50	Most patients
<40	If sterilized
<30	If haemorrhage uncontrolled by drugs

Baltoyannis 1988). Ablation can be performed under local anesthetic with sedation, but the lithotomy position may still be difficult for a patient with severe respiratory disease. Of particular importance are chronic bronchitis/emphysema, coronary artery disease, hypertension (especially with cardiomegaly), insulin-dependent diabetes and chronic renal disease with impaired renal function.

Morbid obesity always causes both anaesthetic and surgical complications but, in a grossly obese woman, ablation is preferable to hysterectomy because the complications of the latter may be very serious. The main problem with obese patients is that other pelvic pathology may not be detected and an enlarged uterus may not be recognized. Medically unfit patients are at a particular risk of complications from fluid absorption into the circulation. Very careful measurements of fluid input and outflow must be kept and even if a small deficit is detected the anaesthetist should be alerted and, possibly, the operation terminated. Radio frequency ablation does not use fluid to distend the uterine cavity and may offer an alternative treatment in women with menorrhagia and severe cardiopulmonary disease (Phipps et al 1990).

FERTILITY

Successful ablation or resection removes all the endometrium, including the basal layers and the superficial myometrium, resulting in amenorrhoea or sterility. Postoperative hysteroscopy shows either a small, white, atrophic, empty cavity or thick adhesions which almost obliterate the cavity. This result is perfectly acceptable in older women but young patients must be carefully counselled so that they fully understand the implications for fertility. There is no evidence that ectopic pregnancy rates are increased but the possibility of a tubal pregnancy cannot be discounted even in women who are amenorrhoeic.

In contrast, women who bleed cyclically, no matter how slight the amount, are at risk of pregnancy (Mongelli & Evans 1991). If an embryo implants on a preserved island of endometrium, there is a high possibility that the pregnancy will progress to term. There is also the theoretical possibility that the placenta may become morbidly adherent, resulting in placenta accreta with major third-stage difficulties. This event has not yet been reported (Hallez et al 1987). These patients should therefore be counselled to use appropriate contraception. It may be appropriate to offer laparoscopic sterilization at the time of ablation. Sterilization should be performed prior to ablation rather than the other way round, because clips on the tubes prevent glycine or saline entering the peritoneum. Table 3.2 summarizes the factors to be considered in selecting patients for endometrial ablation.

SYMPTOMS

Bleeding

Patients who respond well to ablation complain of heavy cyclical bleeding. Women with intermenstrual bleeding or premenstrual or postmenstrual loss or spotting, should be carefully evaluated in order to exclude other pathology such as endometrial hyperplasia or polyps. The volume of blood lost is critical but this is difficult to measure because the loss is subjective and may vary monthly. A patient with chronic hypochromic microcytic anaemia is probably bleeding in excess. A history of clots and flooding uncon-

Table 3.2 Factors influencing patient selection for Endometrial Ablation

A. *May be more suitable for ablation*
  1. Sterilized or family complete
  2. Dysfunctional bleeding with small uterus, <12 cm cavity
  3. No severe dysmenorrhoea suggesting endometriosis
  4. Benign histology
  5. Failed medical treatment
  6. Obesity
  7. Respiratory and cardiovascular disease which precludes major surgery.
  8. Submucous or single intramural fibroid

B. *May be more suitable for hysterectomy*
  1. Coexisting pelvic pathology
     Stress incontinence
     Prolapse
     Endometriosis
     Adenomyosis
  2. Adenomatous hyperplasia or adenocarcinoma in situ
  3. Menorrhagia with cervical intraepithelial neoplasia
  4. Multiple intramural or large subperitoneal fibroids
  5. Sterilized or family complete

trolled by pads is significant. Menorrhagia in excess of the upper limit of 80 ml will rarely be controlled by vaginal tampons. Objective measurement of the blood loss, however, is difficult and time-consuming (Chimbira et al 1980).

Pain

Heavy blood loss is often associated with severe colicky pain caused by the uterus extruding clots. The pain is usually limited to the lower abdomen, suprapubic area and the upper thighs. It is rarely unilateral and almost never causes low backache. The pain reaches a climax as the clot passes through the endocervical canal. The colic may be impossible to distinguish from the pain caused by a submucous myoma or polyp without a hysterosalpingogram or a diagnostic hysteroscopy.

In contrast, hormonal dysfunction is almost painless or is associated with a premenstrual ache in the lower abdomen probably due to pelvic congestion.

The most important alternative diagnosis is endometriosis or adenomyosis, which causes premenstrual, intramenstrual or postmenopausal pain and often severe low backache. The distinction is important because ablative techniques will not cure the patient with endometriosis or adenomyosis. Indeed, the patient may have complete amenorrhoea following surgery but may have crippling cyclical dysmenorrhoea which can only be cured by hysterectomy.

Clinical signs

All patients must have a physical examination, including a careful pelvic bimanual examination. A patient with functional bleeding will have a small mobile non-tender uterus with no ovarian enlargement. A fixed retroverted uterus, or a tender adnexal mass, should suggest endometriosis. Tender nodules in the posterior fornix suggest endometriotic deposits in the recto-vaginal septum, and a tender bulky uterus may indicate adenomyosis. Adenomyosis can sometimes cause generalized uterine hyperplasia to such an extent that it feels like a fibroid.

An irregular uterine outline suggests multiple myomas, which are much more difficult to treat

by laser or resectoscope than a solitary fibroid. The best type of fibroid to remove endoscopically is the submucous fibroid, which should be suspected if the external cervical os is patulous because of attempts by the uterine muscle to extrude the myoma.

Finally, chronic pelvic inflammatory disease causes pain and tenderness and may alter the menstrual pattern. This condition does not improve with ablation.

PREOPERATIVE INVESTIGATIONS (TABLE 3.3)

Size of the Uterus

The single most important indicator for successful ablation is the size of the uterus — specifically the size of the uterine cavity. A uterus greater than the size of a 12 week pregnancy or a cavity greater than 10 cm in length is more difficult to resect or ablate and the operative time is prolonged. Prolonged surgery increases the risk of fluid intravasation and cardiovascular overload. The size of the uterus must therefore be carefully evaluated (Loffer 1990, Lomano 1991).

Ultrasound

Transabdominal ultrasound is helpful but vaginal ultrasound is more comfortable for the patient because she does not need a full bladder and greater detail can be seen. The length of the cavity can be assessed and the distance between the cornua measured. The thickness of the endometrium is important and the scan is best repeated after drug therapy to confirm the thinning effect. Vaginal ultrasound can also detect focal lesions, especially fibroids, and can confirm the number of fibroids, their size and their position in the uterine cavity.

Table 3.3 Preoperative investigations

Haemoglobin and full blood count
Abdominal or vaginal ultrasound
Diagnostic panoramic hysteroscopy
Endometrial biopsy
Hysterosalpingogram — sometimes
Laparoscopy — sometimes

Careful attention should be paid to the adnexa because ovarian enlargement suggests the presence of endometriosis and benign and malignant cysts. Endometriosis of the rectovaginal septum is much more difficult to see.

Diagnostic hysteroscopy

Diagnostic hysteroscopy using a small volume of Hyskon, normal saline or carbon dioxide gas from a specially designed hysteroflator is easy to perform and is an alternative to vaginal ultrasound (Lewis 1990). Sometimes both diagnostic methods are needed.

Hysteroscopy can easily be performed in an out-patient or office setting without the need for any anaesthetic or analgesia. A small-diameter telescope is needed which can be passed through the os with minimal discomfort. The operation is best performed in the postmenstrual phase of the cycle because bleeding interferes with vision. Hysteroscopy provides accurate information on the uterine size, shape of the cavity and the presence of fibroids, and the extent which they intrude or distort the uterine cavity. Hysteroscopy also allows directed punch biopsies of suspicious areas of endometrium (Hamou & Lewis 1990).

Endometrial biopsy

It is absolutely essential to obtain a sample of endometrium for histological examination to exclude atypical hyperplasia. The risk of atypical hyperplasia Grade II or III, progressing to carcinoma in perimenopausal women, is about 20–25% and therefore the patient is best treated by simple hysterectomy rather than ablation (Gusberg et al 1988). Frank invasive carcinoma is rare in premenopausal women, but must always be considered. Sarcomatous change in a fibroid is even less common, but should be suspected if the myoma bleeds excessively or is unduly friable during resection.

An endometrial biopsy should always be obtained before laser ablation or radio frequency ablation because both methods destroy the endometrium and leave no tissue for histology. It is not unreasonable to delay histology until surgery during electroresection because the large chips of endometrium provide ample samples for the pathologist. Moreover, the thermal damage to the endometrium is minimal and does not create problems of interpretation.

Good-quality endometrial samples may be obtained with a number of devices such as the Novak curette, Vabra aspirater or the Pipelle de Cornier (Laboratoire CCD, Paris).

The Pipelle is particularly useful because it is made of plastic with a flexible but blunt end. It can therefore easily negotiate the cervical canal in most patients with minimum trauma and little discomfort. The sample is obtained by withdrawing the inner rod, which creates a vacuum. Samples of endometrium are then drawn into fine holes near the tip of the catheter before being preserved in formal saline.

Hysterosalpingography

Radiographic examination of the uterus by hysterosalpingography is an alternative method of assessing uterine size. It is less accurate than vaginal ultrasound in assessing intramural or subperitoneal fibroids, but gives a good estimate of uterine size and shape. However, air bubbles may cause artifacts, and incomplete filling of the cavity with dye is a cause of failure to detect pathology inside the cavity (Nisolle et al 1991).

Laparoscopy

Preoperative or intraoperative laparoscopy is only rarely needed but should be used if there is any possibility of ovarian pathology, endometriosis, intramural or subperitoneal fibroids, or chronic pelvic inflammatory disease. It may be helpful for inexperienced surgeons to have the laparoscope in the abdomen, because, when the light of the resectoscope is seen through the uterine wall, further resection or laser ablation should cease (Hallez et al 1987).

Other investigations

Standard preoperative investigations include haemoglobin and full blood count, urine analysis, blood pressure recording and, in selected patients, chest radiography and electrocardiography. Serum should be saved for blood grouping and cross-matching, but it is not necessary to have blood immediately available.

PREOPERATIVE PREPARATION

There is considerable discussion whether to thin the endometrium with drugs prior to surgery in order to produce an atrophic endometrium. The alternative approach is to operate in the immediate postmenstrual phase of the cycle. This saves both time and money, because the cost of drugs is considerable, but is more difficult to organize on a busy operating schedule. The four classes of drugs available are the combined oral contraceptives, progestogens alone, danazol and luteinizing-hormone-releasing hormone (LH-RH) agonists.

Progestogens

In low doses most progestogens do not inhibit ovulation and the endometrium remains thick. In higher doses the majority of women develop atrophic changes in the endometrium but a considerable proportion continue to bleed irregularly and have a thick oedematous vascular endometrium. Women in general tolerate progestogens quite well, but some develop weight gain, fluid retention and discomfort from mastalgia. The drugs most commonly used are norethisterone acetate 15–30 mg daily and medroxyprogesterone acetate 30–50 mg daily.

Danazol

Danazol is still probably the most widely used drug to suppress the endometrium but the compound is expensive and causes side-effects which are dose-dependent. In order to produce a good clinical effect, the dose needs to be a minimum of 400 mg daily. Many women need 600 mg daily and a few require 800 mg daily to stop bleeding and cause atrophy. These doses cause weight gain, mild hirsutism, especially excess facial hair, acne, oily skin changes and, occasionally, voice changes. Sometimes muscle pains develop that can be severe, so that the patient voluntarily stops the drug (Barbieri & Ryan 1981).

LH-RH agonists

LH-RH agonists are increasingly used for preoperative endometrial thinning and are probably the drugs of choice. Surgery should be scheduled to occur about 4–6 weeks after the drugs are commenced. In the USA the drug most widely used is leuprolide 1 mg (Lupron Tapp Pharmaceuticals, Chicago; Prostap Lederle), which is accepted for this purpose by the US Food and Drug Administration. In the UK the drugs available are buserelin (Suprefact Hoechst), nafarelin (Synarel, Syntex Pharmaceuticals) and goserelin (Zoladex, ICI Pharmaceuticals). The last drug has the significant advantage that it is given by a single preloaded subcutaneous injection. Although goserelin is being used at the present time in a few units for endometrial preoperative preparation on a named patient basis, it has not yet formally been accepted for this purpose.

The advantages of the LH-RH agonists are that they produce excellent endometrial atrophy (Brooks et al 1991), they have fewer side-effects than danazol and can be given in a single dose so there is no risk of decalcification or osteoporosis. Menopausal symptoms are induced but these are rarely severe. Cost is a significant factor because the manufacturing costs of these complicated drugs are high.

PREVIOUS SURGERY

The main hazards of endometrial ablation are fluid overload and trauma caused by forcible dilatation of the cervix and perforation. Perforation of the uterus occurs in about 1–2% of the patients according to the surveys from the American College of Obstetricians and the Audit Unit from the Royal College of Obstetricians (personal communication). Most perforations occur during insertion of the resectoscope or laser, during collection of endometrial chips or excessive resection, especially at the cornua. A very high intrauterine pressure also increases the risk of intrauterine 'blow out', especially if the myometrium is already thin. A previous history of uterine surgery is therefore important, and should be recorded on the preoperative assessment. The two main operations which predispose to perforation are myomectomy, especially if the uterine cavity was opened, and caesarian section, so that special care should be exercised when operating on these women.

LONG-TERM EFFECTS

Endometrial carcinoma

There is much concern but very little information on the problem of carcinoma developing after ablative procedures. If all the endometrium, including the basal layers, are removed, the risk of subsequent cancer should be eliminated but the concern relates to the fact that if a small island of endometrium is inadvertently preserved it has the potential to develop malignant changes. Moreover, it is not known if the surgical insult applied to the endometrium stimulates increased cellular activity. If amenorrhoea is induced there is a theoretical possibility that if cancer develops in a preserved fragment of endometrium it will not cause visible bleeding if the endocervical canal is obliterated. The other worrying possibility is that the tumour might grow deeply into the myometrium and only present at a clinically advanced stage.

These risks are unknown, but as yet there is no recorded patient who has developed cancer after ablation, although there are reports of malignancy discovered at resection, but the time-scale is very short because there are no long-term follow-up studies. It is hoped that if a British National Register is established, all patients undergoing ablation can be flagged by the National Cancer Registry, which will then detect patients who develop endometrial cancer should it occur in the future. A Scottish National Register has just commenced and a multicentre trial of resection funded by the British Medical Research Council has also just started, although the number of patients is still small and long-term follow-up studies are awaited.

HORMONE REPLACEMENT THERAPY

The questions which need to be discussed are whether hormone replacement therapy is indicated in the postmenopausal patient, and is ablation justified in women taking hormone replacement therapy who do not wish to have cyclical bleeding?

In women who are amenorrhoeic following ablation, most authorities would agree that hormone replacement therapy can be given if there are severe menopausal symptoms. There is no unanimity of opinion about the need to add progestogens to the oestrogen preparation. Progestogens should not be needed if all the endometrium is destroyed but there is concern about the risk of inducing malignancy with unopposed oestrogen in women with preserved islands of endometrium. Moreover, even if the patient is amenorrhoeic, there could be a dormant fragment of basal endometrium which might be stimulated by hormone replacement therapy. At present, therefore, it is generally recommended that women should be given oestrogen and progestogens. Tibolone (Livial, Organon) might be advantageous in these women because it does not cause endometrial stimulation but gives adequate relief of the symptoms of oestrogen lack.

In the UK ablation for postmenopausal women with cyclical bleeding due to hormone replacement therapy is not a recognized indication. In the USA where more women are being treated with cyclical steroids, some practitioners advise endometrial ablation if bleeding is troublesome. Long-term studies of these women are anxiously awaited.

Recurrence of bleeding

The immediate failure rate of ablation in women who report no improvement 6 months after the operation is between 5 and 15%. These women can either be offered a hysterectomy, or have the ablation repeated. The cure rate in women following a second ablation is high and will be preferred by many women because of the simplicity of the operation and rapid recovery from surgery. Early results suggest that, as time passes, bleeding recurs in some women, and this can happen even after 2 or 3 years following an initially good result (Derman et al 1991). If patients are carefully selected, however, i.e. women in the fifth decade who would otherwise be offered a hysterectomy, even a 25% long-term failure rate is acceptable, especially as these patients will be approaching the menopause.

Haematometra

Occasional patients will develop a haematometra because of preserved functioning islands of endometrium with a stenotic cervix. The risk of this happening can be reduced if the endocervical canal is left untreated, but this increases the risk of cyclical bleeds and reduces the incidence of amenorrhoea (Nisolle et al 1991). If a patient presents with cyclical pain a haematometra should be considered and an ultrasound scan performed (Dwyer et al 1991). Blood accumulating in the uterus can be readily detected but a hysterectomy will be necessary if the uterus cannot be drained.

POSTOPERATIVE TREATMENT

Antibiotics

Infection after ablation is not common but can occur in the presence of large amounts of necrotic tissue in the uterus. The risk can be reduced by removing all the chips after resection but some dead tissue inevitably remains and could provide a nidus for infection. It is probably wise to prescribe a broad-spectrum antibiotic for a few days after surgery and the addition of metronidazole for Gram-positive anaerobes is useful (Derman et al 1991). In practice, infection is uncommon and many surgeons prefer to avoid prophylaxis and only treat established sepsis after swabs and blood cultures.

Pain

There is considerable pain for a few hours in a minority of women. Usually, simple analgesics are sufficient but opium alkaloids may occasionally be needed for postoperative pain. Within a few hours the pain improves and very rarely prevents early hospital discharge.

Vaginal discharge

It is usual for women to experience pelvic discomfort and an offensive blood-stained discharge as the necrotic debris in the uterus is expelled. The vaginal loss often continues for 2 or 3 weeks and this should be explained to the patient prior to surgery. The first or second menstrual period can be heavy, so the patients should be warned of this possibility and told that the final result cannot be expected for at least 4 months, because this is the time it takes for fibrosis to develop.

Counselling

Good counselling is the key to patient satisfaction. Detailed explanations should be given with regard to fertility, bleeding, long-term results, short-term complications and the possibility of recurrence, and the need for eventual hysterectomy. It should be pointed out that, although bleeding may be significantly improved, a small proportion of women will be left with or develop cyclical pain which can be severe. They should also be warned that endometrial ablation is not a cure for the premenstrual tension syndrome because ovarian function is unaffected, although there have been isolated reports that both primary dysmenorrhoea and the premenstrual syndrome improve (Lefler 1989). A written explanation is useful in ensuring that the patient fully understands the implications of the operation and is thus able to give the true informed consent.

CONCLUSIONS

The choice between laser ablation, endometrial electroresection or radio frequency ablation depends largely on the preference of the surgeon and the availability of equipment; the success and complication rates of each approach appear to be broadly similar. Long-term studies are not available although laser ablation has been in use 13 years and there is an 8 year follow-up study of electroresection in women with submucous fibroids. The best results and the most satisfied patients will be women who have been carefully counselled and in whom ablation is the only alternative to hysterectomy because other less invasive procedures have failed.

REFERENCES

Baggish M S, Baltoyannis P 1988 New techniques for laser ablation of the endometrium in high risk patients. American Journal of Obstetrics and Gynecology 159: 287–292

Barbieri R L, Ryan K J 1981 Danazol: endocrine pharmacology and therapeutic applications. American Journal of Obstetrics and Gynecology 141: 453–463

Brooks P G, Serden S P, Daves I 1991 Hormonal inhibition of the endometrium for resectoscopic endometrial ablation. American Journal of Obstetrics and Gynecology 164: 1601–1608

Chimbira T H, Anderson A, Turnbull AC 1980 Relationships between menstrual blood loss and patients subjective assessment of loss, duration of bleeding, number of sanitary towels used, uterine weight and endometrial surface area. British Journal of Obstetrics and Gynaecology 87: 603–609

DeCherney A H, Polan M L 1983 Hysteroscopic management of intrauterine lesions and intractable uterine bleeding. Obstetrics and Gynecology 70: 668–670

Derman S G, Rehnstrom J, Neuwirth R S 1991 The long term effectiveness of hysteroscopic treatment of menorrhagia and leiomyomas. Obstetrics and Gynecology 77: 591–594

Dwyer N, Fox R, Mills M, Hutton J 1991 Haematometra caused by hormone replacement therapy after endometrial resection. Lancet 338: 1205

Hallez J, Nettera A, Cartier R 1987 Methodical intrauterine resection. American Journal of Obstetrics and Gynecology 156: 1080–1084

Hamou J, Lewis B V 1990 Hysteroscopy and Microhysteroscopy. In: Bonnar J (ed) Recent advances in obstetrics and gynaecology. Churchill Livingstone, Edinburgh, vol 16, p 185–197

Gusberg S B, Shingleton H M, Deppe G 1988 Female genital cancer. Churchill Livingstone, New York

Lefler H T 1989 Premenstrual syndrome improvement after laser ablation of the endometrium for menorrhagia. Journal of Reproductive Medicine 34: 905–906

Lewis B V 1990 Hysteroscopy for the investigation of abnormal uterine bleeding. British Journal of Obstetrics and Gynecology 97: 283–284

Lockwood M, Magos A L, Bauman R, Turnbull A C 1990 Endometrial resection when hysterectomy is undesirable, dangerous or impossible. British Journal of Obstetrics and Gynaecology 97: 656–658

Loffer F D 1990 Removal of large symptomatic intrauterine growths by the hysteroscopic resectoscope. Obstetrics and Gynecology 76: 836–840

Lomano J 1991 Endometrial ablation for the treatment of menorrhagia: a comparison of patients with normal, enlarged or fibroid uteri. Lasers in Surgery and Medicine 11: 8–12

Mongelli J M, Evans A J 1991 Pregnancy after transcervical endometrial resection. Lancet 338: 578–579

Nisolle M, Grandjean P, Gillerot S, Donnez J 1991 Endometrial ablation with the Nd-Yag laser in dysfunctional bleeding. Minimally Invasive Therapy 1: 35–39

Phipps J H, Lewis B V, Roberts T, Prior M V, Hand J W, Elder M, Field S B 1990 Treatment of functional menorrhagia by radio frequency-induced thermal endometrial ablation. Lancet 335: 374–376

Rutherford A J, Glass M R, Wells M 1991 Patient selection for hysteroscopic endometrial resection. British Journal of Obstetrics and Gynaecology 98: 228–230

4. Preoperative diagnostic hysteroscopy

N. C. W. Hill

INTRODUCTION

Visual examination of the uterine cavity is reputed to have been first performed by Pantaleoni in 1865, who used a small tube inserted through the external cervical os with a kerosene lamp as a light source (Lindemann 1973). However, it is only in the past 25 years with the development of the new telescope lens systems and fibreoptic light sources that the use of hysteroscopy has become more widespread. Hysteroscopy, the direct visualization of the inside of the uterine cavity, is possible with both panoramic and contact techniques. Panoramic hysteroscopy requires distension of the uterine cavity with either a gaseous or liquid medium and, after insertion of the hysteroscope, the uterine cavity can be fully inspected for abnormality. Contact hysteroscopy, as the name implies, is performed with the objective lens of the telescope in direct contact with the structure under observation and does not necessarily require uterine distension.

The normal physiological condition of the endometrial layers is one of contact; therefore, in order to perform hysteroscopy the cavity must be distended with a medium. This results in the endometrial layers being separated by 1.5–2.5 cm. The visual impression obtained provides an indication of colour, contour and of compliance, and must be related to knowledge of uterine anatomy, physiology and pathology. At hysteroscopy it is only possible to visualize the uterine cavity; therefore, myometrial conditions such as adenomyosis and intramural myoma are beyond the scope of the instrument. It is also important to understand the limitations of hysteroscopy because, unless the entire uterine cavity has been

visualized, an incomplete examination may result in missed pathology.

With the development of powerful fibreoptic light sources, it has become possible to perform hysteroscopy using much smaller-diameter instruments. This in turn means minimal or no cervical dilatation is required, and the technique is suitable for an out-patient procedure without routine use of anaesthesia. Although few UK gynaecological clinics are set up to perform invasive out-patient investigations (Lewis 1990), extensive experience of many clinics in other European countries shows this is perfectly acceptable given time, adequate explanation and sympathetic support during the procedure. This is particularly so as the alternative in most centres is dilatation and curettage performed under general anaesthesia.

INSTRUMENTS

The basic equipment required for hysteroscopy includes a viewing system, a system for providing gaseous or liquid distension, and ancillary instruments for operative procedures.

Viewing system

The panoramic hysteroscope consists basically of a modified cystoscope (Fig. 4.1a). The telescope is usually 4 mm in diameter and, depending on the type of hysteroscope, is equipped with a 0 or 30° fore-oblique view with a Hopkins lens system consisting of special glass rods placed at intervals along the axis of the telescope. This system has the advantage of providing high resolution and contrast, natural colour tones, and a wide operative view. The telescope is surrounded by a

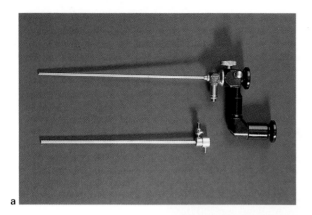

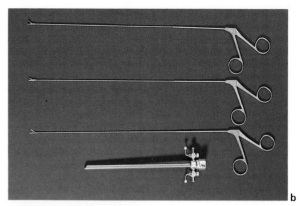

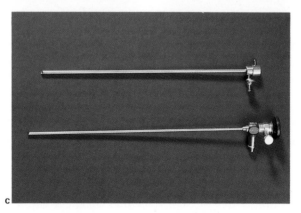

Fig. 4.1   **a** The Hamou I microcolpohysteroscope and diagnostic sheath; **b** operative sheath and auxillary instruments for diagnostic hysteroscopy (scissors, grasping forceps, biopsy forceps); **c** the Hamou II microhysteroscope and diagnostic sheath.

detachable 5–6 mm sheath, which has a proximal valve through which gas or fluid can be insufflated, providing distension of the uterine cavity. Most hysteroscopes also have a wider 7–8 mm operative sheath which when inserted over the telescope allows passage of scissors, biopsy or grasping forceps through a separate channel for minor surgical procedures (Fig. 4.1b). These instruments can be flexible or semiflexible in design, the semiflexible instruments being sturdier and easier to use than their flexible counterparts.

Many different types of hysteroscopes are available and for further information the reader is referred to Valle & Sciarra (1983) or Lewis (1989). A popular hysteroscope is the Hamou I microcolpohysteroscope, which consists of a 4 mm Storz telescope with a direct occular and an offset occular each offering two different magnifications (Hamou 1981). Direct vision allows conventional panoramic hysteroscopy but, when a small lever is depressed on the handle, the offset occular provides a ×20 magnification of the uterine cavity. If the tip of the hysteroscope is placed in direct contact with the endometrium, the magnification increases to ×60 or ×150 with the direct and offset occulars, respectively. This instrument can also be used as a colpohysteroscope. In this mode the squamocolumnar junction of the cervix can be examined, especially if it lies within the endocervical canal as often occurs in postmenopausal patients. At the very high magnifications possible with the instrument, contact hysteroscopy can be performed and the glandular, cellular and vascular layers of the endocervix and endometrium inspected. Hamou & Taylor (1982) recommend staining the epithelium with Waterman blue ink, methylene blue or Lugol's iodine to make the images less difficult to interpret. Although contact hysteroscopy has its advocates (van Herendael 1987), it is seldom required in most hysteroscopies, and is clinically less useful than panoramic hysteroscopy. As very high magnification is unnecessary for panoramic hysteroscopy, the Hamou II (Storz) and the microview telescope (Wolf), which do not have an offset second eyepiece laterally, are probably among the best hysteroscopes currently available (Fig. 4.1c). In both these telescopes the degree of magnification increases as the tip of the hysteroscope approaches the endometrium, and a focusing wheel adjusts the focus at the various focal lengths.

Although all the hysteroscopes considered so far are rigid, recently small flexible hysteroscopes have been developed, which are basically modified choledochoscopes (KeyMed-Olympus) (Fig. 4.2). The 6 mm telescope, with its channel for gaseous or fluid distension, can be introduced through the cervix with minimal or no dilatation, and the tip of the telescope can be angled through 180° by a wheel on the proximal end. The instrument by its very flexible nature provides good views of the cornua, which may be important for localization of intratubular contraceptive devices. Generally, the view obtained is of an inferior quality compared to a conventional hysteroscope, probably related to the increased numbers of optical fibres required by the instrument. In practice the flexible instruments have little advantage over the rigid systems and are much more expensive (Lewis 1988). It remains to be seen whether even smaller flexible hysteroscopes will be better tolerated by the patients compared with the rigid instruments.

Illumination for hysteroscopy can be obtained using a standard 150 W light source transmitted along a fibreoptic cable. However, if closed-circuit television or photography is being used, a xenon light source provides better illumination. Excellent results are obtained when the images are viewed on a high-resolution colour monitor using a chip camera. Although this increases the basic price of the system, the images produced can be recorded on video tape and are therefore available for future viewing. The position of the operator is more comfortable and the patient is also able to see the pictures, which they often find reassuring. All the major instrument manufacturers have their own systems for closed-circuit television, and these should be tried before purchasing. Photographs can be obtained with a standard camera, providing an appropriate coupling system for the hysteroscope is available. Best results are obtained with high speed films of 400 ASA and a motor drive (Lewis 1989). Alternatively, excellent quality photographs can be obtained using a computerized system which electronically controls the duration of the flash. Although it is useful to record pathological findings either on video or film for reference purposes, neither is an essential requirement for hysteroscopy.

Distending the uterine cavity

Normally the anterior and posterior walls of the uterine cavity are in close proximity, and have to be separated before panoramic hysteroscopy. The cavity can be distended using either gas or fluid,

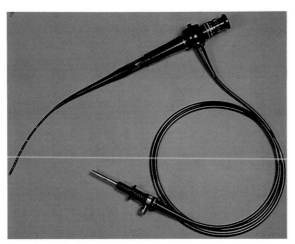

Fig. 4.2 Flexible diagnostic hysteroscope.

which enters the uterus under pressure via a side channel in the telescope sheath. Usually the distending medium is prevented from leaking around the cervix because of the tight fit between the endocervix and the hysteroscope. Occasionally with a very patulous cervix inadequate uterine distension results from cervical leakage of the medium; however, this can be partly prevented by the application of a portio applicator onto the cervix. Although both gas and fluid leak into the peritoneal cavity, in practice this is rarely a problem, especially if the flow rate is not excessive and the examination time short.

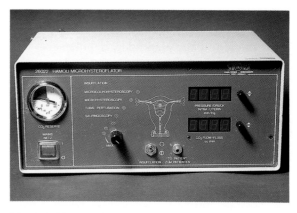

Fig. 4.3   Hamou electronic carbon dioxide insufflator.

Gaseous distension

Carbon dioxide provides a readily available, inert and rapidly absorbed medium for hysteroscopy. The gas provides perfect transmission of the image, has a long history of safety, and the continuous flow of gas provides a good cervical dilator to allow passage of the hysteroscope. The gaseous pressure should not exceed 100 mmHg, but usually only pressures of the order of 20–30 mmHg are required, and flow rates should not exceed 60 ml/min (Taylor & Hamou 1983). It is exceedingly dangerous to attempt to use a laparoscopic insufflator, as the flow rates will be exceeded and gas embolism may occur. Carbon dioxide must therefore be delivered by a special hysteroflator (Storz) or by the Metromat (Wolf) (Fig. 4.3). In both these machines the pressure and flow rates are clearly visible and both can be adjusted easily as appropriate. Another safety feature built into the machines is a reducing valve which ensures that the gas flow rate cannot be excessive. Carbon dioxide is an extremely safe medium for gaseous distension of the uterus, and no change in arterial pH or pCO_2 has been reported after hysteroscopy provided these precautions are taken (Lindemann 1974). The average hysteroscopy takes less than 10 minutes and the average volume of carbon dioxide used does not exceed 400 ml (Hamou & Salat-Baroux 1984).

Although carbon dioxide hysteroscopy gives excellent images, it requires expensive insufflating equipment, good cervical occlusion and, occasionally, bubbles may form inside the uterine cavity which may obscure the view. If the uterus is distended too rapidly or if the intrauterine pressure is too high the uterus will start contracting, which may cause discomfort to the patient and make observation more difficult. Shoulder tip pain secondary to diaphragmatic irritation from intraperitoneal carbon dioxide is a relatively frequent complaint when hysteroscopy is performed without general anaesthesia. This can often be prevented by a slight Trendelenburg position during hysteroscopy. However, undoubtedly the major drawback of carbon dioxide is the very poor image obtained in the presence of blood in the uterine cavity, and in such patients fluid distension may be required.

Fluid distension

High-molecular-weight dextran (dextran 70 or Hyskon) and 5% dextrose are the fluid media most often used during hysteroscopy (Rioux 1984). The major advantages of fluid distension media are that they do not require expensive insufflation machines and clear images are obtained in the presence of blood in the uterine cavity.

Dextran 70 is a colourless liquid with a high viscosity and excellent optical qualities. The technique involves slowly injecting about 20–30 ml of dextran into the uterus via a syringe attached to the perfusion channel of the sheath.

Manual pressure is maintained on the syringe to ensure a continuous flow, preventing accumulation of blood and mucus. Dextran 70 has the advantage of being non-miscible with blood, which forms droplets in the medium and flows slowly out of the tubal ostium, allowing a good visual field. Although hysteroscopy using dextran 70 to distend the uterine cavity is probably the simplest technique for hysteroscopy, there are a number of disadvantages with the medium. Due to its high viscosity the sheath and valves will rapidly become blocked if dextran is allowed to dry in the instrument. This can be prevented by a thorough cleaning of the hysteroscope in warm water immediately after use. Also, the rate of reabsorption and reactivity in the abdominal cavity is unknown, and occasional allergic reactions have been reported.

5% dextrose in water also provides adequate uterine distention without the need for an insufflator. Although of low viscosity, 5% dextrose mixes less readily with blood than normal saline (Valle 1983). The dextrose is delivered by placing a pressure cuff around a 500 ml bag of the solution on a drip stand. The end of the giving set is attached to the sheath, and the blood pressure cuff inflated to approximately 100 mmHg. Dextrose flows freely out of the end of the hysteroscope, which can then be inserted into the uterine cavity. The volume of fluid required for the procedure is small, typically 150 ml of 5% dextrose being used during a 10 minute examination (Taylor & Hamou 1983), and therefore fluid absorption is not a problem. Similar results can be achieved with other solutions such as normal saline. Pumps have been developed to regulate inflow and outflow of these low-viscosity fluids automatically, to maintain a clear image.

The choice between carbon dioxide or fluid distension of the uterus depends on individual preference and availability of equipment. For out-patient hysteroscopy, carbon dioxide insufflation is probably superior because of its simplicity and convenience. Although the insufflators are expensive, they are well worth the outlay and if resources are limited it is better to have a good insufflator than a camera. For diagnostic hysteroscopy, fluid distension is probably only essential when there is intrauterine bleeding.

INDICATIONS FOR PANORAMIC HYSTEROSCOPY

Whenever there is an indication for dilatation and curettage, hysteroscopy is an alternative. Indeed, the traditional operation of dilatation and curettage perhaps could now be replaced by hysteroscopy and biopsy. Although endometrial biopsy performed as an out-patient procedure using flexible plastic curettes has an efficacy similar to dilatation and curettage (MacKenzie 1985), most patients in the UK presenting with abnormal uterine bleeding still have curettage performed under general anaesthesic. An alternative for these patients is out-patient diagnostic hysteroscopy, which has been shown to have a higher sensitivity compared to curettage (Brooks & Serden 1988, Gimpelson & Rappold 1988, Loffer 1989). However, although more units in the UK are following the example of other European countries of performing out-patient hysteroscopy, most hysteroscopies are still performed under general anaesthesia (Lewis 1989). This is because hysteroscopy is usually followed by a formal curettage which obviously requires an anaesthetic, rather than a simple biopsy which does not. In multiparous premenopausal patients, hysteroscopy and endometrial biopsy can usually be completed in minutes without dilatation of the cervix or anaesthesia. In nulliparae or postmenopausal patients cervical dilatation may be required more often, but this can be performed under local anaesthesia. When the wider operative sheath is used, local anaesthesia, either intra- or paracervically, is required, but general anaesthesia may rarely be needed (Hill et al 1992).

In a recent review of out-patient panoramic hysteroscopy practice the indications for hysteroscopy included menorrhagia (45%), intermenstrual or postcoital bleeding (21%), postmenopausal bleeding (10%), irregular menstruation (9%), subfertility (6%) and recurrent miscarriages (4%) (Hill et al 1992). The hysteroscope is also valuable in the diagnosis of congenital uterine abnormalities, intramural or submucous fibroids, cervical and endometrial polyps, endometrial carcinoma, postmenopausal endometritis, uterine synechiae and retained products of conception. Operations which can be performed using a diagnostic hysteroscope include endometrial target biopsy or polypectomy, removal of lost intra-uterine contraceptive devices (IUCDs), division of intrauterine adhesions and sterilization. The hysteroscope is ideal for removing lost IUCD, where the device is easily visualized, examined in full and grasped prior to removal. If a piece of an IUCD is missing, hysteroscopy can also deter-mine if the fragment is still retained within the uterus.

THE TECHNIQUE OF PANORAMIC HYSTEROSCOPY

Hysteroscopy using carbon dioxide as a distend-ing medium is ideally performed during the follicular phase of the menstrual cycle. It can still be performed premenstrually or during men-struation, but often blood will obscure the view and an incomplete examination may result. In this situation, distension with a fluid medium rather than carbon dioxide usually permits a clear view.

The patient is placed in a modified lithotomy position using urology or Lloyd–Davies stirrups. The vulva is washed with a warm antiseptic and a bimanual examination performed to assess the size and position of the uterus. A Sims' speculum is then inserted, and the cervix visualized. The cervix is washed with further warm antiseptic, and usually grasped with a vulsellum forceps which is used to steady the cervix. The direction and length of the uterine cavity is measured with a uterine sound. The technique of hysteroscopy using carbon dioxide as the distending medium then involves the introduction of the hystero-scope into the external cervical os, removal of the Sims' speculum, the light source being switched on and gaseous insufflation commenced. Whilst the images are viewed on the monitor, the tele-scope is gently steered through the endocervical canal into the cavity of the uterus. As noted in Chapter 2, it is essential to take account of the fore-oblique view of the hysteroscope lens during this stage of the procedure. If the uterus is anteverted the image of the endocervical canal is kept at 6 o'clock on the monitor. However, if the uterus is retroverted the hysteroscope lens is rotated through 180° and the image of the canal

kept at 12 o'clock on the monitor. If at any stage the image of the canal is lost, it can usually be relocated by withdrawing the hysteroscope slightly. The gas gently distends the endocervical canal and allows free passage of the telescope through the internal os into the uterine cavity. Once inside the uterus, the illumination is increased to provide a brighter picture, and the cavity is systematically inspected for any abnor-mality. The telescope is then slowly withdrawn from the uterus and the cervical canal viewed in its entire length.

Routine analgesia need not be given to patients, as most women describe the pain as acceptable and 90% report the discomfort being no greater than menstruation (De Jong et al 1990). However, if the hysteroscopy is uncom-fortable, local anaesthetic can be given intra- or paracervically. Intracervical anaesthesia is simple to administer and probably less likely to produce systemic effects than paracervical anaesthesia. It also helps to soften the cervix, which may decrease the need for cervical dilatation in some cases. It is administered by injecting 10 ml of 1% lignocaine with 1:200 000 adrenalin at 1, 5, 7 and 11 o'clock positions of the cervix. Local anaesthetic is required in approximately 30% of patients, and is more common if the cervix needs dilatation or the operative sheath used (Hill et al 1992). The need for local anaesthetic appears not to be affected by parity or menopausal status of the patient. Cervical dilatation to about Hegar size 6 is necessary in less than 20% of patients. Although not affected by parity, cervical dila-tation is required more often in postmenopausal compared to premenopausal women (28.6 versus 16.6%) (Hill et al 1992). If cervical dilatation is required, the dilators should not be inserted too deeply in the uterine cavity as bleeding or pain will occur.

Cervical preparation

Perhaps part of the reluctance to the more wide-spread use of out-patient hysteroscopy is the concept that the procedure is too painful and, as passage of the hysteroscope through the cervix is probably the most painful part of the procedure, various cervical pretreatments have been tried. In postmenopausal patients, Hamou (1986) reported that a small daily dose of ethinyloestradiol for 8 days prior to hysteroscopy facilitates the passage of the telescope through the relatively tight cervix which is more commonly encountered in these patients. However, despite this treatment cervical stenosis precluding successful completion of hysteroscopy occurred in 2.3% of postmeno-pausal patients (Hamou & Taylor 1984). Townsend & Melkonian (1990) reported the use of laminaria tents for cervical preparation 2–3 hours prior to hysteroscopy. This provided sufficient dilatation to permit a virtually painless inspection of the uterine cavity. However, it was less effective in postmenopausal patients and bleeding occurred in a significant number. Recently, Gupta & Johnson (1990) have shown that the oral administration of the antiproges-terone steroid mifepristone results in significant softening and dilatation of the cervix in non-pregnant patients. It is possible that this drug could be given to patients before office hystero-scopy, although, again, endometrial bleeding may be a problem if the dose of mifepristone is too high. Studies on the use of an antiprogesterone steroid prior to hysteroscopy are awaited.

THE NORMAL APPEARANCE

The normal appearance of the endometrium depends on the menopausal state of the patient, phase of the menstrual cycle and on the choice of distension medium.

In postmenopausal patients the endometrium appears pale, flat and atrophic, with small tubal ostia (Fig. 4.4). This pale, thin appearance also occurs if patients have been treated with danazol or a gonadotrophin-releasing hormone (GnRH) analogue prior to endometrial resection. In pre-menopausal women the endometrium is usually a light pink or red colour, but its appearance changes with the menstrual cycle, and with experience it is possible to hysteroscopically date the endometrium (van Herendael et al 1987). In the proliferative phase the endometrium is pink or tan and has few blood vessels, with the endometrial gland openings appearing as pale, punctate, whitish areas (Fig. 4.5). The tubal ostia are clearly visible and the overall appearance is similar to that of postmenopausal patients. Secretory endometrium appears much thicker, velvety and red, with many small submucous blood vessels clearly visible (Fig. 4.6). At this

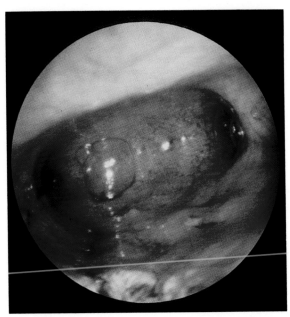

Fig. 4.4 The normal postmenopausal appearance of the uterine cavity.

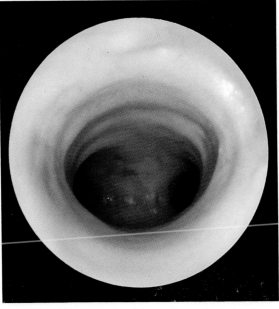

Fig. 4.5 The appearance of the uterine cavity during the proliferative stage of the cycle.

stage of the cycle, if fluid is used as the distending medium, the endometrium appears almost like coral with multiple small fronds. This appearance is lost if carbon dioxide is used for distending the uterus, when the endometrium appears relatively flat. If hysteroscopy is performed premenstrually, the endometrium is much redder and more vascular (Fig. 4.7). If menstruation has occurred, the degenerating endometrium can be seen peeling off the basal layer. Using microhysteroscopic techniques these changes are even more evident and van Herendael et al (1987) have described these features in more detail.

ABNORMALITIES SEEN ON HYSTEROSCOPY

Benign polyps

Benign polyps occur in approximately 5–10% of all patients with abnormal uterine bleeding (Hill et al 1992), and 20–25% of women presenting with postmenopausal bleeding (Cronje 1984, Walton and Macpheil 1988). Hysteroscopy can be useful in the diagnosis and management of both endocervical and endometrial polyps,

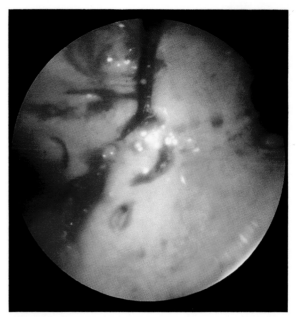

Fig. 4.7   The premenstrual appearance of the endometrium.

especially for identifying the site of origin of the polyp, as one-third of endometrial polyps may protrude through the cervix and appear as endocervical polyps (David et al 1978). If these polyps are removed by the conventional twisting technique, partial excision may occur with possible recurrence of symptoms.

Endometrial polyps are easiest diagnosed during the proliferative phase of the cycles (Fig. 4.8) and, if hysteroscopy is performed in the luteal phase, strips of dislodged endometrium occasionally appear like polyps. Small polyps can be removed using the diagnostic hysteroscope fitted with an operative sheath and grasping forceps, and should be confirmed histologically. Larger polyps may need to be removed using the resectoscope.

Fibroids

Fibroids occur in almost one-quarter of patients presenting with abnormal uterine bleeding (Fig. 4.9). They can be differentiated from endometrial polyps as they are firmer, appear fixed and, unlike polyps, do not move in response to changes in the pressure of the distension medium (Taylor & Hamou 1983). Fibroid polyps are also

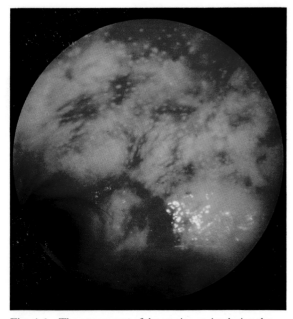

Fig. 4.6   The appearance of the uterine cavity during the secretory stage of the cycle.

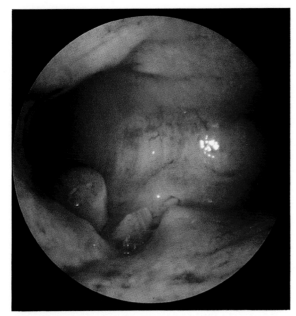

Fig. 4.8 A typical benign endometrial polyp.

recognized by their pedicle, smooth surface and white appearance. Small pedunculated fibroids can occasionally be removed during diagnostic hysteroscopy. As described in Chapter 13, intramural or large intracavity fibroids require different instruments and techniques for their removal.

Occasionally, in cases of multiple fibroids or large intracavity fibroids, the whole uterine cavity will not be visualized. In this situation an incomplete hysteroscopic examination results, and the limitation of hysteroscopy must be understood, as endometrial carcinoma can only be excluded with certainty if the whole of the uterine cavity has been inspected.

Intrauterine adhesions

Intrauterine adhesions (Fig. 4.10) have been reported at hysteroscopy in 3–15% of women with primary infertility and 30–40% of women with secondary infertility (Valle 1980). A spectrum of symptoms exists in these patients, with Sugimoto (1978) reporting amenorrhoea in 12%, oligomenorrhoea in 50% and normal menstruation in 38% of patients. However, intrauterine adhesions may also be associated with infertility and recurrent miscarriages. They should be suspected in any case of secondary amenorrhoea, especially if there is a history of surgical curettage. In these patients it is advisable to check that the patient has normal gonadotrophin levels and fails to withdraw after a progesterone challenge test before performing a hysteroscopy.

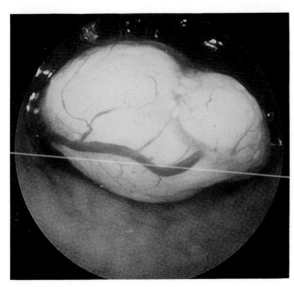

Fig. 4.9 A large intracavity fibroid.

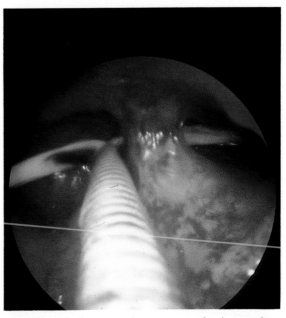

Fig. 4.10 The hysteroscopic appearance of an intrauterine adhesion in a patient with an IUCD in situ.

Hysteroscopically, it is possible to identify three different types of intrauterine adhesions by their surface appearance and force required to effect separation. The severest forms are fibrous, and occurred in 16% of 192 cases of intrauterine adhesions described by Sugimoto (1978). In the same study 53% had myofibrous and 31%, endometrial adhesions.

Once the diagnosis has been established, the traditional treatment of intrauterine adhesions is dilatation and curettage followed by the insertion of an intrauterine contraceptive device, which has been reported to improve the successful delivery rate in patients with recurrent miscarriage (Oelsner et al 1974). The adhesions can also be treated hysteroscopically, but this does depend on their severity. Simple pressure with the hysteroscope or using a fine pair of scissors via the operative sheath is effective in 60% of cases of intrauterine adhesions (Sugimoto 1978). Denser adhesions require hysteroscopic dissection, occasionally with accompanying laparoscopy, or abdominal synechiotomy. As hysteroscopy provides direct vision, the operator is able to cut only scar tissue during the dissection; therefore, the normal endometrium is not traumatized as occurs with curettage, and hence the risk of adhesion reformation may be decreased (Taylor & Hamou 1983). Adhesiolysis may be followed by oestrogen and progesterone therapy to stimulate a withdrawal bleed or, alternatively, clomiphene to induce ovulation (Lewis 1989).

Congenital uterine abnormalities

A bicornuate uterus or a uterine septum can be diagnosed hysteroscopically, and these abnormalities occur in approximately 5% of patients undergoing hysteroscopy for subfertility or recurrent miscarriage (Hill et al 1992). Occasionally, particularly when carbon dioxide is used as the distension medium, the normal uterine cavity can appear saddle shaped, which can be mistaken for a uterine fusion defect. Intrauterine adhesions may also be confused with a congenital uterine abnormality.

Hysteroscopy should now be considered an essential investigation for all women who have had more than two consecutive spontaneous miscarriages to exclude congenital uterine malformation. The procedure is more accurate and less painful than conventional hysterosalpingography (Taylor & Hamou 1983). If a septum is discovered it can be resected hysteroscopically, which is aided by an assistant observing the dissection laparoscopically, thereby reducing the risk of uterine perforation, or under ultrasound control. With increasing surgical experience, the operation has now been advocated as a replacement to conventional laparotomy and metroplasty (March and Israel 1987, Perino et al 1987).

Postmenopausal endometritis

The normal hysteroscopic postmenopausal appearance of the endometrium is pale, whitish pink and atrophic. However, in some patients with postmenopausal bleeding, the atrophic endometrium becomes vascularized by fine capillaries which can coalesce to form vascular patches (Fig. 4.11). This atrophic endometritis can only be diagnosed hysteroscopically and

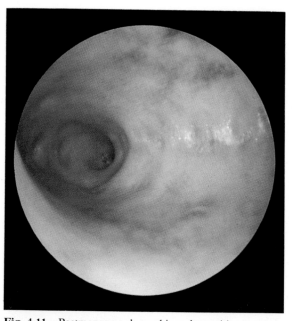

Fig. 4.11 Postmenopausal atrophic endometritis.

occurs in 75% of women with postmenopausal bleeding (Walton & Macphail 1988). This characteristic appearance of menopausal atrophy and bleeding capillaries is probably an important aetiological factor in many women with postmenopausal bleeding (Lewis 1987).

Endometrial hyperplasia

The incidence of endometrial hyperplasia in premenopausal women undergoing hysteroscopy for abnormal uterine bleeding varies from 4% (Sciarra & Valle 1977) to 20% (Barbot et al 1980, Hamou & Salat-Baroux 1984). The wide variation in incidence may reflect the difficulty in the hysteroscopic diagnosis of this condition. Although in its severest form the diagnosis is evident (Fig. 4.12), milder forms of the disease are difficult to distinguish from premenstrual endometrium. Performing the hysteroscopy in the early proliferative phase of the cycle, when the endometrium is thin, makes the diagnosis of endometrial hyperplasia more obvious. Like all hysteroscopic findings, the diagnosis of endometrial hyperplasia should be confirmed by biopsy and histology.

Endometrial carcinoma

Hysteroscopy is particularly useful in the diagnosis of endometrial carcinoma. If patients presenting with abnormal uterine bleeding,

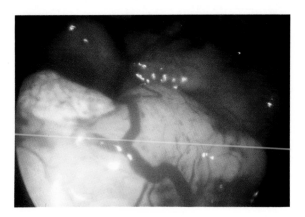

Fig. 4.12 The hysteroscopic appearance of endometrial hyperplasia.

especially postmenopausal, are treated by conventional dilatation and curettage alone, a proportion of carcinomas will be missed (Walton & Macphail 1988). This will result in inappropriate, incorrect and delayed management. Ideally, all patients should have a hysteroscopy performed prior to curettage, and in certain centres, such as that of the author, hysteroscopy has now almost totally replaced dilatation and curettage. In patients with endometrial carcinoma, hysteroscopy has the added advantage over dilatation and curettage in that it can be used to assess the size and the site of origin of the tumour, and thus its stage. This can be important, especially in cases of endometrial carcinoma involving the endocervix, which may be inappropriately treated unless correct staging has occurred. Hysteroscopy also allows a more conservative approach in patients presenting with the worrying symptom of recurrent postmenopausal bleeding. In the past, hysterectomy may have been recommended due to the fear of a missed underlying carcinoma. Today, hysteroscopy is able to exclude any intrauterine lesion and the patient can be continued to be managed conservatively.

The incidence of carcinoma at hysteroscopy depends on the indication for the procedure. In all patients attending an out-patient hysteroscopy clinic, endometrial carcinoma occurred in 0.6–0.8% of women (Hamou & Salat-Baroux 1984, Hill et al 1992). In postmenopausal patients the incidence of endometrial carcinoma at hysteroscopy rises to 5–7% (Deutschmann & Lueken 1984, Walton & Macphail 1988). The typical hysteroscopic features of an endometrial carcinoma are illustrated in Fig. 4.13. The tumour often appears like a necrotic papillomatous or exophytic lesion, usually partly obscured by haemorrhage. Multifocal, isolated or extensive satellites may also be observed in the cornua (Taylor & Hamou 1983). In its early stages endometrial carcinoma may appear polypoid in nature, and therefore may be difficult to differentiate from a benign endometrial polyp. Although endometrial carcinoma may be diagnosed hysteroscopically, biopsy should always be performed for histological confirmation.

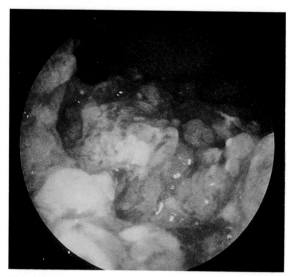

Fig. 4.13   The hysteroscopic appearance of endometrial carcinoma.

Hysteroscopy has the theoretical risk that cancer cells may be dispersed through the fallopian tubes during the procedure (Joelsson et al 1971). However, this has never been reported and Parent et al (1985) reviewed 30 patients with proven endometrial carcinoma who had hysteroscopy performed immediately prior to hysterectomy. In none of the patients were neoplastic cells recovered from the peritoneal fluid in the pouch of Douglas. Although large series have not been reported, at this time there does not appear to be an increased risk of peritoneal spread of tumour cells from hysteroscopy.

CONTRAINDICATIONS AND COMPLICATIONS OF HYSTEROSCOPY

As touched on in Chapter 2, the contra-indications and complications of hysteroscopy are few. Probably the only absolute contraindication to hysteroscopy is carcinoma of the cervix. Hysteroscopy should not be performed in the presence of proven pelvic infection, but may be necessary to remove a retained placental fragment or when infection is associated with a lost IUCD (Lewis 1989). Hysteroscopy should

be avoided in pregnancy, but the procedure has been used for recovery of lost IUCDs or even chorionic villus sampling.

Hysteroscopy is a very safe procedure. Perforation of the uterus is a rare complication, and occurs in 0.10–0.15% of cases (Salat-Baroux et al 1984). This may be caused by failing to recognize a retroverted uterus, blindly inserting the hysteroscope up to the fundus of the uterus, or applying too much force if resistance is encountered during passage of the hysteroscope through the cervix, thereby creating a false passage or tract. Perforation is more likely in cases of cervical stenosis, severe intrauterine adhesions or if operative hysteroscopy is performed. It is very unlikely provided the hysteroscope is inserted into the uterus without excessive force and under direct vision, especially if the significance of the fore-oblique view of the hysteroscope lens is appreciated. If uterine perforation occurs the intestines quickly come into endoscopic view. The hysteroscope should be gently withdrawn and the patient observed for symptoms and signs of shock. Bleeding from hysteroscopic uterine perforations is usually minimal and if necessary a laparoscopy can be performed to assess the damage. Cervical lacerations can also occur during hysteroscopy and these are usually caused by the tenaculum, or by the dilators during cervical dilatation, especially if excessive force has been used.

Salat-Baroux et al (1984) reported that mild pelvic infection occurred in 0.7% of 1000 patients undergoing hysteroscopy. Although hysteroscopy is contraindicated in acute pelvic disease, patients who give a history of recurrent pelvic infections perhaps should have the hysteroscopy performed under antibiotic cover to prevent an acute flare up of the condition.

Complications may also occur related to the distension medium. A small risk of anaphylactic reaction to dextran may occur if this is used for uterine distension, and complications can occur related to carbon dioxide if the flow rate of gas used is too high or the gas is insufflated under high pressure. This is virtually impossible with modern insufflators, but will occur if laparoscopy equipment is mistakenly used for hysteroscopy.

THE FUTURE FOR PANORAMIC HYSTEROSCOPY

New flexible hysteroscopes undoubtedly will be developed and with increasing optical technology these will become smaller in diameter and eventually may replace the rigid telescopes. Sterilization using intratubular devices placed hysteroscopically may in the future offer a safe, simple and efficient method of reversible birth control. Although out-patient hysteroscopy is widely accepted throughout most of Europe, the procedure seems less popular in the UK. The future for panoramic hysteroscopy in this country lies in the greater awareness of the advantages of the technique among gynaecologists. With this awareness must come the introduction of the procedure into more gynaecological units, for it must surely be time to abandon dilatation and curettage under general anaesthesia as the initial screening test for women with abnormal uterine bleeding.

REFERENCES

Barbot J, Parent B, Dubisson J B 1980 Contact hysteroscopy: Another method of endoscopic examination of the uterine cavity. American Journal of Obstetrics and Gynecology 136: 721–726

Brooks P G, Serden S P 1988 Hysteroscopic findings after unsuccessful dilatation and curettage for abnormal uterine bleeding. American Journal of Obstetrics and Gynecology 158: 1354–1357

Cronje H S 1984 Diagnostic hysteroscopy after postmenopausal uterine bleeding. South African Medical Journal 66: 773–774

David A, Mettler L, Semm K 1978 The cervical polyp: a new diagnostic and therapeutic approach with CO_2 hysteroscopy. American Journal of Obstetrics and Gynecology 130: 662–664

De Jong P, Doel F, Falconer A 1990 Out-patient diagnostic hysteroscopy. British Journal of Obstetrics and Gynaecology 97: 299–303

Deutschmann C, Lueken R P 1984 Hysteroscopic findings in postmenopausal bleeding. In: Siegler A M, Lindemann H J (eds) Hysteroscopy principles and practice. Lippencott, Philadelphia, p 132–134

Gimpelson R J, Rappold H O 1988 A comparararive study between panoramic hysteroscopy with directed biopsies and dilatation and curettage. The American Journal of Obstetrics and Gynecology 158: 489–492

Gupta J K, Johnson N 1990 Effect of mifepristone on dilatation of the pregnant and non-pregnant cervix. Lancet 335: 257–258

Hamou J 1981 Microhysteroscopy. Journal of Reproductive Medicine 26: 375–382

Hamou J 1986 Hysteroscopie et Microcolpohysteroscopie. Masson, Paris

Hamou J, Taylor P J 1982 Panoramic, contact and microcolpohysteroscopy in gynaecological practice. Current Problems in Obstetrics Gynecology and Fertility. Year Book Medical Publishers, Chicago

Hamou J, Salat-Baroux J 1984 Advanced hysteroscopy and microhysteroscopy in 1000 patients. In: Siegler A M, Lindemann H J (eds) Hysteroscopy principles and practice. Lippencott, Philadelphia, p 63–79

Hill N C W, Broadbent J A M, Baumann R P, Lockwood G M Magos A L, 1992 Local anaesthesia and cervical dilatation for out-patient diagnostic hysteroscopy. Journal of Obstetrics and Gynaecology 12: 33–37

Joelsson I, Levine R U, Moberger G 1971 Hysteroscopy as an adjunct in determining the extent of carcinoma of the endometrium. American Journal of Obstetrics and Gynecology 111: 696–702

Lewis B V 1987 Panoramic hysteroscopy in the diagnosis of postmenopausal bleeding due to atrophic endometritis. Journal of Obstetrics and Gynaecology 8: 151–152

Lewis B V 1988 Hysteroscopy in clinical practice. Journal of Obstetrics and Gynaecology. 9: 47–55

Lewis B V 1989 Hysteroscopy. In: Studd J (ed) Progress in Obstetrics and gynaecology. Churchill Livingstone, Edinburgh, Vol 7, p 305–317

Lewis B V 1990 Hysteroscopy for the investigation of abnormal uterine bleeding. British Journal of Obstetrics and Gynaecology 97: 283–284

Lindemann H J 1973 Historical aspects of hysteroscopy. Fertility and Sterility 24: 230–242

Lindemann H J 1974 A symposium on advances in fibreoptic hysteroscopy. Contemporary Obstetrics and Gynaecology 3: 115–134

Loffer F D 1989 Hysteroscopy with selective endometrial sampling compared with D&C for abnormal uterine bleeding: the value of a negative hysteroscopic view. Obstetrics and Gynecology 73: 16–20

MacKenzie I Z 1985 Routine out-patient diagnostic uterine curettage using a flexible plastic aspiration curette. British Journal of Obstetrics and Gynaecology 92: 1291–1296

March C H, Israel R 1987 Hysteroscopic management of recurrent abortion caused by septate uterus. American Journal of Obstetrics and Gynecology 156: 834–842

Oelsner G, David A, Insler V et al 1974 Outcome of pregnancy after treatment of intra-uterine adhesions. Obstetrics and Gynaecology 44: 341–344

Parent B, Guedj H, Barbot J, Nodarian P 1985 Hysteroscopie panoramique. Maloine, Paris

Perino A, Mencaglia l, Hamou J, Cittadini E 1987 Hysteroscopy for metroplasty of uterine septa. Fertility and Sterility 48: 321–323

Rioux J E 1984 Methods of uterine distension. In: Siegler A M, Lindemann H J (eds) Hysteroscopy principles and practice. Lippencott, Philadelphia, p 37–40

Salat-Baroux J, Hamou J E, Maillard G, Chouraqui A, Verges P 1984 In: Siegler A M, Lindemann H J (eds) Hysteroscopy principles and practice. Lippencott, Philadelphia, p 112–117

Sciarra J J, Valle R F 1977 Hysteroscopy: a clinical experience with 320 patients. American Journal of Obstetrics and Gynecology 127: 340–344

Sugimoto O 1978 Diagnostic and therapeutic hysteroscopy for traumatic intrauterine adhesions. American Journal of Obstetrics and Gynecology 131: 539–547

Taylor P J, Hamou J E 1983 Hysteroscopy. Journal of Reproductive Medicine 28: 359–389

Townsend D U, Melkonian R 1990 Laminaria tent for diagnostic and operative hysteroscopy. Journal of Gynecologic Surgery 6: 271–274

Valle R F 1980 Hysteroscopy in the evaluation of female infertility. American Journal of Obstetrics and Gynecology 137: 425–431

Valle R F 1983 Hysteroscopy for gynecologic diagnosis. Clinical Obstetrics and Gynaecology 26: 253–276

Valle R F, Sciarra J J 1983 Current status of hysteroscopy in gynecologic practice. Fertility and Sterility 32: 619–632

van Herendael B J, Stevens M J, Flakiewicz-Kula A, Hansch C H 1987 Dating of the endometrium by microhysteroscopy. Gynecologic and Obstetric Investigation 24: 114–118

Walton S M, Macphail S 1988 The value of hysteroscopy in postmenopausal and perimenopausal bleeding. Journal of Obstetrics and Gynaecology 8: 332–336

5. Fluid infusion during hysteroscopic surgery

J. Davis   C. Miller

INTRODUCTION

Satisfactory and safe resection or ablation depends on an appropriate choice of distending medium and a correct manner of infusing it. Trial and error have led to a variety of suitable systems and there is sufficient reported information to enable any new practitioner to safely infuse the uterus and minimize the risks to the patient.

This chapter will deal firstly with the fluids and instruments suitable for hysteroscopic surgery, secondly with the procedures for infusing and retrieving the fluid and thirdly with the problems of fluid infusion and how to deal with them.

CHOICE OF FLUID

Any fluid used should have good optical qualities and if infusion into the bloodstream occurs it should cause the minimum physiological disturbance.

Transcervical resection of the endometrium (TCRE)

Solutions that conduct electricity are valueless when performing resection or rollerball coagulation. Saline is thus of no use. Urologists use glycine when performing transurethral resection of the prostate (TURP), so this is the usual choice of infusion fluid when carrying out TCRE.

1.5% glycine

Glycine is an amino acid, has good optical qualities and is poorly miscible with blood. It is a poor conductor of electricity and is not caramelized by electrocautery. It was initially used in TURP as long ago as 1947, solutions of 2.1% or 1.1% being used as these prevented haemolysis of the blood if systemic infusion occurred (Nesbit & Glickman 1948).

1.5% glycine has the disadvantage that it is non-physiological and hypotonic (Weiner & Gregory 1990), consequently a significant infusion into the circulation causes a dilutional hyponatraemia as well as risking fluid overload, with pulmonary and cerebral oedema, convulsions, coma and death. This is equivalent to a condition well known to urologists — the TURP syndrome.

Systemic absorption of small quantities of glycine is generally well tolerated; however, there is increasing evidence that glycine absorption and products of its metabolism cause specific symptoms which may contribute to the TURP syndrome (Ovassapian et al 1982, Roesch et al 1983, Alexander et al 1986, Casey et al 1988, Hahn et al 1989). Furthermore, a report indicating a possible risk of myocardial stress during TURP (Coppinger & Hudd 1989) is cause for concern and deserves further study.

3 or 5% sorbitol

5% sorbitol is an iso-osmotic solution. This is used for TURP (Rao 1987). It is rapidly converted in the liver to fructose and probably glucose, its half-life being 35 minutes (Norlen et al 1986). The value of sorbitol in TCRE has yet to be assessed fully, but McLucas (1990) and Lefler et al (1991) describe its successful use during electrocoagulation of the endometrium.

5% Mannitol

This isotonic solution of mannitol is used by some urologists (Rao 1987), but there are no reports of its use in gynaecological resection. It has a longer half-life than sorbitol of 127 minutes (Norlen et al 1986).

Hysteroscopic endometrial ablation by laser (HEAL)

Normal saline, 5% dextrose, dextrose–saline, Ringer's lactate

Normal saline (Daniell et al 1986, Lomano 1986, Davis 1989), 5% dextrose (Goldrath 1981), dextrose–saline (Goldrath 1986) or Ringer's lactate solution (Loffer 1988) have all been used. These have sufficient optical qualities for safe ablation. If bleeding occurs the blood mixes with these fluids and may lead to loss of visibility unless fluid infusion pressure or throughput is increased.

With the exception of 5% dextrose, these fluids do not cause dilutional hyponatraemia if they enter the circulation, although the danger of fluid overload and pulmonary oedema still exists (Feinberg et al 1989, Morrison et at 1989). Goldrath (1981) abandoned the use of dextrose because of the occurrence of dilutional hyponatraemia. He has subsequently been using dextrose–saline. Normal saline is the usual choice as this is the cheapest and is readily available in 3 litre bags.

1.5% glycine

Glycine 1.5% is used by some surgeons as its optical properties are superior to saline (Dequesne 1987). Severe dilutional hyponatraemia has been reported (serum sodium 115 mmol/1) during laser ablation using this medium (van Boven et al 1989).

Hyskon (32% dextran 70 in 10% dextrose)

Dextran 70 consists of polymers of glucose of an average molecular weight of 70 000. It is used, in a 6% solution, as a plasma volume expander. Dextran as a 35% w/v solution in 10% dextrose was introduced for use in diagnostic hysteroscopy over 20 years ago (Edstrom & Fernstrom 1970).

Hyskon is a commercial preparation (Pharmacia Ltd) of a 32% solution of dextran in 10% dextrose specifically designed for use with the hysteroscope. It is a very hypertonic solution (approximately six times the plasma osmolality), resulting in a viscosity which allows optimum distension of the uterus, without too rapid flow or escape from the cavity and does not mix with blood. Its optical qualities are excellent.

This medium has been successfully used for laser ablation by Baggish and Baltoyannis (1988). Very little is required during a single case. However, it is essential to wash the instruments immediately after use with hot water otherwise crystallization inside the channels and stopcock occurs.

Fluids not to use

Hypertonic solutions of dextrose should not be used as these can cause a severe osmotic expansion of the circulation.

Water should never be used as it causes haemolysis, the products of which can result in renal damage.

The properties of the various fluids discussed above are outlined in Table 5.1.

CHOICE OF INSTRUMENTS

The essential requirement for safe resection or ablation is that the operator can see at all times. Clear fluid circulating through the uterus, under sufficient pressure, creates good visibility by washing blood and debris away and distends the uterus sufficiently to allow manipulation of the instruments.

Initially, laser ablation was carried out after dilating the cervix widely to allow a good intrauterine circulation (Goldrath 1981). This has the disadvantage that careful calibration of the flow rate and pressure is not possible and the quantities of fluid escaping from the cervix cannot be controlled. The inevitable result is that larger volumes of fluid are used than is really necessary (Davis 1989). Furthermore, easy collection of

Table 5.1 Summary of fluid properties

	H$_2$O	1.5% Glycine	5% Mannitol	5% Sorbitol	0.9% NaCl	5% Dextrose	Hyskon
Optical qualities	+++	++	++	++	+	+	+++
Electrical conductivity	–	–	–	–	+	–	++
Crystallizes on instruments	–	+	+	+	–	–	
Haemolytic	+	–	–	–	–	–	–
Tonicity compared to plasma	Hypotonic ++	Hypotonic +	Isotonic	Isotonic	Isotonic	Isotonic	Hypertonic +++
Hyponatraemia on absorption	+	++	+++	+++	–	+++	–
Plasma expansion on absorption	+	++	+++	+++	+++	+++	++++++
Specific central nervous system toxicity	–	+	–	–	–	–	–
Allergic potential	–	–	–	–	–	–	+

discharged irrigating medium is not possible and errors in calculating fluid discrepancies are more likely. With a hysteroscope that allows fluid to circulate only through the uterus, via separate inflow and outflow channels, it becomes much easier to control the intrauterine pressure and the volumes of fluid used. Only one instrument appears to meet these specifications for laser ablation (Baggish 1988).

For TCRE the continuous irrigation resectoscope with a suction channel is the correct instrument to use and not the single-channel resectoscope still used by some urologists. As the demand for endometrial resection is rapidly increasing it is appropriate that gynaecologists should purchase their own dedicated gynaecological resectoscope.

FLUID ABSORPTION

The debate regarding fluid control would be unnecessary were it not for the possibility that the infused fluid can enter the patient's circulation (Goldrath 1981). This can have dire consequences if the fluid volume absorbed is large or the fluid used is inappropriate.

Route of absorption

Via uterine veins

During either resection or ablation, myometrial blood vessels are opened and fluid under pressure can enter the circulation.

The uterus has to be distended to enable surgery to be carried out and, as the uterus is thick and muscular with a small internal volume, the risks of circulatory infusion would seem to be higher than in TURP, where the large volume of the compliant bladder gives some measure of protection. Conversely, there are no large venous sinuses in the uterus and if it is suitably prepared beforehand, with danazol or similar agents, the endometrial vascularity is further reduced. Extrapolations from the experience of urologists to the principles of hysteroscopic surgery therefore seem inappropriate as the circumstances are really very different. Gynaecologists must make their own rules and recognize the unique problems of hysteroscopic surgery.

Transtubal loss and intraperitoneal absorption

In unsterilized women undergoing hysteroscopic surgery there is the possibility that fluid will enter the peritoneal cavity through the fallopian tubes. Laparoscopy, if it is performed after endometrial ablation, will invariably reveal fluid in the pouch of Douglas and Baumann et al (1989) have demonstrated in one case at least that this fluid contains glycine. During an initial assessment of HEAL prior to hysterectomy, significant quantities of fluid were found in the abdominal cavity (Davis 1987).

Lomano (1986), with respect to HEAL, failed to show that patients previously sterilized absorbed any less saline. Whereas Magos et al (1990a) showed that prior tubal occlusion reduced the absorption of fluid by 20%, this was not statistically significant.

Peritoneal fluid is quite rapidly absorbed and will therefore contribute to the problems of fluid overload. The question of its contribution is only relevant because it is potentially preventable by bilateral tubal occlusion prior to resection. There is no consensus of opinion regarding this problem and it seems that transtubal infusion is not regarded as a great clinical problem. The best advice is to consider tubal occlusion in high-risk cases (Baumann et al 1990). During laser ablation the tubal ostia can be closed by coagulating around them at the beginning of the operation.

CONTROL OF FLUID INFUSION

Several factors control the risk of fluid infusion into the patient's circulation. These are:

1. Experience of the operator
2. Duration of the procedure
3. Surgical technique
4. Size of the uterine cavity
5. Intrauterine pressure during surgery.

The first four factors are to some extent inter-related and only positive intrauterine pressure can be controlled. It serves to distend the uterus to maintain visibility and also has the secondary effect of preventing bleeding. The ideal pressure is the minimum required to achieve these two aims.

Endometrial capillary pressure is only a few millimetres of mercury but, as the aim of treatment is to destroy the basal endometrium, then vessels at a much deeper level will be opened. These deeper vessels are the terminal branches of the radial and basal arteries where the pressure is unlikely to be more than 30 mmHg. Intrauterine pressure if it is above this pressure will control bleeding, but will also lead to infusion of irrigating fluid into the uterine veins.

Unfortunately, it seems that pressures higher than this theoretical minimum are necessary to achieve adequate distension of the uterine cavity. Schroeder, as long ago as 1934, measured intrauterine pressure during diagnostic hysteroscopy and found that measurements were of the order of 25–35 mmHg. Quinones-Guerrero (1983) meas-

ured intrauterine pressure during hysteroscopy using a 5% glucose solution. A pressure of 'no less that 40 mmHg' was required to obtain a panoramic view. To see the tubal orifices clearly the pressure had to be increased to 100–110 mmHg. Magos et al (1990b) agreed with this observation. Such a pressure is 'essential to ensure proper uterine distension during hysteroscopic surgery to reduce the risks of perforation and other accidents as a result of poor visualisation'.

A more recent study by the authors of intrauterine pressure during laser ablation has not confirmed that such pressures are necessary. The intrauterine pressures were recorded using a fluid-filled transducer connected directly to the uterine cavity. Pressures varying from 39 to 69 mmHg were needed for dilatation of the cavity and were sufficient to see the ostia and perform ablation (Table 5.2). In some cases adequate visualization can be achieved at even lower pressures, but 40 mmHg seems to be the minimum necessary to control bleeding and to maintain visibility.

There are probably two reasons that explain this discrepancy. Firstly, Quinones-Guerrero was performing diagnostic procedures and did not examine uteri pretreated with danazol. The thickened endometrium under ovarian control may interfere with visibility during hysteroscopy using fluid distension media, whereas the relatively avascular and atrophic endometrium seen after 6 weeks of danazol therapy enables easy examination of the uterus. Secondly, laser ablation probably does not require the same degree of uterine distension as does resection. The laser fibre is less bulky and more manouvreable than the loop of the resectoscope. Furthermore, a complete panoramic view is not so necessary during laser ablation provided the area undergoing treatment can be adequately visualized.

Bleeding is rarely a problem with laser ablation and this is possibly due to the excellent coagula-

Table 5.2   Intrauterine pressure measurements during laser ablation

12 cases
Intrauterine pressure: 39–69 mmHg
Gravity feed system, outflow closed
Stobhill Hospital, Glasgow, 1990

tive properties of the neodymium:yttrium aluminum garnet (Nd:YAG) device, which produces localized ablation with an extensive area of coagulation around it. Experimental studies have shown that it can coagulate vessels up to 4 mm in diameter, this being in part due to the shrinkage of tissue surrounding a vessel (Lehata & Gorisch 1975). Much of the potential for fluid absorption is perhaps limited by this feature of the laser and Reid (1989) has shown that the maximal size of vessels within 5 mm of the surface of the endometrium pretreated with danazol is no larger than 450 μm. However vessels exposed in the myometrium will be of a greater diameter than this.

The pressure requirements will vary from case to case and, therefore, rather than use standard settings for treatment, the operator should set up the equipment to provide the minimum pressure that will produce the appropriate distension to allow safe surgery. The pressure can be increased if bleeding occurs.

Methods of instilling fluid

There are a variety of methods for the instillation and regulation of fluid during resection or ablation. A pump may be used or a gravity feed system may be adequate with the bags of fluid elevated above the patient or compressed with a pressure cuff.

Pressurizing the fluid infusion bags

The infusion bag can be placed inside a blood pressure cuff and compressed to a predetermined setting. However, the pressure falls as the bag empties and an assistant has to maintain the pressure periodically. Only 1 litre bags of fluid can be used and this leads to the constant changing of bags during the operation. This unsophisticated approach carries the risk of creating unnecessarily high pressures.

This problem can be overcome if an orthopaedic pneumatic tourniquet is attached to the blood pressure cuff instead of the bulb that usually is used to inflate the cuff. The appropriate pressure can be preset and this pressure is maintained until the 1 litre bag is empty (Loffer 1988).

Pumps

Peristaltic pumps are the type most commonly used. These act externally on the drip tube carrying fluid to the hysteroscope. A rotating roller compresses the tube and pushes pulses of fluid into the uterus. The flow rate can be varied by increasing the rate at which the roller arms rotate. Some devices can produce very high rates of flow of up to 500 ml/min. Although the infusion pressure is low, these pumps can generate very high pressures against a resistance. The pump initially used by the authors (Watson Marlow, Belmont Instruments, Glasgow) could continue to irrigate fluid against a resistance of 200 mmHg and one of the pumps used by Loffer (personal communication) could generate pressures up to 300 mmHg. These pressures are dangerous, so preset limitations must be introduced.

The Hamou Hysteromat (Karl Storz, Tuttlingen, Germany) and the Staflo (Litechnica, Manchester, UK) have a built-in pressure-limiting facility, although they measure pressures in the inflow channel and not in the uterus. This is probably the safest type of pump to use (Magos et al 1991).

Garry et al (1992) have demonstrated the value of using this pressure-controlled device by comparing two groups of patients. The first group of 105 patients had fluid instilled into the uterus with a simple peristaltic pump, while in a later series of 92 patients the fluid infusion was controlled with the Hysteromat. There was a mean 85% reduction in the fluid absorbed by the second group compared with the first (1386 versus 209 ml). In a small randomized study these authors showed that infusion volumes could be reduced to zero using the continuous-pressure variable-flow Hysteromat compared to a mean of over 1300 ml using a continuous-flow variable-pressure peristaltic pump.

If Hyskon is used during laser surgery, a special carbon dioxide-driven pump can be used to maintain pressure (Baggish 1990), which eliminates having to drive the viscous fluid manually into the uterus with syringes.

Gravity feed systems

Goldrath (1986) in his initial series injected dextrose– saline into the uterus via the hysteroscope using 50 ml syringes. This complicated the procedure and made treatment unnecessarily labour-intensive. Furthermore, such a system means that control of the pressure within the uterus is not possible.

The development of appropriate laser hystero-scopes with dual channels, for inflow and out-flow, has made it possible to rely on a gravity feed system. 3 litre bags of irrigating medium are connected by a Y-tube to the hysteroscope, and the uterine distension created by raising the bags to a suitable height above the patient. Regulation of the uterine pressure and therefore of the uterine distension can be made in this way. The loss of pressure caused by the gradual reduction of the fluid column during surgery can lead to a slow collapse of the uterus. The bag therefore has to be raised a few centimetres as the operation progresses and is lowered again if a second bag has to be used.

Outflow control

Many practitioners recommend that a conti-nuous flow is maintained by keeping the outflow tap open. This allows any blood, debris or bub-bles to be flushed out of the uterine cavity. This practice may lower the pressure inside the uterus and create difficulties in establishing uterine distension. This can be overcome by partially closing the tap. Alternatively, a simple suction device attached to the outflow can be used to control intrauterine flow.

A gravity feed system with outflow suction can be used quite adequately for endometrial resec-tion, using a column of fluid of 100 cm and adjusting the outflow suction to the minimum (West & Robinson 1989).

Another way of maintaining a continuous flow is to place the peristaltic pump in the outflow arm of the system and rely on gravity to provide the pressure. Because the rollers of the pump are constantly squeezing the outflow tubing the system remains closed, and it has been suggested, provided flow rates are not high, that there is no loss of pressure in the system.

This does not seem to be the case. Fine control cannot be achieved with a roller pump and even when switched off fluid still escapes past the

stationary rollers if inappropriate tubing is used. Even slow rates of rotation lead to significant rates of flow with consequent loss of intrauterine pressure (Table 5.3).

It seems that simple roller pumps will lead to the use of excessive volumes of fluid whether used in the inflow or outflow arm.

In cases where a laser is to be used the tap can be closed altogether and, by inserting an aspira-tion cannula into the uterus through a subsidiary channel of the hysteroscope, any blood, or bubbles, is removed by intermittent suction from a syringe. A Buchanan cholangiogram cannula (Stoke on Trent type, Portex) with its tip cut off is used by the authors. An alternative is an epidural catheter.

This method is suitable for nearly all cases of laser ablation. The authors have used far less fluid than before and have not had a single case of fluid overload since the inception of this method in their unit (Table 5.4).

Table 5.3 Flow rates and loss of pressure with the roller pump on hysteroscope outflow tubing

Roller pump		Reduction in pressure within the uterus (mmHg)
Setting[a]	Measured extraction rate (ml/min)	
5	55	5
10	115	9
20	220	17

[a]Relates to the rotation rate levels of the roller pump (Watson Harlow, Belmont Instruments, Glasgow, UK).

Table 5.4 Influence of fluid infusion system on quantities of fluid used and lost per case

	Average fluid infused per case (litres)	Average fluid lost per case (litres)	
1986–1987 29 patients	15.8	1.8	Peristaltic pump widely dilated cervix
1988 37 patients	9.4	1.25	Peristaltic pump Dual-channel scope
1990 59 patients	3.1	0.48	Gravity feed Dual-channel scope Suction cannula

Stobhill Hospital, Glasgow, 1986–1990

Estimating fluid absorption

Direct measurements

An essential requirement in hysteroscopic endo-metrial ablation is that of keeping account of the volumes of fluid being infused and comparing them with the volumes retrieved. The difference should equal the volume absorbed by the patient, either directly into the circulation, through the fallopian tubes, or both.

Estimating fluid infused should be a relatively simple procedure if the containers are gradated allowing volumes to be measured.

Collecting the fluid may present more problems. Firstly, it is essential to use a dual-channel hysteroscope or resectoscope with the tubing from the outflow leading to a graded collection chamber (Fig. 5.1). Fluid will often escape around the endoscope in varying amounts and trickle out

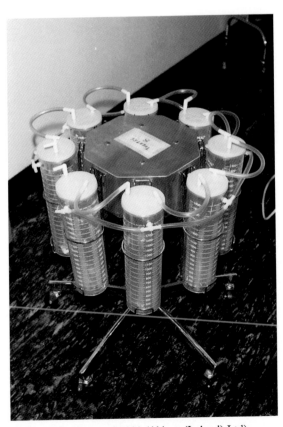

Fig. 5.1 The Receptal 2000 (Abbott (Ireland) Ltd), known as the 'octopus'.

into the vagina. Placing a urology collection bag or perineal pouch (Fig. 5.2) under the buttocks of the patient will catch most of this. Fluid aspirated from the uterus must be measured as well. Simple addition and subtraction will give the fluid discrepancy.

These precautions are essential and, if simple rules are applied and rigidly adhered to, it should be possible to avoid significant fluid infusion.

Accounting should be done at regular intervals throughout the operation — ideally every 5 minutes by a named member of the theatre team.

There is no safe upper limit to irrigant absorption. Most patients undergoing ablation or resection are fit and can safely tolerate fluid infusion of up to a maximum of 2 litres of hypotonic or isotonic irrigant and considerably less for the hypertonic irrigant Hyskon (a theoretical maximum being 250 ml). It is important that the limits of infusion are set and agreed by the anaesthetist. Patients with medical problems can be treated, but the acceptable levels of fluid infusion will be very much lower than in a healthy woman.

If the agreed level is reached the operation should stop. It is better to consider completing therapy at a second session rather than risking the patient's well-being. Abandoning surgery is an infrequent event, but it is a wise precaution to warn patients that this may be necessary, so that misunderstanding is avoided postoperatively.

Rules for avoiding fluid overload

1. Maintain the minimum intrauterine pressure for safe surgery
2. Have an efficient system for retrieving fluid circulated through the uterus
3. Keep a regular account of fluid volumes infused and retrieved during the operation
4. Set a maximum allowable fluid discrepancy for each case
5. Maintain constant liaison with the anaesthetist and nursing staff throughout the procedure
6. Stop surgery once the preset limit is reached
7. Warn patient of the possibility of foreshortening the operation
8. Adhere to these rules.

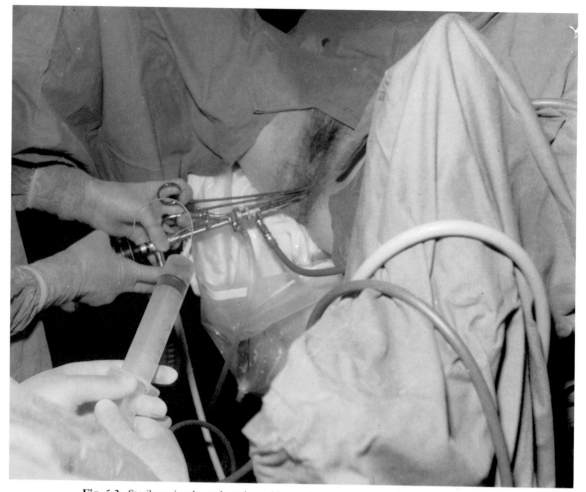

Fig. 5.2   Sterile perineal pouch set in position at the start of surgery (Steridrape 1016, 3M).

For most practical purposes, simple measurement of the fluid used and retrieved is adequate. Even so, various laboratory methods can be a useful adjunct to monitoring fluid infusion.

Indirect measurements

Haematocrit

The extent of haemodilution is assessed by measuring the change in the haematocrit. This can be done in the theatre with a minicentrifuge, but requires frequent blood sampling and will be affected by fluid lost from the intravascular space or by fluid gained by intravenous infusions.

End-expiratory alcohol concentration

The irrigant solution is labelled with 1% alcohol and the end-expiratory alcohol concentration measured. This method has only been used during endoscopic prostatic surgery using 1.5% glycine (Hahn 1988). It is a sensitive method and has the advantage of being non-invasive and less subject to arithmetical error.

Cardiovascular parameters

The blood pressure, heart rate or central venous pressure is measured to assess changes in the intravascular volume. These methods will be most sensitive when used with isotonic or hypertonic irrigants containing large molecules, which are confined to the intravascular space, i.e. dextran. When hypotonic or rapidly excreted or metabolized fluids are used these methods will be less sensitive as the initial expansion of plasma volumes disappears when the absorbed fluid rapidly moves out of the intravascular space into the extracellular and intracellular spaces or urine.

Furthermore, cardiovascular responses are effected by general anaesthesia, sympathetic blockade during regional anaesthesia or sedation.

Off-site laboratory methods

Methods that demand off-site laboratory analysis require a longer turnaround interval and will not be useful to identify or prevent irrigant absorption before symptoms develop. They are useful in diagnosing and managing symptomatic fluid infusion or in research. These methods include measuring changes in blood haemoglobin, serum osmolality, glycine levels, sodium, chloride, creatinine or albumin levels, and of radioactive tracers previously injected into the bloodstream. Intravascular probes are available for the continuous monitoring of plasma sodium concentrations, but these are currently experimental.

PROBLEMS OF FLUID ABSORPTION

When clinically significant volumes of irrigant are absorbed, the symptoms and signs will depend on the nature and volume of the fluid absorbed and on the type of anaesthetic.

The effect of the irrigant fluid depends on:

1. Tonicity
2. Molecular weight
3. Speed of metabolism and excretion
4. Sodium content
5. Specific solute characteristics
6. Temperature.

The first three characteristics will determine the pattern of fluid shift following absorption. Hyperosmolar irrigants draw water into the intravascular space from the interstitial space and ultimately the intracellular spaces. Conversely, hypo-osmolar solutions will dilute the extravascular space in a manner dependent on their osmolality. As the irrigant osmolality decreases

proportionately, more extravascular dilution occurs and thus the net change in plasma osmolality is reduced (Norlen 1985).

The molecular weight will determine whether the fluid is retained in the vascular space or distributed throughout the extracellular space. High-molecular-weight dextran will remain mostly in the vascular compartment, while glycine, mannitol, saline or glucose, having low molecular weights, will eventually be distributed throughout the extracellular space. Freely filtered solutes, such as mannitol or glucose, will act as osmotic diuretics and will decrease solute redistribution.

Acute hyponatraemia can only follow absorption of hyponatraemic solutions. Thus, when normal saline is used, signs and symptoms of absorption are those of intravascular expansion rather than hyponatraemia.

The irrigating fluid should not be cooled, because if large volumes of cold irrigant are used the patient's temperature will fall. This may cause hypoxia during rewarming, when the patient's metabolic rate and oxygen demand rises.

Circulatory overload with isotonic fluids (normal saline)

There are several reports of fluid overload during the laser ablation, but few give sufficient details to identify the volumes at which problems occur. Goldrath (1986) describes that 'several patients had evidence of fluid overload' and noted that out of a series of 261 patients two developed pulmonary oedema. He does not provide any data regarding fluid volumes in these cases.

Loffer (1988) carefully monitors fluid input and output and states that in a series of 60 cases there was never more than a 1000 ml deficit of irrigating fluid (Ringer's lactate).

Daniell et al (1986) in a small series had no fluid infusion problems and had a fluid discrepancy of, on average, only 300 ml (range 100–800 ml). Lomano (1986) in his first reported series of ten cases found the measured loss varied from 600 to 4800 ml. The average was 2045 ml, yet none of his patients had any signs or symptoms of fluid overload. In a later study (Lomano 1988) of 62 cases the results were similar, except that for patients treated by the non-contact coagulation technique, fluid absorption was reduced to an average of 846 ml per case (range 100–3300 ml). The greatest discrepancy between fluid infused and retrieved, and consequently presumed absorbed, was 7300 ml. Although this study does not refer to problems with fluid overload, it seems inconceivable that absorption of such quantities of normal saline in a short time should have no clinical sequelae. Lomano dilated the cervix to allow egress of fluid around the hysteroscope, which makes for difficulties in collecting and calculating the retrieved fluid. It is possible that he has overestimated the fluid lost.

There is one detailed report of a case of fluid overload (Feinberg et al 1989). In this report a 44-year-old hypertensive patient absorbed 6550 ml of normal saline during a 70 minute procedure; 14 litres of saline had been infused under a pressure of 100 mmHg. Pulmonary oedema was recognized before extubation and the patient was ventilated until the next day. Diuretic therapy produced a urinary output of 6000 ml within 12 hours. Her immediate postoperative haematocrit value fell by 20%. The patient made a good recovery thereafter.

Garry et al (1991) in the largest series of cases of laser ablation to date (859 cases) report an incidence of pulmonary oedema of 0.4%, but give no biochemical details. In a later paper, Garry et al (1992) compared six patients, where fluid infusion was controlled by the continuous-pressure variable-flow Hysteromat, with six patients where infusion was provided by a peristaltic pump. Significant changes in the haematocrit (mean fall 19%), total protein (mean fall 19%) and colloid osmotic pressure (mean fall 26%) were recorded only in the group infused with the peristaltic pump.

Morrison et al (1989) reported on the problems of fluid absorption during their first 12 cases. These patients were monitored extensively. As well as taking standard pre- and postoperative haematological and biochemical measurements, the study involved recording of the central venous pressure, and radioisotope studies were used to identify plasma volume changes. The most significant variables were an increase in the serum chloride level and a decrease in the haematocrit and the plasma protein and albumin levels. In five cases there was a marked rise in the central venous pressure, with one patient developing pulmonary oedema. The plasma volume studies were inconclusive, probably because the fluid absorbed was rapidly redistributed into the interstitial space. This work demonstrated the potential for fluid infusion across the endometrium during HEAL. It is, however, no more than a reminder that a careful technique with close monitoring of fluid volumes are essential aspects of laser ablation. These 12 cases were the first patients treated by laser ablation in the authors' department. The procedure took considerably longer than they do now, fluid recording during surgery was not as tightly controlled, no limit on pressures was set and, because the cervix was widely dilated, rapid flow rates were necessary to maintain distension of the uterus. An average of 15.8 litres of irrigating saline was used during the cases at an average flow rate of 173 ml/min. In one case with a widely dilated cervix 55 litres of fluid were used. Such prodigious quantities of irrigating fluid are quite inappropriate and, with a continuous-flow system, relying on lower intrauterine pressures and having a foolproof system for retrieving fluid, there is no reason for significant fluid absorption to occur.

Infusion of hypotonic irrigating fluid (1.5% glycine)

Rao (1987) in an excellent review of fluid absorption during TURP clearly describes the problems with glycine. The absorption of significant quantities of glycine causes both fluid overload and hyponatraemia. Hyponatraemia causes bradycardia and hypotension. Cerebral oedema occurs, due to a shift of fluid from the intravascular to the intracellular space, which leads to delayed recovery from anaesthesia and confusion. Furthermore, glycine and its metabolites, especially ammonia, may be toxic. The consensus in the literature is that toxic levels are rarely reached during TURP. Ammonia is a central nervous system depressant and its effects include nausea and vomiting, agitation and even coma.

Several gynaecologists have studied the risks and effects of glycine infusion during TCRE. West and Robinson (1989) reported on 100 cases of TCRE. In only three cases was fluid absorption in excess of 1000 ml and none of these had symptoms and signs of fluid overload or of hyponatraemia. Baumann et al (1990) studied glycine infusion in ten patients undergoing TCRE. A mean of 4948 ml (range 1750–8900 ml) of irrigating fluid was used with a mean deficit of 643 ml (range 100–2030 ml). They recorded a negative correlation between the fluid absorbed and the fall in the plasma sodium concentration. These changes were paralleled by falls in the haematocrit, and the haemoglobin, total protein and albumin levels. No clinical problems occurred in these ten patients and no specific measures seem to have been necessary even in the patient who absorbed over 2 litres of glycine. In this same paper the authors refer to an additional case, who absorbed 4350 ml of glycine with a fall in the plasma sodium level to 117 mmol/l. An induced diuresis brought the serum sodium concentration back to normal within 24 hours.

In response to this report, Boto et al (1990) published their experience of 26 cases in whom serum electrolyte concentrations and plasma osmolality had been measured. Values before and after treatment showed no significant difference at a 5% level. They attributed this to keeping infusion pressure levels low at no more than 60 cm H_2O. They recommended that surgery should be stopped if more than 500 ml of glycine was absorbed.

In later correspondence, Magos et al (1990b) reviewed their experience of 139 procedures. The medium volume of glycine absorbed was 350 ml, with 11 patients absorbing over 1 litre. They stated that relatively young and fit patients could tolerate fluid loads of up to 2 litres well, but if this level of fluid absorption occurs then surgery should be stopped. These results are summarized in Table 5.5 and include the latest data from Magos et al (1991).

Boubli et al (1990) studied 100 patients undergoing hysteroscopic resection, examining the haematological and biochemical effects of glycine infusion. Most of these patients required surgery for intrauterine myomas (57) or polyps (34). Their average age was 40.9 years.

The most important variations were in haematocrit and protein levels, which fell by values of greater than 5% in 44.9% and 57.1% of patients, respectively. Only 11% of patients had a 5% change in serum sodium levels, even so there was a correlation between the variations in all three measurements. The factors that influenced these changes were the height and weight of the patient, taller and heavier patients being more at risk of absorbing fluid, but the length of the operation did not influence these changes. Two patients with marked changes had operating times of 22 and 10 minutes only.

Pre- and postoperative glycine levels were also measured. There was an average rise in serum glycine levels by a factor of 4.5. There was no correlation between blood levels of glycine and changes in the haematocrit, or the protein or sodium levels. The rise in glycine levels was directly related to the volume of glycine absorbed. Unfortunately, Boubli et al did not attempt to show any relationship between fluid used and the fall in haematocrit, protein or sodium levels.

An unexplained observation was that nulliparous patients were more likely to experience a fall in the haematocrit and a greater rise in serum glycine levels than were multiparous patients. Perhaps this is due to the effect of pregnancy on the uterine vasculature.

These results leave many questions unanswered. Serum glycine levels relate to the quantity of irrigant used, but changes in haematocrit and biochemical variables will be influenced by compensatory mechanisms, which will vary between patients.

Table 5.5   Fluid infusion volumes and fluid deficit with the incidence of fluid overload in three series of TCRE

	Number of patients	Fluid volumes (ml)	Fluid deficits (ml)	Clinical signs	Cases of hyponatraemia (<130 mmol/l)
Boto et al (1990)	26	1750–8900	Not given	None	None
West & Robinson (1989)	100	1500–15 000	0–1500	None	None
Magos et al (1991)	250	1100–20 900	−250–4350	5	5

This further underlines the problems of comparing TURP and TCRE. Patients undergoing TCRE are younger and generally fitter than those treated by TURP, the vascular anatomy is entirely different and the volumes of irrigant used are of a differing order.

Infusion of 32% dextran 70 (Hyskon)

32% dextran leads to plasma volume expansion by drawing fluid from the extracellular space into the circulation. Although the patient has received little additional fluid, the large fluid shifts can cause circulatory overload and pulmonary oedema. Only small amounts of infused Hyskon are necessary to produce marked shifts of fluid. It has been calculated that 100 ml of infused Hyskon would lead to plasma volume expansion of 860 ml (Lukascko 1985). Because Hyskon is so hypertonic (it contains six times the concentration of dextran used intravenously for the treatment of shock), it is a powerful osmotic expander and so there is the risk of a marked circulatory expansion should even a modest infusion occur (Schinagl 1990).

Baggish and Baltoyannis (1988) did not report any problems with circulatory infusion and used small volumes of Hyskon (mean 350 ml). Even so, scrupulous recording of fluid volumes must be practised if Hyskon is chosen, especially in high-risk cases. Zbella et al (1985) and Mangar et al (1989) have each reported a case of pulmonary oedema associated with hysteroscopic surgery, which emphasize the potential risks of Hyskon. In each report (the first using resection and the second laser ablation) a patient undergoing treatment of a submucosal fibroid developed pulmonary oedema and a coagulopathy. The amounts of Hyskon used in the operations were 700 and 900 ml, respectively. In the first case the preoperative haemoglobin level of 14.1 g/dl fell to 6.5 g/dl and in the second case the haematocrit fell from 41.2 to 23%. The authors attributed this to a toxic effect of dextran on the pulmonary capillaries. However, Schinagl (1990), discussing dextran-induced pulmonary oedema, thought that the effects observed were due to an increase in the capillary hydrostatic pressure secondary to excessive expansion of the intravascular volume. He strongly recommended that the volumes of Hyskon used during intrauterine surgery be limited to 500 ml.

Dextrans can cause anaphylactic reactions (Bailey et al 1967, Borten et al 1983). Such a reaction requires prior sensitization to dextran. A case of anaphylactic shock with a skin rash and successfully reversed asystole in association with Hyskon has been reported (Trimbos-Kemper & Veering 1989).

When intraperitoneal dextran is known (or suspected) to be present and anaphylaxis has occurred, successful treatment and resolution of symptoms may not be achieved until the collection of intraperitoneal dextran has been aspirated (Borten et al 1983).

INFLUENCE OF THE TYPE OF ANAESTHESIA

General anaesthesia

General anaesthesia, by masking the signs of irrigant absorption, can delay early recognition and treatment. This effect will be greatest in the paralysed and ventilated patient when tachypnoea and fitting will be masked. In addition, positive airway pressure will delay the onset of pulmonary oedema. This masking of signs will be less apparent in the ventilated, but not paralysed, patient, and even less so in the spontaneously breathing patient.

Spinal or epidural anaesthesia

Spinal or epidural anaesthesia will allow the conscious patient to communicate symptoms earlier. Local anaesthetic-induced sympathetic blockade causes vasodilatation, which will delay the onset of circulatory overload and allow relatively more irrigant to be absorbed before cardiovascular signs and symptoms develop. However, the development of early specific symptoms of glycine toxicity (visual disturbances, prickling and burning skin sensations and nausea) in the conscious patient can alert the anaesthetist and lead to remedial action being taken, before serious morbidity occurs.

Many anaesthetists prevent the hypotension

caused by spinal or epidural anaesthesia with intravenous fluid, but during hysteroscopic surgery it may be more appropriate to withhold intravenous fluids and treat hypotension with vasopressors.

If laparoscopy is planned then regional anaesthesia is less attractive, as the high block necessary increases the likelihood of intense sympathetic blockade.

Paracervical block with intravenous sedation

Paracervical block with intravenous sedation is routinely used in some centres (Magos et al 1991) and has the advantages of maintaining patient contact and avoiding large changes in autonomic function. This technique, although not universally popular with patients nor necessarily with surgeons, is probably the method of choice in a high-risk patient.

TREATMENT OF FLUID ABSORPTION

Prevention is best. If clinically significant absorption does occur, the treatment will depend on the degree of circulatory overload and the extent of hyponatraemia.

Circulatory overload

Circulatory overload causes acute ventricular failure, which in the fit patient produces tachypnoea, wheezing, frothy oedema, arterial hypertension, raised venous pressure, tachycardia and extreme anxiety. The raised end-diastolic ventricular pressure initially results in an increased stroke volume, but with further rises this beneficial relationship is lost, stroke volume decreases and cardiac output falls. Where there is an imbalance between myocardial oxygen supply and demand, myocardial ischaemia and anginal chest pain can occur. The high venous pressures cause increased movement of serum into the extracellular space, which eventually overcomes the lymphatic system's ability to absorb fluid. In the lungs this causes bronchospasm and an increase in the alveolar–arterial oxygen difference. The resulting hypoxia dramatically increases when the interstitial oedema develops into frank pulmonary oedema. Elsewhere in the body interstitial oedema lengthens the diffusion distance between the capillaries and the cell walls, so the cellular environment becomes increasingly hypoxic and acidotic. A vicious circle of hypoxia and falling cardiac output develops.

Management of circulatory overload

It is critical to treat the pulmonary oedema by reversing the hypoxia and improving cardiac function.

Reversing the hypoxia. All patients will require arterial blood gas monitoring. In mild cases, sitting the patient upright and increasing the inspired oxygen concentrations may be all that is needed. However, when there is frank pulmonary oedema, paralysing the patient and ventilating her, initially with positive end-expiratory pressure (PEEP) will be necessary. This raises the arterial oxygen content by inhibiting the formation of further pulmonary oedema and by removing the oxygen demand due to the work of breathing. In fit patients at rest the work of breathing accounts for about 2% of the body's oxygen demand, but in a highly stressed patient it can account for up to 40% (Nicholls 1990). When high levels of PEEP are used, the resultant fall in cardiac output may offset the increase in the partial pressure of oxygen in the blood and oxygen delivery may fall.

Improving cardiac function. In mild cases an intravenous diuretic may be all that is necessary. The decrease in plasma volume and vasodilatation reduces the cardiac distension, which causes an increase in stroke volume and allows the heart to move back onto a more physiological part of the Frank–Starling curve. In addition, the hydrostatic forces favouring pulmonary oedema formation are reduced.

More severe cases will require additional venodilatory and inotropic support. Nitrates, dobutamine and low-dose dopamine are the most commonly used agents in this situation, although the type 3 phosphiodesterase inhibitors or angiotensin-converting enzyme inhibitors may also be useful. These patients will need central venous pressure monitoring and, if there is doubt about whether the pulmonary oedema is of a cardiogenic origin or if high levels of PEEP are required, a pulmonary flotation catheter should be placed and cardiac output and oxygen delivery monitored.

Hyponatraemia

When a low-sodium irrigant is absorbed the signs and symptoms of acute hyponatraemia will be added to those of circulatory overload. During endoscopic prostatic surgery, the TURP syndrome can develop and information on acute dilutional hyponatraemia is mostly derived from these patients. These cases do not, however, represent purely the problems of hyponatraemia with superadded complications of initial circulatory overload, but also have a lowered plasma oncotic pressure and an elevated serum concentration of glycine and its metabolites.

The presentation and management of isolated severe hyponatraemia is largely based on reports of slow-onset hyponatraemia (over 24 hours), mostly due to thiazide medication (sodium loss), inappropriate secretion of antidiuretic hormone or postoperative infusion of 5% dextrose (water excess). Rapidly developing hyponatraemia will produce symptoms earlier, as the rate of shift between compartments is increased and there is less time for compensatory intracellular changes to develop. When the plasma sodium is less than 120 mmol/l, symptoms of hyponatraemia are more likely to develop. This can present with agitation, nausea. vomiting, headache and incontinence. However, in a significant number of patients minor symptoms can suddenly change into seizures and respiratory arrest.

Management of hyponatraemia

The specific treatment of severe symptomatic hyponatraemia is to raise the plasma sodium level into the mildly hyponatraemic range (121–134 mmol/l).

In slow-onset hyponatraemia the primary treatment is to infuse, intravenously, hypertonic saline to raise the plasma sodium level by a rate of up to 2 mmol/l per hour into the mildly hyponatraemic range and to avoid raising the plasma

sodium level by more than 25 mmol/l in the initial 48 hours of therapy (Ayus et al 1987). A loop diuretic, usually frusemide, is often given to increase water loss. Osmotic diuresis with hypertonic mannitol will initially exacerbate intravascular expansion. Frequent monitoring of the plasma sodium level is essential as rapid sodium replacement and hypernatraemia are implicated in causing brain damage (Sterns et al 1986).

Lesser degrees of rapid-onset hyponatraemia following irrigant absorption are often asymptomatic and resolve over 24 hours, after a spontaneous diuresis. When significant infusion is suspected, the plasma sodium level should be measured and if below 120 mmol/l the hyponatraemia should be treated actively, irrespective of whether symptoms are present or not. This involves:

1. Stopping any sodium-free intravenous solutions.
2. Parenteral administration of a loop diuretic.
3. Administration of intravenous hypertonic saline. This may not be needed in the asymptomatic patient, but is required when symptoms occur — bradycardia, hypertension followed by hypotension, chest pains, respiratory distress, mental confusion, seizures or cardiorespiratory collapse.
4. Transfer to an intensive care unit where facilities for invasive monitoring and rapid resuscitation are easily available.

ONCOTIC PRESSURE CHANGES

The reduction in the plasma albumin level and hence oncotic pressure, following irrigant absorption, is slight and should not cause symptoms. Similarly, small increases in the serum potassium level are described, but these are not clinically significant (Norlen 1985).

GLYCINE ABSORPTION AND TOXICITY

Glycine absorption is thought to contribute significantly to the symptomatology of the TURP syndrome (Roesch et al 1983). This is not a feature of sorbitol or mannitol absorption (Norlen 1985). Glycine is normally metabolized to serine, but when present in higher concentrations is metabolized via several pathways to various other amino acids and to ammonia, which have been implicated in causing encephalopathy and coma (Norlen 1985). There may be a subgroup of the population that is more likely to develop hyperammonaemia after glycine absorption (Hoekstra et al 1983). L-Arginine may have a protective or therapeutic role in the treatment of glycine toxicity (Fahey 1957), but there is no data on this application during endoscopic bladder or uterine surgery.

CONCLUSION

The risk of significant fluid infusion during hysteroscopic surgery is small, but the scope for disaster has been amply described in the literature.

The risk seems greatest at the beginning of an operator's experience, during the learning curve. So, although vigilance must be maintained at all times, it is especially important at the beginning of a gynaecologist's hysteroscopic surgical career.

The anaesthetist's understanding of the procedure and its risks is just as important as is the surgeon's, so there must be close liaison between them.

Much of the discussion on the effects of fluid overload and hyponatraemia has been derived from the extensive experience of studying patient's undergoing TURP, but the authors believe it is relevant to women who develop these problems during hysteroscopic surgery.

ACKNOWLEDGEMENT

Our thanks go to Mr Paul Kaszubski, Senior Medical Photographer at Stobhill Hospital.

REFERENCES

Alexander J F, Polland A, Gillespie I A 1986 Glycine and transurethral resection. Anaesthesia 41: 1189–1195
Ayus J C, Krothapalli R K, Arieff A I 1987 The treatment of symptomatic hyponatraemia and its relationship to brain damage. New England Journal of Medicine 317: 1190–1195
Baggish M S 1988 New laser hysteroscope for neodymium – YAG endometrial ablation. Lasers in Surgery and Medicine 8: 99–103
Baggish M S 1990 Hysteroscopic laser surgery. In: Baggish M S (ed) Endoscopic laser surgery, Clinical practice of gynaecology 2(1): 187–206
Baggish M S, Baltoyannis P 1988 New techniques for laser ablation of the endometrium in high-risk patients. American Journal of Obstetrics and Gynecology 159: 287–292
Bailey G, Strub R, Klein R C, Salvaggio F 1967 Dextran induced anaphylaxia. Journal of the American Medical Association 200: 185
Baumann R, Magos A L, Kay J D S, Turnbull A C 1990 Absorption of glycine irrigating fluid during transcervical resection of the endometrium. British Medical Journal 300: 304–305
Borten M, Seibert C F, Taymor M L 1983 Recurrent anaphylactic reaction to intraperitoneal dextran 75 used for prevention of postsurgical adhesions. Obstetrics and Gynecology 61: 755–757
Boto T C A, Fowler C G, Cockroft S, Djahanbakch O 1990 Absorption of irrigating fluid during transcervical resection of endometrium. British Medical Journal 300: 748–749
Boubli L, Blanc B, Bautrand E, Achilli Cornesse M E, Houvenaeghel M, Manelli J C, Aquaron R 1990 Le risque metabolique de la chirurgie hysteroscopique. Journal de Gynecologie Obstetrique et Biologie de la Reproduction 19: 217–222

Casey W F, Hannon V, Cunningham A, Heaney J 1988 Visual evoked potentials and changes in serum glycine concentration during transurethral resection of the prostate. British Journal of Anaesthesia 60: 525–529
Coppinger S W V, Hudd C 1989 Risk factor for myocardial infarction in transurethral resection of the prostate. Lancet 333: 859
Daniell J, Tosh R, Meisels S 1986 Photodynamic ablation of the endometrium with the Nd:YAG laser hysteroscopically as a treatment of menorrhagia. Colposcopic and Gynecologic Laser Surgery 2: 43–46
Davis J A 1987 The principles and use of the neodymium–YAG laser in gynaecological surgery. In: Monaghan J M (ed) Gynaecological Surgery. Bailière's Clinical Obstetrics and Gynaecology 1(2): 331–352
Davis J A 1989 Hysteroscopic endometrial ablation with the neodymium–YAG laser. British Journal of Obstetrics and Gynaecology 96: 928–932
Dequesne J 1987 Hysteroscopic treatment of uterine bleeding with the Nd–YAG laser. Lasers in Medical Science 2: 73–76
Edstrom K, Fernstrom I 1970 The diagnostic possibilities of a modified hysteroscopic technique. Acta Obstetrica Gynecologica Scandinavica 49: 327
Fahey J L 1957 Toxicity and blood ammonia rise resulting from intravenous amino-acid administration in man: the protective affect of L-arginine. Journal of Clinical Investigation 36: 1647–1655
Feinberg B I, Gimpleson R J, Godier D E 1989 Pulmonary edema after photocoagulation of the endometrium with the Nd:YAG laser. Journal of Reproductive Medicine 34: 431–434
Garry R, Erian J, Grochmal S A 1991 A multi-centre collaborative study into the treatment of menorrhagia by Nd–YAG laser ablation of endometrium. British Journal

of Obstetrics and Gynaecology 98: 357–362

Garry R, Hasham F, Kokri M S, Mooney P 1992 The effects of controlling intrauterine pressure on fluid absorption during endometrial ablation. In press

Goldrath M 1986 Hysteroscopic laser ablation of the endometrium. In: Sharp F and Jordan J A (eds) Gynaecological laser surgery. Proceedings of the fifteenth study group of the Royal College of Obstetricians and Gynaecologists. Perinatology Press, Ithaca, p 253–269

Goldrath M H, Fuller T A, Segal S 1981 Laser photovapourisation of the endometrium for the treatment of menorrhagia. American Journal of Obstetrics and Gynecology 140: 14–19

Hahn R G 1988 Ethanol monitoring of irrigation fluid absorption in transurethral prostatic surgery. Anesthesiology 68: 867–873

Hahn R G, Stalberg H P, Gustafsson S A 1989 Intravenous infusion of irrigating fluid containing glycine or mannitol with and without ethanol. Journal of Urology 142: 1102–1105

Hoekstra P T, Kahnoski R, McCamish M A, Bergen W, Heetderks D R 1983 Transurethral prostatic resection syndrome — a new perspective: encephalopathy with associated hyperammonia. Journal of Urology 130: 704–707

Lefler H T, Sullivan G H, Hulka J F 1991 Modified endometrial ablation: electrocoagulation with vasopressin and suction curettage preparation. Obstetrics and Gynaecology 77: 949–953

Leheta F, Gorisch W 1975 Coagulation of blood vessels by means of argon ion and Nd:YAG laser radiation. Proceedings of the 1st international symposium on laser surgery. Jerusalem Academic Press. Jerusalem, p 178–184

Loffer F D 1988 Laser ablation of the endometrium. Obstetrics and Gynaecology Clinics of North America 15(1): 77–89

Lomano J M 1986 Photocoagulation of the endometrium with the Nd:YAG laser for the treatment of menorrhagia. Journal of Reproductive Medicine 31: 148–150

Lomano J M 1988 Dragging technique versus blanching technique for endometrial ablation with the Nd:YAG laser in the treatment of chronic menorrhagia. American Journal of Obstetrics and Gynecology 159: 152–155

Lukascko F 1985 Noncardiogenic pulmonary edema secondary to intrauterine distension of 32% dextran 70. Fertility and Sterility 44: 560–561

McLucas B 1990 Endometrial ablation with the roller ball electrode. Journal of Reproductive Medicine 35: 1055–1058

Magos A L, Baumann R, Turnbull T C 1990a Safety of transcervical endometrial resection. Lancet 335: 44

Magos A L, Lockwood G M, Baumann R, Turnbull A C, and Kay J D S 1990b Absorption of irrigating solution during TCRE. British Medical Journal 300: 1079

Magos A L, Baumann R, Lockwood G M, Turnbull A C 1991 Experience with the first 250 endometrial resections for menorrhagia. Lancet 337: 1074–1078

Mangar D, Gerson J I, Constantine R M, Lenzi V 1989 Pulmonary edema and coagulopathy due to Hyskon (32% dextran-70) administration. Anesthesia and Analgesia 68: 686–687

Morrison L, Davis J A, Sumner D 1989 Absorption of irrigating fluid during laser photocoagulation of the endometrium in the treatment of menorrhagia. British Journal of Obstetrics and Gynaecology 96: 346–352

Nesbit R M, Glickman S I 1948 The use of glycine solution as an irrigating medium during transcervical resection. Journal of Urology 59: 1212–1217

Nicolls M G 1990 Heart failure. In: Oh T E (ed) Intensive care manual, 3rd edn, Butterworths, Sydney

Norlen H 1985 Isotonic solutions of mannitol, sorbitol and glycine and distilled water as irrigating fluids during transurethral resection of the prostate and calculation of irrigating fluid influx. Scandinavian Journal of Urology and Nephrology (Supplement) 96: 1–50

Norlen H, Allgen L, Wicksell B 1986 Sorbitol concentrations in connection with transurethral resection of the prostate using sorbitol solution as an irrigating fluid. Scandinavian Journal Urology and Nephrology 20: 9–17

Ovassapian A, Joshi C, Brunner E A 1982 Visual disturbance: an unusual symptom of transurethral prostatic resection. Anesthesiology 57: 332–334

Quinones-Guerrero R 1983 Liquid distension media. In: van de Pas H, van Herendael B J, van Lith D A F, Keith L G (eds) Hysteroscopy. MTP Press, Lancaster, p 29–32

Rao P N 1987 Fluid absorption during urological endoscopy. British Journal of Urology 60: 93–99

Reid F 1989 Nd:YAG laser endometrial ablation. MD thesis, Faculty of Medicine, Manchester University, p 161

Roesch R P, Stoetling R K, Lingeman J E, Kahnoski R J, Bakes D J, Gephard S A 1983 Ammonia toxicity resulting from glycine absorption during a transuretheral resection of the prostate. Anesthesiology 58: 577–579

Schinagl E F 1990 Hyskon (R) (32% Dextran 70) hysteroscopic surgery and pulmonary edema. Anesthesia and Analgesia 70: 223–224

Schroeder C 1934 Ueber den Ausbau und die Leistunger der Hysteroskopie. Archiv für Gynekologie 156: 407

Sterns R H, Riggs J E, Schochet S S 1986 Osmotic demyelination syndrome following correction of hyponatraemia. New England Journal of Medicine 314: 1535–1542

Trimbos-Kemper T C M, Veering B T 1989 Anaphylactic shock from intracavity 32% dextran 70 during hysteroscopy. Fertility and Sterility 61: 1053–1054

van Boven M J, Singelyn F, Donnez J, Gribomont B F 1989 Dilutional hyponatremia associated with intrauterine endoscopic laser surgery. Anaesthesiology 71: 449–450

Weiner J, Gregory L 1990 Absorption of irrigating fluid during transcervical resection of endometrium. British Medical Journal 300: 748–749

West J H, Robinson D A 1989 Endometrial resection and fluid absorption. Lancet ii: 1387–1388

Zbella E A, Moise J, Carson S A 1985 Noncardiogenic pulmonary edema secondary to intrauterine instillation of 32% dextran 70. Fertility and Sterility 43: 479–480

6. Anaesthesia for endometrial ablation

C. J. R. Elliott   V. P. Page

INTRODUCTION

Currently, endometrial ablation is performed by electrocautery, laser and radio frequency methods. These procedures can be carried out under general anaesthesia or with local anaesthetic agents administered either by infiltration or regional block. As with other operative procedures the anaesthetist is concerned with reducing patient anxiety and eliminating intra- and postoperative pain. In this chapter methods are described which are based on general anaesthesia, local infiltration plus sedation and regional epidural block combined with general anaesthesia.

The first part of the chapter deals mainly with general considerations and management details of ablation with electrocautery. Some aspects of ablation by laser are also considered. The second part is concerned with principles and management in ablation using radio frequency.

PART 1
GENERAL AND LOCAL ANAESTHESIA FOR ENDOMETRIAL ABLATION
C. J. R. Elliott

The nerves of the pelvic organs are particularly suited to local or regional block techniques and ablation can be carried out by these methods instead of general anaesthesia. The decision is influenced by a number of considerations:

1. **Patient preference**. Some patients choose general anaesthesia simply because they do not want to be awake in the theatre. Others choose local anaesthesia because they are frightened or wish to watch the operation on the video screen (Fig. 6.1).

2. **Surgeon preference**. Surgeons will be influenced by training, experience of regional anaesthesia and the wish to converse freely when teaching a junior colleague.

3. **Length of operation**. The efficiency of local anaesthetic injections is limited to a maximum of 2 hours. If a prolonged procedure is anticipated, e.g. for large or multiple fibroids, general anaesthesia may be preferable to avoid the discomfort of returning sensation and prolonged immobility on the operating table.

4. **Accompanying laparoscopy**. Although diagnostic laparoscopy can often be performed under local anaesthetic, patients who are awake may experience discomfort from gas distension, shoulder tip pain from diaphragmatic irritation and breathing difficulties from excessive head down tilt. In these circumstances an additional ablation procedure is unacceptable and general anaesthesia should be chosen.

5. **Day surgery**. Endometrial ablation does not always demand an overnight stay, and discharge from hospital on the same day is possible provided pain relief and nausea are controlled. The Royal College of Surgeons guidelines (RCS 1985) advise that operations under general anaesthesia should not exceed 30 minutes if the patients are discharged on the same day. No patient should be expected to travel a long distance after either regional or general anaesthesia.

6. **Medical fitness**. Young premenopausal women undergoing endometrial ablation are

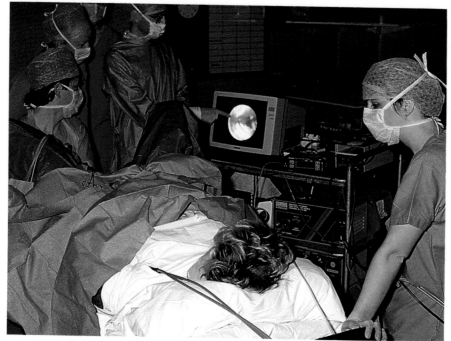

Fig. 6.1   Transcervical resection of the endometrium (TCRE) with local anaesthesia and sedation. The patient is watching the operation on the video screen.

usually healthy. However, patients may be selected for transcervical resection of the endometrium (TCRE) because of medical conditions which make them unfit for hysterectomy and in some instances also for general anaesthesia. Preoperative assessment by the anaesthetist can identify which patients should have local or general anaesthesia. Combined local anaesthesia such as a paracervical block administered by the gynaecologist and sedation by the anaesthetist is often convenient.

Table 6.1, although not exhaustive or exclusive to TCRE operations, includes relative and absolute contraindications to general anaesthesia.

Patients with arrhythmias and hypertension require special care, bearing in mind that local anaesthetic solutions containing adrenalin can be absorbed into the circulation. Patients with bleeding disorders or who are receiving anticoagulants should not be given epidural blocks because of the risk of extradural haematoma formation, but infiltration blocks are permissible.

Table 6.1   Contraindications to general anaesthesia

Local anaesthetic preferable

Gross obesity
Unstable diabetes
Hiatus hernia
History of heavy smoking with productive cough
Upper respiratory tract infection

Contraindications to general anaesthesia

Family history of malignant hyperthermia under general anaesthesia
Porphyria
Myasthenia gravis
Dystrophia myotonica
Patients with predictable intubation problems:
   Cervical spondylitis
   Rheumatoid arthritis affecting temporomandibular joints and cervical spine
   Fit patients with distorted oromandibular anatomy which may interfere with intubation

LOCAL ANAESTHESIA

The sensory nerve supply

Afferent uterine nerves enter the spinal cord via networks called, in ascending order, the lower hypogastric plexus, the hypogastric nerve and upper hypogastric plexus. They enter the cord through the posterior roots of the 11th and 12th thoracic and, possibly, first lumbar spinal nerves. They are joined by afferent nerves in anatomical proximity with the ovarian vessels. Pain pathways from the cervix enter the spinal cord via second, third and fourth sacral nerve roots.

Local anaesthesia for diagnostic or operative hysteroscopy is usually performed by the surgeon with a paracervical block and intracervical injection containing a solution of 1% lignocaine with 1:200 000 adrenalin. After dilating the cervix to Hegar size 10 and inserting the hysteroscope, further injections can be given under direct vision by a fine needle inserted directly into the uterine muscle close to the cornua. Up to 40 ml of local anaesthetic can be administered. The uterus and cervix are rich in blood vessels and aspiration should always be performed to prevent intravascular injection. However, even if the test is negative, transient tachycardia, rise in systolic blood pressure and facial pallor can occur on occasion. Therefore, electrocardiograph and blood pressure readings should always be recorded and prominently displayed on a monitor.

In a series of 94 patients treated under local anaesthesia in Oxford and in London, the mean amount of local anaesthetic was 36.3 ml (standard deviation 7.73 ml).

Local anaesthesia with sedation

Sedation is employed to allay anxiety in patients undergoing operative procedures under local anaesthesia.

Sedation is a state of calm or reduced nervous activity. Clinically, this description is often used in a broad sense to describe or be synonymous with anxiolytic, hypnotic or neuroleptic effects. The term 'sedative' should be strictly applied only to the older drugs, such as phenobarbitone, which allay anxiety and induce sleep by depressing the cerebral cortex. Most of the modern sedative drugs also possess hypnotic effects which induce drowsiness at a higher dose.

Different sedative techniques using a variety of drugs can be given, each technique having its own terminology.

The lytic cocktail

This old method uses a combination of pethidine, promethazine and chlorpromazine, which induces a deep sedative effect and in combination with local anaesthesia provides an alternative to general anaesthesia. The method was particularly applicable to cataract surgery when coughing or vomiting after extubation could compromise the successful result of surgery. Disadvantages of the technique are hypotension and a prolonged recovery time.

Neuroleptanalgesia

This method combines the neuroleptic effect of droperidol on dopamine receptors of the brain and the analgesic properties of fentanyl. Reports of restlessness and agitation have reduced the popularity of the technique.

Subanaesthetic doses of anaesthetic agents

Intravenous infusions of thiopentone and methohexitone were once popular in providing sleep levels of anaesthesia for surgical procedures carried out under epidural analgesia.

Intermittent intravenous methohexitone in small increments gained widespread popularity for several years, particularly to remove anxiety in dental patients undergoing conservation treatment. However, small additional doses can induce deep general anaesthesia and the introduction of benzodiazepine anxiolytic drugs reduced demand for this technique.

Anxiolysis

This is a relatively new term, by which is meant a reduction of anxiety resulting in a reduced state of awareness during which verbal contact with the patient is retained. Drugs which are commonly used for this purpose are the benzodiazepines in low dosages. Lunn (1986) describes anxiolytic agents as drugs which reduce circulating catecholamine levels but should not depress patients to the point of causing sleep. Jacobsen et al (1990) have demonstrated a reduction of anxiety, stress and trauma by β-adrenergic blockade in controlled trials comparing metoprolol, diazepam and a placebo.

Sedoanalgesia

This term is used to describe a technique in which fentanyl and a benzodiazepine are used in combination. This is the technique favoured by Magos et al (1989), who use fentanyl with midazolam to sedate their patients.

Fentanyl. This is a drug structurally related to pethidine but 1000 times more potent. It is also 50–100 times more potent than morphine. Although its half-life is 3–6 hours, the duration of action of 100 μg is only 30 minutes due to a rapid tissue uptake of the drug. In a dose of 1–2 μg/kg there is minimal hypnotic effect but the respiratory rate may be reduced although the tidal volume is increased. In doses exceeding 3 μg/kg, both the tidal volume and rate are depressed. The pulse and blood pressure are maintained but bradycardia may sometimes occur.

Midazolam. This benzodiazepine is water-soluble and does not cause pain or phlebitis on intravenous injection. It possesses both sedative and amnesic effects and is used for the intravenous induction of anaesthesia in doses of 0.1–0.3 mg/kg. In common with other anaesthetic agents, respiratory depression is caused in higher doses. In doses of 0.15 mg/kg given to healthy patients there is a moderate reduction in systolic and diastolic blood pressure and an increase in heart rate. In higher doses the drug causes similar cardiovascular changes seen following administration of thiopentone.

In healthy adults a dose of 0.075 mg/kg can be given intramuscularly without respiratory depression. When given intravenously, 1–2 mg increments may be given but 2–3 minutes must be allowed before repeating the dose. The onset of hypnosis or sedation may be slightly delayed and the difference between a sedative and an anaesthetic dose is small. The drug works for a short time only and the elimination half-life is between 1.7 and 4 hours.

Fentanyl and midazolam combination. Because each drug individually causes respiratory depression, this effect is magnified when consecutive doses of each are given. It is good practice to observe the effect of fentanyl first and watch carefully for further changes in respiratory rates when midazolam is given 5 or 6 minutes later. Bailey et al (1988) reported hypoxaemia and apnoea in healthy male volunteers even with careful observation with this technique.

Sedoanalgesia for TCRE. TCRE under local anaesthesia was performed in 33 patients in London. The majority of cases were admitted to hospital the day before operation and discharged the day following surgery. Seven patients were treated on a day care basis. Most patients knew of the availability of local anaesthesia and sedation before admission but some finally agreed only when details of the procedure were explained at a preanaesthetic assessment visit. Following the practice of Magos et al (1989), the women were premedicated with temazepam 10–20 mg and mefenamic acid 500 mg orally*, 1 hour before surgery followed by fentanyl and midazolam given by the anaesthetist. During surgery, further amounts were infused according to need. When a patient wished to view the surgery on the video screen the dose was reduced. Sedation was more readily achieved in the absence of background noise and activity within the theatre. The correct dosage was sometimes difficult to judge with very nervous patients. It was important to be aware that in some of these cases patient alertness, when stimulated by conversation, could have misled the anaesthetist into administering a larger dose than was necessary. When this stimulus ceased the patient could have then lapsed into respiratory depression.

Because sedation of this nature causes hypoventilation, 30% oxygen was given continuously through a face mask to all patients. The respiratory rate was monitored by clinical observation and the oxygen saturation was recorded with a pulse oximeter. Aitkenhead & Smith recommend that the alarm of the monitor should be set at 94% saturation.

In the series of 94 cases undertaken under local anaesthesia and sedation in Oxford and in London, the mean dose of midazolam was 5.7 mg (standard deviation 2.85 mg) and that of fentanyl was 125 μg (standard deviation 58.04 mg).

---

* Another option, not used in this series, is to use diclofenax 100mg per rectum instead of mefenamic acid orally in the premedication.

GENERAL ANAESTHESIA

General anaesthesia was given to 59 patients undergoing TCRE in London. The majority of cases were admitted the day before operation and discharged the day after surgery. Seven patients were treated on a day care basis.

When planning anaesthesia the following must be taken into consideration:

1. **Length of the operation.** The operative time in 250 TCRE procedures carried out in Oxford and London under both general and local anaesthesia was 33.6 minutes (standard deviation 14.2 minutes) (Magos et al 1991).

2. **Position of the patient.** Surgery was carried out with the patient in a modified lithotomy position, the legs being supported by knee rests with the thighs at 45° to the horizontal. In this position intra-abdominal pressure is lower than in the full lithotomy position and respiration is less affected.

3. **Surgical stimulation.** Dilation of the cervix, intrauterine manipulation and possibly stretching and burning of the uterine muscle causes considerable pain. This in turn modifies the amount of anaesthetic agent required.

4. **Muscle relaxation.** Reduction of muscle tone was needed only to position the limbs in the lithotomy position.

5. **Intravascular absorption of the irrigating fluid.** Absorption of glycine into the circulation can result in electrolyte disturbance and hyponatraemia (see Ch. 5). Large volumes of irrigating fluid are used and the balance between input and output must be closely monitored for deficits which may suddenly arise. Ideally, the theatre team member who is delegated to change the infusion bags and suction bottles should chart the running totals and inform the surgeon and anaesthetist of the current balance. If the deficit exceeds 1500 ml, the serum sodium level should be measured and frusemide 20–80 mg administered intravenously. However, other causes of fluid imbalance must be considered, such as leakage around the cervix.

6. **Day surgery.** If patients wish to go home soon after general anaesthesia, sufficient recovery time is necessary. This means that surgery should be scheduled for morning lists and a bed made available if recovery is delayed. Adequate postoperative analgesia and antiemetic drugs also facilitate early discharge from hospital.

7. **Haemorrhage.** Major blood loss is not usually encountered during endometrial ablation, but because of the small risk of trauma the preoperative haemoglobin level should be measured and serum kept in reserve should cross-matching of blood be necessary.

General anaesthetic agents used and the airway

For patients of lean or moderate build, anaesthesia is based on the administration of propofol for induction and maintenance, fentanyl and nitrous oxide – oxygen. A clear airway is provided by a laryngeal mask (see p. 62).

Propofol

This intravenous agent is a phenol derivative presented in a white emulsified form which contains glycerol, purified egg phosphate, sodium hydroxide, soya bean and water. The drug has been available since 1986.

Anaesthesia occurs about 30 seconds after injection and is usually accompanied by temporary respiratory depression or apnoea. In healthy young adults there is only moderate depression of cardiovascular function, which may cause mild hypotension. The outstanding feature of propofol is its rapid metabolism and elimination, which make it an ideal agent for continuous infusion. When the infusion is stopped the patient wakes up rapidly.

The incidence of laryngospasm is low. Caution is required when the drug is administered to patients with epilepsy. The induction dose is 2–2.5 mg/kg and maintenance infusion rates are between 6 and 12 mg/kg.h. Blood propofol levels of approximately 3 µg/ml are needed to supplement nitrous oxide–oxygen for surgical anaesthesia.

The laryngeal mask

This device (Fig. 6.2) has recently been introduced into clinical practice. It comprises a wide bore silicone tube and an eliptical mask with a cuff which encloses the posterior aspect of the

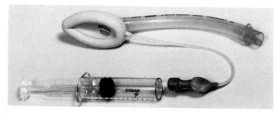

Fig. 6.2   The laryngeal mask.

larynx when inflated (Fig 6.3). It can be used with spontaneous or controlled respiration. The seal formed by the cuff does not guarantee against aspiration of regurgitated gastric contents. The laryngeal mask is introduced blind over the back of the tongue until resistance is felt. Correct positioning is confirmed if the lungs can be easily ventilated without leaks after the cuff has been inflated.

Details of a general anaesthetic technique

The patients were given temazepam 10–20 mg 1 hour prior to surgery.

Induction of anaesthesia was performed with the patient positioned on the theatre operating table. Fentanyl 25–50 μg and propofol 2 mg/kg were given sequentially through a 21 gauge Wallace Y cannula sited on the dorsum of the

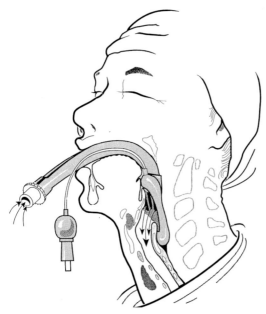

Fig. 6.3   The laryngeal mask in position. (Courtesy of Intavent Ltd, Reading, UK)

hand. Time was allowed to observe the effect of each drug before the next was given. After injection of propofol, jaw relaxation permitted inflation of the lungs with oxygen and introduction of the laryngeal mask. A single antibiotic injection of cephradine 500 mg was given.

Anaesthesia was maintained with nitrous oxide–oxygen supplemented by propofol infused from an Ohmeda pump (Fig. 6.4). Spontaneous respiration was maintained with a Bain breathing system. The end-tidal carbon dioxide level was monitored by capnography and the fresh gas flow adjusted to prevent rebreathing. This arrangement required a high gas flow. J. Scott (1990 personal communication), anaesthetizing for laser ablation with propofol infusion, alfentanyl and a laryngeal mask, maintains carbon dioxide homeostasis with more economic fresh gas flow using controlled respirations.

The infusion rate of propofol administered was influenced by considerations which have been discussed by Sear et al (1988) and Roberts et al (1988). The initial rate was normally set at 10 mg/kg.h. Patients in the lithotomy position are vulnerable to aspiration if vomiting occurs. This can be provoked by light anaesthesia and the presence of a laryngeal mask. For this reason, subsequent time-related reductions aimed at maintaining a constant blood propofol level were avoided in case the anaesthetic inadvertently became too light. Instead, the infusion was adjusted near to the initial rate according to clinical needs and the perceived depth of anaesthesia.

The appropriate level was adjusted according to the patient's reaction to cervical dilation and other painful stimuli, the onset of swallowing, the rate, depth and regularity of respirations, interpretations of end-tidal carbon dioxide levels, ocular movements, pupil size and variations of pulse rate and blood pressure. The speed of infusion was controlled by an automatic pump.

Recovery from anaesthesia

The propofol infusion was discontinued when the patient was moved from the lithotomy to the lateral position. When the laryngopharyngeal reflex appeared, and after suction of oropharyngeal secretions, the cuff was deflated and the mask removed.

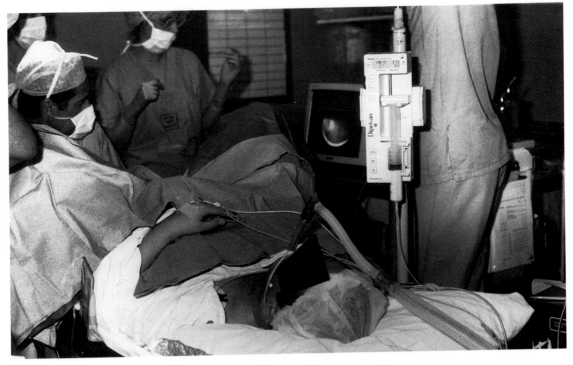

Fig. 6.4 Intravenous propofol anaesthesia with an infusion pump.

Advantages of the technique

1. The airway is maintained without manual elevation of the jaw or endotracheal intubation.

2. Propofol makes it easy to insert the laryngeal mask. Because intubation is not needed, sore throat, laryngotracheitis, laryngospasm and damage to the teeth are unlikely to occur.

3. Reduction of environmental pollution because a predominantly intravenous anaesthetic agent is used.

4. Rapid elimination of propofol allows predictable early recovery from anaesthesia, which is important in planning an operating list.

5. There is minimal drug toxicity.

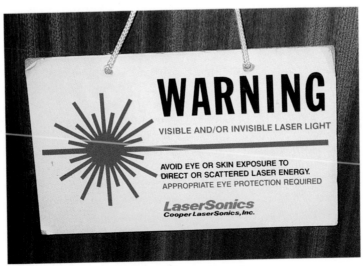

Fig. 6.5 Laser warning notice.

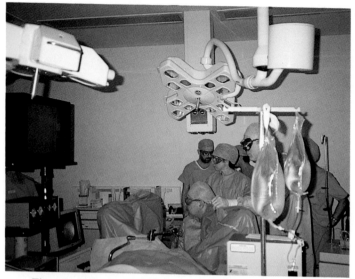

Fig. 6.6   Theatre staff wearing eye protection against laser light.

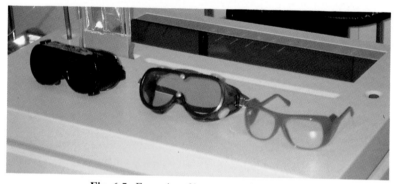

Fig. 6.7   Examples of laser protection glasses.

Disadvantages of the technique

1. Propofol can cause pain following injection into peripheral veins.

2. High fresh gas flows are required if the Bain breathing system is used.

Alternative techniques

Obese patients are not suited to anaesthetic techniques with spontaneous respiration because gas exchange is impaired. These patients should be ventilated with a cuffed endotracheal tube because of the high airway pressures. If a patient has a hiatus hernia she also needs a cuffed endotracheal tube because of the risk of regurgitation of gastric contents.

Postoperative analgesia

Non-steroidal anti-inflammatory drugs can be given alone or with opiates. MacLoughlin et al (1990) used diclofenac for postoperative analgesia in arthroscopy and Kenny (1990) has reviewed the results of studies comparing the efficacy of ketorolac and opiates given separately or together for pain relief after different surgical procedures. Possible side effects of ketorolac were also stated.

Analgesia was provided by diclofenac given intramuscularly immediately postoperatively or as a suppository preceding surgery. Pain after TCRE was variable and sometimes severe according to the extent of surgery, the length of the procedure and the time lapse following the administration of fentanyl. On occasions papaveretum 10 mg given intravenously was needed immediately postoperatively. Milder oral analgesic agents were sometimes sufficient and given additionally later in the ward.

A paracervical block is likely to provide effective postoperative pain relief after general anaesthesia, but further studies are needed to evaluate the best regime for postoperative analgesia following TCRE.

LASER ABLATION AND ANAESTHESIA

Greville & Clements (1990) have described the effect of neodymium:yttrium aluminium garnet (Nd:YAG) laser surgery on anaesthetic departments by noting isolation caused by locked theatre doors, laser proofing of windows with dark non-reflective materials and the restricted access to recovery rooms. Laser procedures are often performed in a darkened theatre, which makes observation of the patient by the anaesthetist more difficult.

Laser light can damage the unprotected retina, and the eyes of all staff and the patient must be protected against accidental exposure. Exposure to laser light can result if the fibreoptic light cables fracture, emphasizing the need for staff to observe safety precautions at all times (Fig. 6.5 and 6.6).

Until recently, laser safety glasses were green or green-grey in colour and could distort the anaesthetist's view of the dials on the monitors. Clear safety glasses are now available (Fig. 6.7). Absten & Joff (1989) have recommended that all safety glasses should be inspected for the wavelength marking of 1060 nm and optical density matching the Nd:YAG laser.

ACKNOWLEDGEMENT

Mr J. Erian is thanked for permission to take the photographs that appear in Fig. 6.5–6.7 during his operating list.

REFERENCES

Absten S T, Joff S N 1989 Lasers in medicine — an introductory guide, 2nd edn. Chapman and Hall, London

Aitkenhead A R, Smith G 1990 Textbook of anaesthesia, 2nd edn. Churchill Livingstone, Edinburgh
Bailey P L, Moll J W B, Pace N L, East K A, Stanley T H 1988 Respiratory effects of midazolam and fentanyl: potent interaction producing hypoxaemia and apnea. Anaesthesiology 69(3A): abstract 813
Greville A C, Clements E A F 1990 Anaesthesia for laparoscopic cholecystectomy using Nd:YAG laser. The implication for District General Hospitals. Anaesthesia 45: 944–945
Jacobsen C-J, Blom L, Bron M, Jerg D B, Lenler-Peterson A 1990 Metoprolol and Diazepam. Anaesthesia 45: 40–43
Kenny G N C 1990 Ketorolac trometamol — a new non-opioid analgesic. British Journal of Anaesthesia (Editorial) 65: 445–447
Lunn J N 1986 Lecture notes on anaesthesia, 3rd edn. Blackwell Scientific, Oxford
MacLoughlin C, Mackinney M S, Fee J P, Boules Z 1990 Diclofenac for day-care arthroscopy surgery: comparison with a standard opioid therapy. British Journal of Anaesthesia 65: 620–623
Magos A L, Bauman R, Cheung K, Turnbull A C 1989 Intrauterine surgery under intravenous sedation as an outpatient alternative to hysterectomy. Lancet ii: 925–926
Magos A L, Bauman R, Lockwood Gill M, Turnbull A C 1991 Experience with the first 250 endometrial resections for menorrhagia. Lancet i: 1074–1078
R C S 1985 Guidelines for day case surgery. Royal College of Surgeons
Roberts F L, Dixon J, Lewis G T R, Tackley R M, Prys-Roberts C 1988 Induction and maintenance of propofol anaesthesia. A manual infusion scheme. Anaesthesia 43(Supplement): 14–17
Sear J W, Shaw I, Wolf A, Kay N H 1988 Infusion of propofol to supplement nitrous oxide–oxygen for the maintenance of anaesthesia. A comparison with halothane. Anaesthesia 43(suppl): 18–22

FURTHER READING

Wood M, Wood A J J 1990 Drugs and anaesthesia. Pharmacology for anestheologists, 2nd edn. Williams and Wilkins, Baltimore

PART 2
ANAESTHESIA FOR RADIO FREQUENCY ENDOMETRIAL ABLATION
V. P. Page

INTRODUCTION

Radio frequency endometrial ablation (RaFEA) is the most recent technique for selectively destroying the endometrium (Phipps et al 1990). A conductive probe is placed in the uterine cavity and selectively destroys the endometrium by heating, using radio frequency energy. Hence the patient is charged with a high-intensity electric field.

PATIENT SELECTION

Most patients are fit women aged 35–50 years and are treated as day cases. Increasingly, however, patients are referred because of the potential difficulties that might occur if these women were offered hysterectomy. In particular, this includes obese patients and those with severe medical disorders. These women require admission for assessment before an appropriate anaesthetic is given. The anaesthetic described here assumes a fit patient.

FEATURES

It is essential that the anaesthetist is aware of basic radio frequency physics and the special precautions necessary for safe practice. An electrical field is set up around the active tip of the probe. The heating effect falls off inversely with distance so that penetration beyond 7 mm is negligible (Phipps et al 1990). Because the patient is 'radio frequency energized', any contact of the patient with an earth results in current flow and heating in the same way as standard diathermy. So whenever the anaesthetist touches the patient some warming of the examining fingers will be noticed; the patient's body temperature is not elevated. This phenomenon results from current flowing to earth in the same way as in standard diathermy. Because of the relationship between current density and area, a finger becomes warmer than a palm. This is harmless, although prolonged contact may eventually become uncomfortable for the anaesthetist — the patient remains unaffected.

Where the above effect does present a hazard is if the patient comes into contact with any metallic surface that is earthed, e.g. stirrup pole frames, the operating table frame or any metal tube connectors. It is important that this does not occur. Should contact occur and be maintained, severe burns may result.

Bearing these features in mind, as day cases, the induction agent of choice is propofol. A laryngeal mask is inserted and anaesthesia is maintained with nitrous oxide–oxygen and a volatile agent. The earth for the radiofrequency energy is provided in the form of a belt around the patient's waist. This is placed on the patient before placing her in the lithotomy position. In this way the risk of contact with metal equipment is minimized. After positioning of the patient a check is made by three members of staff as to the protection of the patient.

MONITORING

The high-volume radio frequency causes a very low signal-to-noise ratio and can drown the electrocardiograph signal, depending on the monitor used. At Hammersmith Hospital, London, a fully screened four-pin lead is used with a specially constructed filter (Menostat ECG filter, Rocket of London, Watford) and a Hewlett Packard monitor, and the electrocardiogram trace is unaffected. It is important that the electrocardiograph leads are insulated as they can melt with use. The filter itself becomes warm during the procedure but this does not affect performance or patient safety. Some monitors can be used without adaptation. It must be ensured that the pulse oximeter design should not become earthed. Burns can result at the site of the instrument.

REFERENCES

Phipps J H, Lewis B V, Roberts T et al 1990 Treatment of functional menorrhagia by radio frequency-induced thermal endometrial ablation. Lancet 335: 197–198

7. Endometrial laser ablation

R. Garry

With contribution from A. Gallinat

The endometrium possesses amazing powers of regeneration. The epithelium is repaired each month after menstruation by cellular regrowth from glands in the basal layers of the endometrium. Successful local treatment of menorrhagia requires complete destruction of these basal glands. It is surprisingly difficult to destroy the deepest layers of the endometrium and a wide variety of chemical, physical and surgical techniques have been found to be ineffective. Lasers can vaporize, coagulate and destroy tissue to a considerable depth. This chapter reviews the effectiveness of hysteroscopically directed laser energy in producing relief of menorrhagia by endometrial laser ablation.

LASERS IN GYNAECOLOGY

Laser radiation can cause thermal, mechanical and chemical damage to living tissue. When a laser beam strikes a tissue, part of the beam will be reflected from the surface, while some of the incident energy will be transmitted through the tissue, and some will be bounced off tissue molecules and cells and scattered. Most of the absorbed energy is converted to heat and is conducted from the site of impact but some may be converted to mechanical energy and produce tissue disruption. All medical lasers produce an area of tissue vaporization at the site of impact, surrounded by a zone of coagulation necrosis, the extent of which depends on the wavelength of the laser and the absorptive properties of the particular tissue (Huether 1989) (Fig. 7.1).

The carbon dioxide laser produces light with a wavelength of 1060 nm in the far-infrared region of the electromagnetic spectrum, which is almost

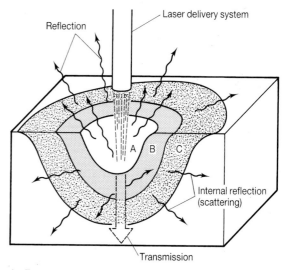

A Zone of vaporization
B Zone of thermal necrosis
C Zone of oedema and recovery

Fig. 7.1 Reflection, scattering, absorption and transmission of laser energy within tissue and zones of injury reduced. (Reproduced with permission from Huether (1989).)

completely absorbed by intra- and extracellular water with little transmission to the surrounding tissues (Fig. 7.2). These physical properties produce excellent and precise tissue cutting with little spread of damage into adjacent tissues. This 'what you see is what you get' type of tissue destruction has been found to be of considerable value in the treatment of cervical dysplasia and for the intra-abdominal treatment of endometriosis and adhesions. The carbon dioxide laser is not, however, appropriate for intrauterine surgery. There is at present no convenient flexible fibre which can transmit its energy into the uterine cavity and very complex and cumber-

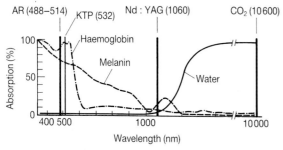

Fig. 7.2 Absorption as a function of wavelength for medical lasers. (Reproduced with permission from Huether (1989).).

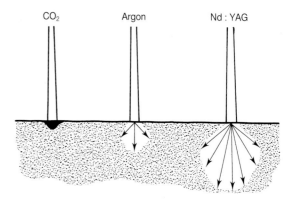

Fig. 7.3 Beam penetration and scattering of different lasers in tissue.

some articulated arms and wave guides are clinically impractical in this situation. Carbon dioxide lasers release considerable amounts of smoke 'plume' during vaporization, and in the small closed cavity of the uterus this can rapidly obscure vision and produces poor operating conditions. Carbon dioxide laser energy is completely absorbed by water, and fluid distension media cannot therefore be used in conjunction with this laser wavelength.

Argon and potassium titanyl phosphate (KTP) lasers produce light of wavelengths that are close together (500 nm and 532 nm respectively) in the visible blue-green region of the electromagnetic spectrum. Several clinical properties are shared by these lasers (Fig. 7.2). The laser radiation from both can be transmitted through small-diameter flexible fibres and is effective in both gaseous and fluid environments. Tissue can only be penetrated to a depth of 1–2 mm as there is little internal tissue scatter of the beam and only a limited zone of tissue coagulation. Both of these laser wavelengths are absorbed to some degree by melanin and haemoglobin. These properties limit the effectiveness of these lasers for endometrial ablation, for they are unable to penetrate sufficiently deep to destroy the basal glands.

The neodymium:yttrium aluminium garnet (Nd:YAG) laser possesses properties which make it the most suitable of the currently available lasers for intrauterine destructive surgery. This laser was first developed in 1961 by Snitzer. Convenient commercial Nd:YAG lasers of up to 100 W in power are available. The energy is transmissible down flexible quartz fibres and is not significantly absorbed by clear fluids, haemoglobin or melanin. There is considerable intratissue scatter of

the beam, producing tissue coagulation necrosis for about 4–5 mm in all directions (Fig. 7.3). Such spread of Nd:YAG laser energy should ensure that when it is applied to the surface of appropriately prepared endometrium, the full thickness of the endometrium including the regenerative basal glands are destroyed without threatening the integrity of the external layers of the myometrium, which is 20 mm thick.

In certain intra-abdominal situations this wide zone of tissue destruction is a disadvantage. In these circumstances synthetic ceramic tips can be attached to the quartz fibre. These sapphire probes 'focus' the beam and significantly reduce intratissue scatter. Artificial sapphire tips must withstand very high temperatures and require coaxial cooling with either fluid or carbon dioxide. Such tips should not be used for laser ablation of the endometrium and are contraindicated for both practical and safety reasons. Tips significantly reduce the zone of tissue necrosis produced by the Nd:YAG laser, thereby reducing the main clinical benefit of this wavelength. Cooling these tips with gas under pressure may force gas into the circulation with the grave consequence of massive gas embolism. 'Bare' quartz fibres give superior clinical results and should have no coaxial channel so that such air embolism is impossible.

LASER SAFETY

Lasers, in common with most surgical devices, are potentially dangerous and it is most important that all members of the surgical team using them should be familiar with the possible hazards associated with their use and the appropriate protocols designed to avoid such problems. The laser surgeon must have had didactic instruction and attended specific practical courses in endoscopic laser surgery. The laser distributors must ensure that equipment is correctly installed and that operating personnel are familiar with the correct working procedures for the equipment. The key must be kept by the nominated laser safety officer and issued only to staff accredited to use the laser.

Nd:YAG, KTP and argon lasers are all class IV lasers and the main hazard to both staff and patients is eye damage. The beams from these lasers will pass through the sclera and the anterior chamber of the eye and will be focused onto the macula, resulting in catastrophic damage to vision. To reduce this risk the operating room should be a restricted area and all personnel in that area must wear protective goggles with side protectors of a suitable colour and optical density to absorb the appropriate laser wavelength when the laser is in use. For the Nd:YAG laser this will be blue-green. Unfortunately, such glasses may alter colour vision and reduce the quality of the field of vision. The patient must also wear such goggles or have their eyes covered with padding and reflective foil. If closed-circuit video is not used then an appropriate filter must also be attached to the hysteroscope. All windows of the laser operating room must be obscured with appropriate absorbent material and a warning sign must be hung from each door. A sign must advise when the laser is in operation and entry forbidden when it is illuminated to those not wearing protective eyewear. The laser must not be directed at flammable materials and only non-flammable skin preparations should be used. Alcohol, ether and combustible anaesthetic gases should be avoided. Some authorities place a moistened sponge in the rectum to minimize the risk of a methane explosion. A trained laser operative who must have no other responsibilities must be assigned to remain at the control panel of the laser throughout the procedure. The laser must remain in the stand-by mode until the gynaecologist gives clear instructions to activate the equipment. This should only be done when the fibre is correctly applied to the tissue to be treated and the laser must never be active when the fibre is outside the patient.

These precautions are essential for the safe operation of any medical laser. Once a satisfactory protocol has been developed and a good team understanding has been acquired, lasers quickly become a non-intrusive and useful addition to the operating room armamentarium.

PREOPERATIVE PREPARATION

Preoperative assessment has been discussed in detail in a previous chapter. In the author's[*] practice, patients considered suitable for endometrial laser ablation are required to have preoperative out-patient hysteroscopy, endometrial sampling, vaginal ultrasound, and a recent negative cervical cytology. These investigations are considered necessary to exclude major structural disease which would contraindicate local ablative treatment. In the absence of any associated pathology the woman should be pretreated to ensure the endometrium is as thin and inactive as possible. This is usually achieved with oral danazol in a dose of 600–800 mg/day for at least 28 days. Alternative preparations such as the luteinizing-hormone-releasing hormone (LH-RH) agonists (e.g. buserelin, goserelin or luprolide acetate) may be effective. If none of these medications are available the ablation should be performed in the immediate postmenstrual phase of the cycle when the endometrium is physiologically at its thinnest.

INSTRUMENTATION AND TECHNIQUES

The flexible quartz laser fibre is introduced into the uterine cavity via the operating channel of a suitably designed multichannel hysteroscope (Fig. 7.4). Cornier has investigated the use of flexible operating hysteroscopes but almost all workers prefer the rigid type of hysteroscope with its larger field of view and better image quality. Such an operating laser hysteroscope should have

---

[*]'The author' refers to R. Garry throughout the chapter.

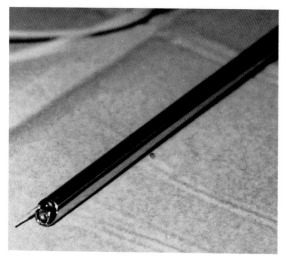

Fig. 7.4   Flexible quartz fibre inserted down a channel of an operating hysteroscope.

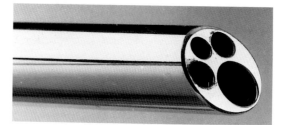

Fig. 7.5   Weck–Baggish operating hysteroscope with a telescope tract and three discrete operating channels.

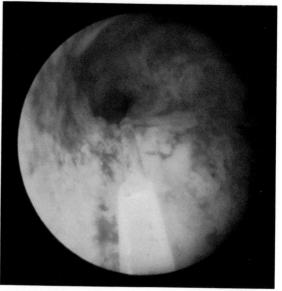

Fig. 7.6   Laser ablation: view of endometrium with fibre in place (Reproduced from Gordon A Lewis B V, (1988) Gynaecological Endoscopy, courtesy of Chapman & Hall, London and Mr. Jonathan Davis.)

very high-quality rod lens optics and be used with an appropriate high-intensity light source so that both close-up and panoramic views of the whole uterine cavity are possible. It is essential that a laser hysteroscope has discrete and totally separate inflow and outflow channels. An ideal laser hysteroscope should be round in cross-section to mirror the shape of the dilated cervical canal and thereby ensure a watertight seal. Many laser hysteroscopes currently on the market do not have all these features, and some betray their cystoscopic antecedents by having an oval cross-section more relevant to the male urethra than the cervical canal. A further common but unsatisfactory feature of some hysteroscopes is the need to insert them with the help of a trocar and canula. This arrangement prevents the hysteroscope being inserted into the uterine cavity in the preferred manner under direct vision. The author recommends the hysteroscope described by Baggish & Baltoyannis (1988), which incorporates the features listed above (Weck, E R Squibb and Sons, New Jersey, USA) (Fig. 7.5). Surgery is best performed using continuous video monitoring.

Two methods of ablating the endometrium have been described. The original 'dragging' technique remains the most widely used (Goldrath et al 1981). The laser fibre is placed on the surface of the endometrium and a series of closely adjacent parallel furrows made (Figs. 7.6–7.8). These furrows consist of a vaporized U-shaped trough with a golden-brown base of char. Unseen beneath this is a zone of coagulation necrosis some 4–5 mm in all directions. With the 'blanching' method of endometrial ablation (Loffer 1987, Lomano 1988) the fibre is held a short distance from the endometrium and moved slowly in a systematic 'airbrushing' back and forward manner over the uterine surface. The ablated areas go white and the surface roughens slightly. It can be quite difficult to determine which areas have been treated with this technique, particularly when the endometrium is very white from the effects of preoperative medication and it is less easy to be sure that every area has been adequately treated. The depth of destruction

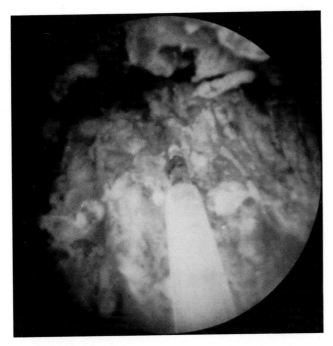

Fig. 7.7 Laser ablation during surgery (Reproduced from Gordon A Lewis B V, (1988) Gynaecological endoscopy, courtesy of Chapman & Hall, London and Mr. Jonathan Davis.).

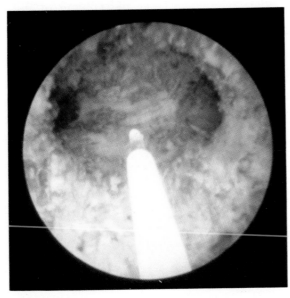

Fig. 7.8 Hysteroscopy view at completion of surgery (Reproduced from Gordon A Lewis B V, (1988) Gynaecological Endoscopy, courtesy of Chapman & Hall, London and Mr. Jonathan Davis.).

achieved is less with this method. For satisfactory blanching it is important to hold the fibre at right angles to the surface, which is relatively easy at the fundus but much more difficult lower down the uterine cavity. Some authorities favour a third technique combining both blanching and dragging methods (Daniell 1989). The author uses the dragging technique throughout because of its greater depth of tissue destruction and more certain demarcation between the treated and non-treated areas.

The power of Nd:YAG laser energy recommended varies. Baggish & Baltoyannis (1988) have suggested that 30 W of power is adequate, Daniell (1986) and Lomano (1988) recommend 40–60 W, whilst Goldrath et al (1981) recommend between 55 and 60 W. Davis (1989) has demonstrated that his results improved in proportion to the power used and he recommends 80 W, which is also the power used by Donnez (1989). The author (R. G) also favours the use of higher powers and finds that 80 W produces a satisfactory depth of tissue destruction with an appropriately short treatment time of about 15–25 minutes.

The 'potential' uterine cavity must be distended by an optically clear medium to permit adequate visualization, and continuous clarity of vision is an essential prerequisite for safe hysteroscopic surgery. As with diagnostic hysteroscopy, either a fluid or a gaseous distension medium may be used. Most gynaecologists favour the use of clear liquid distension media. A major advantage of the Nd:YAG laser over electrical methods of endometrial ablation is that there is no concern about electrolyte solutions and conduction of electricity and so simple and relatively physiological fluids can be used. Most authorities find normal saline convenient and safe, although 5% dextrose, glycine and dextran 70 have also been used.

The author believes that correct control of the distending medium is the most important factor in ensuring quick, effective and, above all, safe hysteroscopic surgery. This matter is discussed in detail elsewhere (Ch. 5) but the principles are becoming clear. It is necessary to achieve a significant intrauterine pressure to distend the uterine cavity and to produce a tamponade effect to control bleeding from vessels which are inevitably disrupted during the ablation. Direct intrauterine pressure studies by the author's team suggest that in most circumstances the minimum pressure needed is between 40 and 75 mmHg. If arterial bleeding is encountered, higher pressures are needed to produce an effective tamponade and maintain clear vision. Fluid must therefore be infused under pressure and this can be achieved:

1. Hydrostatically by suspending a bag of infusion fluid above the patient; it is usual to suspend the bags about 60 cm (45 mmHg) above the patient and this height can be varied to alter the infusion pressure
2. Using syringes for intermittent infusion
3. Using blood pressure cuffs around infusion bottles
4. Using simple roller and pressurized pumps
5. With pressure-controlled pumps (Hamou Hysteromat).

A consequence of raising the intrauterine pressure is that a proportion of the distending fluid may be forced into the patient's circulation and if the amount is excessive clinical fluid overload and pulmonary oedema may occur. Goldrath (1981) reported this complication several times in his first series of cases and most other workers have subsequently encountered this same potentially fatal complication.

Various solutions to this problem have been proposed (Table 7.1). Goldrath (1981), because

Table 7.1 Fluid management systems

Study	Cervical dilatation	Infusion	Outflow	Medium	Laser method
Goldrath (1981)	Wide	Syringe	Free	Saline	Dragging
Lomano (1986)	Wide	?	Free	Saline	Blanching
Loffer (1986)	Minimal	BP cuff	Free	Saline	Blanching
Baggish (1988)	Minimal	Syringe	Syringe	Hyskon	Dragging
Grochmal (1989)	Minimal	BP cuff	Suction	Saline	Dragging
Goldrath (1989)	Minimal	Gravity	Pump	Saline	Dragging
Davis (1989)	Wide	Pump	Free	Saline	Dragging
Davis (1989)	Minimal	Gravity	Pump	Saline	Dragging
Garry (1991)	Minimal	Hamou -Pump	Free	Saline	Dragging

he originally had only a single-channel hysteroscope with a channel for fluid inflow but no route for fluid outflow, suggested that the cervix be hyperdilated to allow the fluid to flow out of the cavity around the hysteroscope. Lomano and Loffer both suggested that blanching the surface of the endometrium rather than dragging the laser fibre across and into the endometrium would minimize vessel damage and hence fluid absorption. This change in technique produced some marginal improvements in the volume of fluid absorbed but was associated with a lower amenorrhoea rate than associated with the dragging technique. Baggish demonstrated that dextran 70, which is much more viscid, entered the circulation less readily, but unfortunately some serious anaphylactic reactions have been reported with use of this medium and most workers find it a difficult fluid to work with (Leak et al 1987).

The Hamou Hysteromat (Fig. 7.9) is a pump designed specifically for intrauterine surgery. It has a rotary pump connected to a pressure transducer. A maximum infusion pressure can be set and the pump and the transducer are connected in such a way so that as the predetermined pressure is approached the pump slows and when the level is reached the pump stops completely. Garry (1990) has shown that the volume of fluid absorbed during endometrial laser ablation can be reduced by 85% using such a pump (Table 7.2). These observations suggest that the intrauterine pressure may be the most important factor controlling extravasation of distending fluid from the uterine cavity. The intrauterine pressure can be measured directly by inserting a fluid-filled catheter into the cavity and connecting it to an appropriate pressure transducer and monitor (Fig.

Table 7.2 Comparison of simple roller pump (constant flow) and a Hamou Hysteromat (constant pressure) as uterine distension systems

	Simple pump	Hamou Hysteromat
Number	105	92
Mean laser time (minutes)	32	23
Mean fluid absorption (ml)	1386	209

Difference between the means 85% (p = 0.00001)

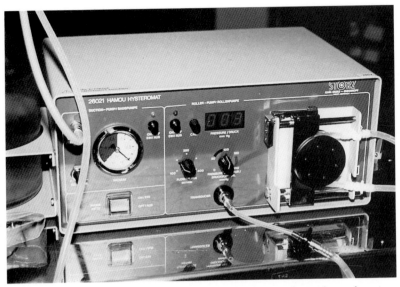

Fig. 7.9   A Hamou Hysteromat with a rotary pump connected to an integral pressure transducer.

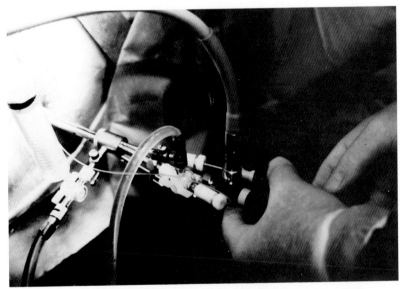

Fig. 7.10   A Weck–Baggish hysteroscope with a laser fibre inserted in the left operating channel, a three-way tap with fluid inflow and a catheter from the uterine cavity to a pressure transducer in the right channel, and a three-way tap for fluid outflow and a syringe for channel flushing in the central channel.

7.10). Using such a system the author has recently shown that in most cases the pressure remains constant throughout the treatment and if it remains below a critical level no fluid absorption will occur. In a number of patients, after a variable period of stability the intrauterine pressure may suddenly rise dramatically (Fig. 7.11). The inflow and intrauterine conditions have usually not altered and investigations indicated that it was in the outflow channel that significant changes had occurred. This channel, even in a properly designed laser hysteroscope, is of limited

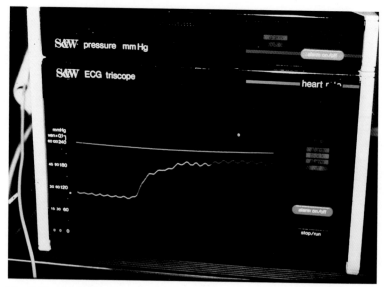

Fig. 7.11   An S&W pressure monitor with the central trace showing a sudden rise in intrauterine pressure.

diameter and is fairly easily blocked completely or partially by small particles of endometrial debris which are often produced during laser ablation (Fig. 7.12). Narrowing the outflow whilst keeping the inflow rate constant invariably produces a sharp rise in intrauterine pressure and if sustained is then inevitably associated with fluid absorption.

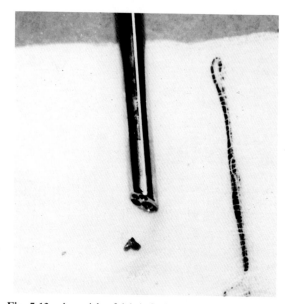

Fig. 7.12   A particle of debris flushed from the outflow channel of the hysteroscope at the end of an endometrial laser ablation procedure.

If the outflow channel is cleared the uterine pressure rapidly returns to normal and fluid absorption does not occur.

The author has also demonstrated that although absorption of distension fluid is related to intrauterine pressure this relationship is not a progressive one. Absorption appears to be an 'all or nothing' phenomenon. If the pressure remains below a certain level no absorption occurs and if the intrauterine pressure rises above this level fluid enters the uterine capillary and venous system directly, rapidly and, in some cases, in considerable volume. This 'all or nothing' phenomenon can be demonstrated by taking a series of hysterosalpingograms at various measured pressure levels upon completion of laser ablation procedure. Such radiographs clearly show how the distending medium is retained in the uterine cavity if the intrauterine pressure is kept below the mean arterial pressure, but if the intrauterine pressure rises above this level a complete pelvic venogram is invariably produced (Figs. 7.13 and 7.14). Such venograms demonstrate unequivocally that the route of fluid absorption is directly into the uterine venous system and demonstrate just how large these pathways can be. In some circumstances several hundred millilitres per minute of distension medium can be absorbed.

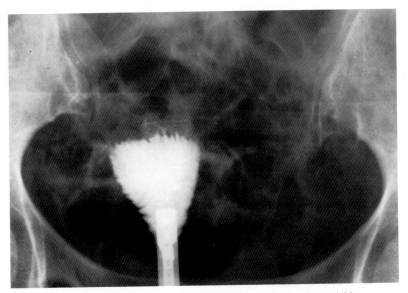

Fig. 7.13 A radiograph of the uterine cavity at the end of an endometrial laser ablation procedure with the uterine pressure maintained at a steady 80 mmHg. Note the irregular uterine outline of the multiple laser furrows and that at this pressure all the radiopaque medium is contained inside the cavity.

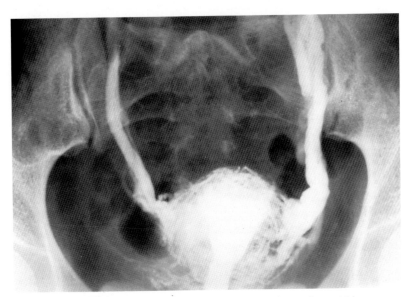

Fig. 7.14 A radiograph of the uterine cavity at the end of an endometrial laser ablation procedure, with the intrauterine pressure in excess of 160 mmHg. Note that much of the radiopaque medium escapes out of the cavity and enters the uterine capillaries and veins and readily outlines the whole of the venous system of the uterus.

In summary, to achieve consistent, clear vision without any significant fluid absorption it is necessary to control the intrauterine pressure and to titrate the intrauterine pressure against the uterine tissue pressure. If the pressure is too low, bleeding into the distending medium will occur with immediate loss of vision. If the pressure is too high the distending fluid will be forced into the circulation. If the pressure is maintained at an optimum level the cavity will be adequately distended without any extravasation of fluid. If the uterine pressure is maintained above 45 mmHg and below the patient's mean arterial pressure, these conditions will be fulfilled. It is important to ensure that both the inflow pressure is maintained below the mean arterial blood pressure and the outflow channel remains completely patent to ensure an adequate and consistent fluid outflow. Continuous measurement of the intrauterine pressure gives early warning of any outflow obstruction, which can readily be cleared by flushing the outflow channel.

With such a closed, pressure-controlled fluid distension system the visual conditions should remain perfect throughout the procedure. There should be no bleeding because of the tamponade effect, bubbles and small particulate matter should be flushed out by the continuous flow, and there should be no large pieces to obscure the view. The hysteroscope should not need to be removed during the ablation and this permits a significant reduction in treatment time. In 250 consecutive cases using this technique the mean treatment time was 22 minutes.

A different approach to uterine cavity distension has been pioneered by Gallinat. He recommends the use of carbon dioxide as the distension medium (Gallinat 1989), believing it to be safer because there is no risk of fluid overload and electrolyte disturbances and no problems with allergic reactions. Carbon dioxide is highly soluble in blood, and providing the infusion pressure is fixed at 150 mmHg and the infusion flow is limited to a maximum rate of 70 ml/min the patient can safely metabolize and excrete what gas is absorbed. These safe operating conditions can be provided conveniently using a special insufflation apparatus with inbuilt smoke extraction filters. A further advantage of this system is that the gaseous distension medium requires lower laser powers to produce an adequate depth of tissue destruction and Gallinat finds a power of 20–40 W adequate (Fig. 7.15). The main disadvantage of this technique is that steam and smoke plumes generated by Nd:YAG laser ablation may obscure vision temporarily. Such steam and smoke will be cleared by the

continuous flow of the distending gas, but this requires intermittent rather than continuous use of the laser. Care must be taken to use equipment which can only deliver carbon dioxide at controlled rates of less than 150 ml/min; higher rates of infusion risk catastrophic air embolism. Few authorities have yet adopted this potentially interesting method of distending the cavity and most prefer the more continuously clear view afforded by fluid distension.

A METHOD OF ENDOMETRIAL LASER ABLATION

As discussed in Chapter 6, endometrial laser ablation may be performed under general, regional or local analgesia. The patient is placed in a modified lithotomy position with the hips abducted as far laterally as possible to maximize the space available between her thighs. This position will improve access to the tubal ostia areas. The perineum is cleaned using a nonflammable preparation and draped in the standard manner. A plastic urological pouch is placed beneath the perineum to collect leaked distension fluid. The bladder is not now routinely catheterized. After a standard bimanual examination, dilatation of the cervix is restricted to that which will just accept the operative hysteroscope and maintain a watertight seal.

The Weck Baggish hysteroscope with three separate operative channels is connected to a powerful balanced light source and a compatible

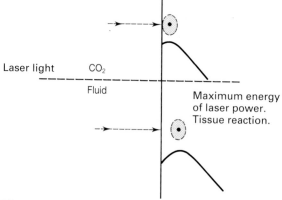

Fig. 7.15   Tissue reaction during laser ablation using gaseous and liquid distension media. The maximum effect of the YAG-Laser light is found using a gaseous medium directly at the surface of tissue. Using a fluid medium, the maximum tissue effect rises beyond the surface.

single-chip video camera. The uterine distension medium chosen is normal saline. Two 3 litre bags suspended from a drip stand are connected by a Y tube to ensure a continuous flow. This inflow tube is led through the peristaltic pump of a Hamou Hysteromat. The rate of inflow is set initially at 100 ml/min and the maximum inflow pressure is set at the level of the patient's mean arterial blood pressure, which is usually about 100 mmHg. From the Hysteromat the fluid is led into the side-arm of a three-way tap connected to one of the operating channels of the hysteroscope. A 16 gauge catheter is placed down the direct arm of this three-way tap. This catheter is filled with normal saline under pressure and is connected to a Viggo Spectramed pressure transducer, which in turn is connected to a Simonson and Weel monitor. The outflow channel of the hysteroscope is also connected to a three-way tap. One channel of this leads to the graduated collecting jar of the Hysteromat. To the other channel can be connected a syringe to flush out the outflow tract. This rather complex closed fluid circuit permits measurement and control of the inflow, cavity and outflow pressures. Such a system provides optimum operating conditions whilst minimizing the risks of absorption of distension fluid.

When clear vision is established the 600 μm quartz laser fibre is inserted in a flexible metal protective sheath into the remaining operative channel. This bare fibre has no connection for a sapphire tip and no coaxial channel. An SLT CL100 laser is used and set at 80 W of power. The regions around the tubal ostia can be the most difficult to visualize and to reach with the fibre. The ablation is therefore begun in these areas and then gradually extended across the fundus until the treated areas join in the midline. The hysteroscope is maintained constantly in the 12 o'clock position and is not rotated. This is helpful to maintain orientation when operating via changed couple device television (CCDTV). The fibre is withdrawn with the right hand. Simultaneously the left hand depresses or elevates the proximal end of the hysteroscope to keep the fibre in contact with the endometrial surface. The glowing tip of the fibre is kept in view throughout the procedure and the laser is only fired when the fibre is being drawn down towards the cervix, never when the fibre is being returned to the fundus. When the fundus has been fully treated, the anterior, both lateral and finally the posterior walls are also ablated down to the level of the internal os. To reduce the risk of cervical stenosis, Gallinat stops the ablation a few millimetres above the internal os.

With careful control of the flow of distension medium the many bubbles released during vaporization and the small particles of endometrial debris inevitably produced by the ablation are rapidly flushed out of the cavity. Bleeding is prevented by careful control of the intrauterine pressure and so excellent vision should be consistently and continuously maintained. The hysteroscope should seldom if ever be removed from the cavity and every effort made to complete the ablation in a single steady-state session. Any blockage which occurs in the outflow channel can readily be cleared by flushing out the channel with a syringe full of normal saline.

RESULTS

Table 7.3 lists the intraoperative and immediate postoperative results of a multicentre study of more than 1000 patients with menorrhagia treated by endometrial laser ablation. After the early learning phase the treatment time fell and the mean time to complete the ablation was 23 minutes (range 11–90 minutes). Almost all the patients were discharged within 24 hours and many went home on the day of surgery. Some complained of menstrual-like cramps for a few hours after ablation but this was almost invari-

Table 7.3 Operative details of a multicentre study of endometrial laser ablation (Garry et al 1991).

	Princeton	Farnborough	Middlesbrough	Total
Number	342	359	318	1019
Operative[a] time (minutes)	17 (11–27)	27 (17–90)	26 (11–90)	23
Mean fluid deficit (ml)	1500	1500	743 (1416[b], 289[c])	1272

[a] Mean with range in parentheses.
[b] 115 cases with a continuous-flow non-pressure-controlled pump.
[c] 170 cases with a pressure-controlled variable-flow-rate pump.

ably relieved by simple analgesia and early post-operative pain was not a problem. A variable serosanguineous loss persists for up to 6 weeks after the endometrial ablation and during this time some women experience a heavy menstrual-like bleed attributed to the shedding of the necrotic endometrium. In those in whom a simple continuous-flow pump was used to distend the cavity the mean volume of normal saline absorbed was 1416 ml. In the 170 patients in whom the fluid was infused with a Hamou Hysteromat the mean volume absorbed was 289 ml, a reduction of 80%.

More than 500 of these cases have been followed up for more than 6 months and the clinical outcomes are shown in Table 7.4. Of the 514 cases studied, 312 (61%) were considered to have an excellent result with either complete amenorrhoea or profound oligomenorrhoea with only vaginal spotting as an outcome. A further 158 (32%) were classified as having a good clinical result associated with continuing menstruation but at a significantly reduced level completely acceptable to the patient as less than 'normal' and much less than pretreatment levels. 39 (8%) were considered initial treatment failures, but 26 responded to a second laser ablation and only 13 (3%) required hysterectomy. When the follow-up period was prolonged and those treated more than 12 months previously were studied, the apparent success rate fell slightly, with 4% of patients who had good early results relapsing. No patient with amenorrhoea at 6 months became worse at 12 months. Overall, 470 (97%) women at 6 month review had a satisfactory clinical response to endometrial laser ablation.

These results are similar to those reported by other workers and the clinical outcomes of more than 1000 patients treated by endometrial laser ablation are now in the literature (Table 7.5). Further details can be found in Chapter 11.

COMPLICATIONS

The principal short-term complications expected following endometrial laser ablation are uterine perforation with damage to bowel, bladder and blood vessels, fluid overload with pulmonary oedema and electrolyte disturbances, intra- and postoperative haemorrhage, and infection. The incidence of these complications in the 1015 patients reported by Garry et al (1991) is shown in Table 7.6. The total short-term complication rate was extraordinarily low at only 1%. This was made up as follows. The uterus was perforated on three occasions, a rate of 0.4%. All of these occurred during insertion of the rigid hysteroscope. When this happened the procedure was discontinued, the patients allowed home within 24 hours and in each case the treatment was successfully repeated within 4 weeks. No uterine perforation was caused by the laser, nor were there any cases of damage to the bowel, bladder or other surrounding structure. None of the women had perioperative bleeding requiring active treatment or blood transfusion and none developed haematometra. All of these women had uterine distension produced by simple non-pressure-controlled pumps. Four women (0.4%) developed symptomatic pulmonary oedema requiring management with postoperative intravenous

Table 7.4 Clinical results of a multicentre trial of endometrial laser ablation (Garry et al 1991).

	Princeton	Farnborough	Middlesbrough	Total
Number	198	213	103	514
Excellent	111 (56%)	139 (65%)	62 (58%)	312 (61%)
Good	74 (37%)	55 (26%)	29 (28%)	158 (31%)
First failure	13 (7%)	19 (9%)	18 (17%)	50 (10%)
Successful second laser ablation	10 (5%)	12 (6%)	6 (6%)	28 (5%)
Hysterectomy	3 (2%)	7 (3%)	5 (5%)	15 (3%)

Overall satisfaction rate of patients[a] 466 (97%)

[a]With one or two endometrial laser ablation procedures.

Table 7.5   Summary of published results of endometrial laser ablation[a]

Study	Number	Excellent results	Normal results	Failures	Overall success
Goldrath (1981)	321	292	7	22	93%
Lomano (1988)	62	47	14	1	98%
Loffer (1987)	55	38	11	6	90%
Baggish (1988)	14	10	3	1	93%
Daniell (1986)	18	13	1	4	78%
Donnez (1989)	50	47	2	1	98%
Bertrand (1989)	22	16	5	1	95%
Multicentre (Lomano et al 1986)	23	18	3	2	91%
Davis (1989)	25	8	5	12	52%
Gallinat (1989)	102	95	4	3	97%
Garry (1991)	479	288	178	13	97%
Total	1171	872 (74%)	233 (20%)	66 (6%)	94%

[a] Some patients treated more than once.

Table 7.6   Complications in a multicentre study

Complication	Princeton	Farn-borough	Middles-brough	Total
Pulmonary oedema	2	2	0	4
Perforation with hysteroscope	1	2	0	3
Perforation with laser	0	0	0	0
Haemorrhage	0	0	0	0
Infection	0	2	2	4
Haematometra	0	0	0	0
Total				11 (1%)

diuretics. Each responded promptly and all left hospital between 6 and 48 hours. None of these cases required intensive care but in other series severe fluid overload problems have been encountered. Significant postoperative pyrexia was noted in four women but only one of these had proven pelvic inflammatory disease.

DISCUSSION

The relative thickness of the myometrium, the ease with which effective uterine tamponade can be produced to arrest haemorrhage, and the fact that endometrial destruction is produced by Nd:YAG laser energy spreading from the quartz fibre placed superficially on the surface layers of the endometrium minimize the risk of serious complications. The large multicentre study reported above was associated with a very low early complication rate of only 1%. However, endometrial laser ablation, like any surgical procedure, is associated with the risk of severe complications. Three cases of uterine perforation and bowel damage have been reported (Perry et al 1990), attributed respectively to an abnormally thin myometrium in a congenitally abnormal uterus, the use of laser power in excess of 90 W, and inexpert use of the laser in an inadequately supervised situation. The inappropriate use of sapphire tips cooled by high-flow carbon dioxide or air under pressure has caused four deaths, and an additional case of severe brain damage due to catastrophic gas embolism has also been reported (Baggish & Daniell 1989). Significant intraoperative haemorrhage is unlikely but major postoperative haemorrhage remains a possibility. Large amounts of necrotic tissue are produced by endometrial laser ablation and this can provide a focus for infection. The author recommends the use of a perioperative broadspectrum antibiotic to reduce this risk.

The most common serious complication of endometrial laser ablation remains excessive extravasation of the distending medium into the systemic circulation with the risk of fluid overload, dilutional problems and pulmonary oedema. This complication was reported in Goldrath's original series and has been noted to a greater or lesser extent in almost every subsequent series. Careful monitoring at frequent intervals of infusion fluid inflow, outflow and deficit is essential. As described in more detail in Chapter 5, the maintenance of a closed-circuit, high-flow, low-pressure distension system with a continuously maintained clear outflow channel will minimize this risk. Using a pressure-controlled infusion system has been shown to reduce fluid absorption and directly measuring the intrauterine pressure and adjusting flow rates appropriately has been shown to virtually eliminate the risk of excessive fluid absorption.

Endometrial laser ablation is a treatment for patients complaining of menorrhagia. Most women suffering from this complaint request relief of the symptom of heavy menstrual loss. They usually do not request amenorrhoea or demand a hysterectomy. In fact many women are delighted to be relieved of their symptoms and yet still retain their uterus. The distinction between absolute amenorrhoea and profound oligomenorrhoea appears to be of greater consequence to the gynaecologist than the patients. Goldrath's original clinical classification of outcome into 'excellent' (which includes both amenorrhoea and oligomenorrhoea), 'good' (with continuing but significantly reduced menstruation) and 'failure' continues to seem relevant. It is the aim of most laser endoscopists to produce amenorrhoea in every case and it is not yet clear why this is achieved in some cases and not others. The precise mechanism by which menstrual reduction is produced is not clear. It is certainly not due to the production of a complete Ashermans syndrome and in most cases a much reduced but still patent cavity can be demonstrated at follow-up hysteroscopy. It is of particular interest that in many cases it takes 3–6 months to achieve the maximal reduction in menstrual flow. Many questions remain to be answered about how this technique works and about its long-term safety and effectiveness.

The endometrium is destroyed, the uterotubal junctions damaged and often occluded and considerable myometrial scarring is produced by endometrial laser ablation. These features all combine to reduce the chances of conception. Pregnancy, however, remains possible and one of the author's series of 318 cases has become pregnant. It is important to counsel the patients appropriately and to offer those at risk alternative contraceptive protection.

Endometrial laser ablation requires a considerable amount of expensive equipment and questions have been raised about the cost effectiveness of the procedure. No meaningful answers can be given until we know the long-term relapse and complication rates. Some facts are, however, already clear. Patients who have had a laser ablation procedure spend less time in the operating room, less time in hospital, and less time off work or away from their family duties than those who have had a hysterectomy (Table 7.7). These savings in time can also lead to considerable financial savings for the hospital service. The magnitude of these savings will depend much more on the number of cases dealt with than on the capital cost of the equipment. We have calculated that if a laser has a working life of 7 years and 500 patients per year can be treated with it the cost per case of providing the laser is only about £22 (Table 7.8). The cost of theatre consumables such as drapes, swabs and suture materials is 45% less for endometrial laser ablation than for hysterectomy. This saving alone, if continued for the life of the laser, is sufficient to pay for the equipment. Thus, Nd:YAG lasers when used frequently in large and busy departments are cost-effective items, and with a small cost per case the capital costs of buying the equipment are very quickly recovered. If the change from long-term in-patient hospital stay associated with hysterectomy to day case surgery permits closure of in-patient beds it is estimated that for every 500 patients treated by endometrial laser ablation rather than hysterectomy there could be a saving of £390 000. The

Table 7.7 Operative details of endometrial laser ablation compared with hysterectomy

	Hysterectomy	Endometrial laser ablation
Time in theatre (minutes)	88	44
Treatment time (minutes)	60	23
Mean hospital stay (days)	7	1
Mean convalescence (days)	56	10
Proportion with noted post-operative complication (%)	45	1
Postoperative pain (<24 hours) (%)	94	0

Table 7.8   Costs of hysterectomy compared with endometrial laser ablation

	Hysterectomy	Endometrial laser ablation
Theatre consumables	£58.09	£27.77
Laser depreciation		£21.42
Laser fibre costs		£9.60
Staff costs	£107.21	£74.07
Total theatre costs	£165.30	£132.86
Ward costs	£800.00	£50.00
Total procedure costs	£965.30	£182.60

financial benefits are even greater if the savings associated with early return to work and reduced social benefit payments are included. In the short-term, endometrial ablation is certainly very popular with patients and with those who pay for their treatment. With an immediate morbidity of only 1% and a patient satisfaction rate in excess of 90% it is a technique worthy of further study. From consideration of both the theoretical mode of action and the clinical evidence currently available, Nd:YAG laser ablation seems to be the safest of the ablative techniques now available. Well-structured studies are, however, required to determine the long-term relapse rate, the effect of the procedure on various genital tract malignancies and the sustained safety and effectiveness of the procedure.

REFERENCES

Baggish M S, Baltoyannis P 1988 New techniques for laser ablation of the endometrium in high risk patients. American Journal of Obstetrics and Gynecology 159: 287–292

Baggish M S, Daniell J F 1989 Death caused by air embolism associated with neodymium:yttrium–aluminum–garnet laser surgery and artificial sapphire tips. American Journal of Obstetrics and Gynecology 161: 877–878

Baggish M S, Bardot J, Valle R F 1989 Diagnostic and operative hysteroscopy. A text and atlas. Year Book Medical Publishers, Chicago

Bertrand J D 1989 Endometrial ablation using Nd–YAG laser for menorrhagia. Proceedings of the Second World Congress of Gynecologic Endoscopy. Clermont-Ferrand, France

Daniell J F Hysteroscopic Laser Surgery. In: Sanfilippo J S, Levin R L (eds) Operative gynecologic endoscopy. Springer-Verlag, New York

Daniell J F, Tosh R, Meisels S 1986. Photodynamic ablation of the endometrium with the Nd–YAG Laser hysteroscopically as a treatment for menorrhagia. Colposcopy and Gynecologic Laser Surgery 2: 43–46

Davis J A 1989 Hysteroscopic endometrial ablation with the neodymium–YAG laser. British Journal of Obstetrics and Gynaecology 96: 928–932

Donnez J, Nisolle M 1989 Laser hysteroscopy in uterine bleeding. Endometrial ablation and polypectomy. In: Donnez J (ed) Laser operative laparoscopy and hysteroscopy. Nauwelaerts, Leuven

Gallinat A 1978 Metromat. A new insufflation apparatus for hysteroscopy. Endoscopy 3: 234

Gallinat A, Lueken R R, Moller C P 1989 The use of the Nd:YAG laser in gynecological endoscopy. MBB-Medizintechnik GmbH, Laser Brief 14, Munich

Garry R 1990 Safety of hysteroscopic surgery. Lancet 336: 1013–1014

Garry R, Erian J, Grochmal S 1991 A multicentre collaborative study into the treatment of menorrhagia by Nd–YAG laser ablation of the endometrium. British Journal of Obstetrics and Gynaecology 98: 357–362

Goldrath M H 1990 Intrauterine laser surgery. In: Keye W R (ed) Laser surgery in gynecology and obstetrics, 2nd edn. Year Book, Chicago, p. 151–165

Goldrath M H, Fuller T, Segal S 1981 Laser photovaporization of endometrium for the treatment of menorrhagia. American Journal of Obstetrics and Gynecology 140: 14–19

Huether S E 1989 Laser physics and light-tissue interaction. In: Keye WR (ed) Laser surgery in gynecology and obstetrics. Year Book, Chicago, p. 14–34

Leake J F, Murphy A A, Zacur H A 1987 Noncardiogenic pulmonary edema: a complication of operative hysteroscopy. Fertility and Sterility 48: 497–499

Loffer F D 1987 Hysteroscopic endometrial ablation with the Nd–YAG laser using a non-contact technique. Obstetrics and Gynecology 69: 679–682

Lomano J M 1988 Photocoagulation of the endometrium with the Nd–YAG Laser for the treatment of menorrhagia. Journal of Reproductive Medicine 31: 148–150

Lomano J M, Feste J R, Loffer F D, Goldrath M H 1986 Ablation of the endometrium with neodymium:YAG laser. A multicentre study. Colposcopy and Gynecologic Laser Surgery 2: 4–6

Perry C P, Daniell J F, Gimpelson R J 1990 Bowel injury from Nd–YAG endometrial ablation. Journal of Gynecologic Surgery 6: 199–203

8. Experimental developments in laser endometrial destruction

M. D. Judd   S. G. Bown

INTRODUCTION

Excessive menstrual bleeding is found in approximately 20% of women during their reproductive years (Jacobs & Butler 1965, Hallberg et al 1966) and hysterectomy still remains the commonest surgical procedure for women whose menorrhagia has failed to respond to medical treatment. Recently, techniques for local endometrial destruction have become more widely used and include the use of the resectoscope (Neuwirth & Amin 1976, Magos et al 1989), laser ablation (Goldrath et al 1981, Lomano 1986, Loffer 1987) and radio frequency-induced ablation (Phipps et al 1990). These techniques are successful but are not without their problems (Gannon et al 1991, Irwin 1991, Sturdle & Hoggart 1991) and include fluid overload (Morrison et al 1989, West & Robinson 1989, Baumann et al 1990), haemorrhage (Goldrath et al 1983), uterine perforation and damage to extrauterine organs (Pittroff et al 1991).

Two experimental techniques are being studied which use either the principle of laser hyperthermia or of photodynamic therapy.

LASER HYPERTHERMIA

Hyperthermia has been used to treat a variety of diseases. Since the last century, fever-inducing infections were used to kill tumours, while whole-body heating was used in patients with resistant gonococcal and non-specific urethritis (King et al 1943, Macdonald 1944). Generalized hyperthermia was not very specific and had a high morbidity and mortality; this technique produced jaundice, deranged liver function and irreversible liver and cardiac failure. Therefore, localized hyperthermia has been directed at specific organs and has attempted to produce uniform heating of tissue to temperatures in the range 42.5–50°C for extended periods of time (often over 1 hour). There is a relationship between temperature and cell death, such that at 42°C and above the temperature required to cause cell death by heating is halved with every increase of 1°C. Canine bladder can be completely destroyed at temperatures ranging from 59 to 69°C and replaced by a fibrous nodule (Linke et al 1972). A number of methods of inducing hyperthermia have been tried, including radio frequency, microwave and ultrasound (Hand & Ter-Haar 1981), but they all produce irregular tissue heating with damaged to surrounding structures.

Laser light can interact with biological tissue in four ways: it can be absorbed, reflected, transmitted or scattered (Fig. 8.1). Transmitted and reflected laser light will produce no biological effect. Scattering of laser light causes it to be

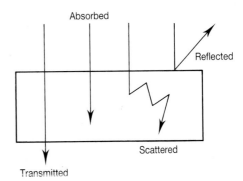

Fig. 8.1   Action of laser light on living tissue.

absorbed by a larger volume of tissue. Neodymium:yttrium aluminium garnet (Nd:YAG) laser light, which has a wavelength of 1064 nm, is poorly absorbed but considerably scattered by biological tissue; therefore, light distribution within irradiated tissue is relatively uniform. Absorbed laser energy is converted to heat and, at low powers, local tissue necrosis is produced without vaporization.

Interstitial laser hyperthermia has been shown to be a safe and predictable technique when used to treat lesions within solid organs. The necrosis produced is well defined and reproducible and resolves by healing with fibrosis or regeneration. Interstitial laser hyperthermia has been used in many experimental models including rat (Matthewson et al 1987) and canine liver (Steger et al 1987a), canine pancreas (Steger et al 1987b), chemically induced rat colon tumour (Matthewson et al 1988) and in an implanted flank fibrosarcoma (Matthewson et al 1989). Single bare quartz fibres placed into a solid structure or organ using low power (1–2 W) produced areas of thermal necrosis up to 16 mm in diameter. These healed by resolution and fibrosis. There was a clear 'dose–response' relationship between energy delivered to the tissue and the final lesion size. A clear border between normal and necrotic tissue existed and there was evidence of a reduction in blood flow in necrosed areas.

Interstitial laser hyperthermia has also been used in small clinical studies to treat solitary liver metastases, inoperable pancreatic carcinoma and metastatic breast tissue (Steger et al 1989, Masters & Bown 1990) using either single or multiple fibres.

Hollow organs like the uterus are not particularly suited to interstitial therapy, and obviously a single bare fibre placed in the endometrium using low power would not be a practical treatment for menorrhagia. However, using a modified fibre tip in which the light is emitted in a suitable distribution has the potential to treat the entire endometrium in a safe and predictable manner. Gentle thermal damage to the entire endometrium would potentially result in safe healing with the structural integrity of the surrounding tissue maintained.

EXPERIMENTAL WORK USING LASER HYPERTHERMIA

An animal model was used to assess the feasibility of destroying and preventing the regrowth of the endometrium using a low-power laser hyperthermia technique (Judd et al 1991). The fibre tip was passed into the uterine horn at laparotomy (Fig. 8.2). The endometrium was exposed to laser light using 1–3 W either to produce single lesions or to destroy the entire endometrium by treating a series of adjacent sites.

A continuous-wave Nd:YAG laser was used at a power of 1–3 W. A modified fibre tip (Fig. 8.3) was used in which the light was incident upon a gold cone and reflected in a disc-shaped distribution, producing circumferential lesions. Gold was used for the tip because it is durable and has a high reflectivity. The tip was securely fixed to a

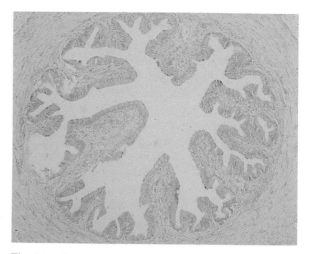

Fig. 8.2   Cross-section of normal uterine horn showing the stellate-shaped endometrial cavity (Haematoxylin & Eosin, magnification ×8).

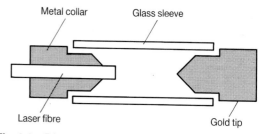

Fig. 8.3   Diagram of the modified fibre tip.

plastic-clad silicone fibre (core diameter 400 μm) which was polished at both ends. The length of the tip was 20 mm and the diameter 3 mm, which allowed it to be passed easily through the cervix into the uterine horn. Its output was measured at the start and finish of each procedure using an integrating sphere power meter. A copper–constantan thermocouple was used in conjunction with a display unit to monitor serosal temperature changes.

Single-lesion procedure

In this part of the study three to four separated lesions were produced in each uterine horn. The power used was 1–3 W with maximum exposure times of 100 seconds. All specimens were examined 6–8 days following treatment, when the maximum amount of damage had occurred. These results are summarized in Table 8.1. Lesions produced using 2 W at exposure times of 100 seconds were symmetrical in 89% of cases. They had a mean serosal length of 6.3 mm (range 5–9 mm) and were easily identifiable, being paler in colour than the untreated tissue. Symmetrical endometrial destruction occurred, causing loss of all villi (Fig. 8.4), and these parameters were used in subsequent experiments to treat the entire endometrium.

Overlapping lesions procedure

When destroying the whole endometrium the tip was passed to the cornual end of the horn and positioned to ensure that it was pressed equally against all parts of the uterine cavity. After each delivery of laser light (2 W for 100 seconds) the

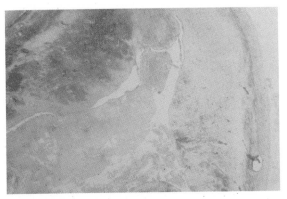

Fig. 8.4 Histological section of the uterine horn exposed to 2 W for 100 seconds 5 days after treatment. The upper layer shows loss of all villi, most glands and incomplete surface re-epithelialization. The lower myometrial and serosal layers are intact. (Haematoxylin & Eosin, magnification ×20.)

fibre was withdrawn approximately 5 mm before the next site was treated. A 5 mm gap would ensure overlap of treated areas because single lesions produced at 2 W for 100 seconds were approximately 6 mm in length.

However, early on in the work it was discovered that areas of endometrium were consistently difficult to treat. Firstly, the upper 5 mm of each horn remained undamaged because its diameter was too narrow to allow the passage of the fibre tip. Secondly, the lowest part of the cervix which had the most complex villi was often only partially destroyed. Therefore, in subsequent animals the upper quarter of each uterine horn was tied off with sutures and only the lower part treated, while the cervix was treated with maximum exposure times of 200 seconds. Animals were killed at intervals from 24 hours to 14 weeks after treatment.

The results are summarized in Table 8.2. From 28 days post-treatment macroscopically the horn was either completely absent except for a thin fibrous strand (Fig. 8.5) or present and distorted by adhesions. In the intact horns endometrial regeneration had occurred but with reduced numbers of glands and abnormal regrowth of villi (Fig. 8.6). There were areas of fibrosis within the myometrium. Histology performed at 2 months post-treatment showed intermittent fibrous occlusion of the uterine cavity and areas completely denuded of glands.

The technique was safe, with other pelvic

Table 8.1 Single lesions produced using a power of 1–3 W. All specimens were examined 6–8 days after laser treatment.

Power (W)	Exposure time (seconds)	Number of lesions	Result
1	50	13	Little effect
	100	9	Little effect
2	50	10	Little effect; few lesions symmetrical
	100	36	Symmetrical lesions
3	50	14	Asymmetrical lesions
	100	7	Asymmetrical lesions

Table 8.2 Results of the horns treated with overlapping lesions. The upper end of each ligated horn was tied off with sutures and only the endometrium below this treated

Survival (days)	Uterine horns	Macroscopic appearance	Microscopic appearance
4–8	Non-ligated: 4 Ligated: 4	Haemorrhagic	Full thickness lesions except upper 5 mm and cervix
14–21	Non-ligated:1 Ligated: 10	Normal Thinned, necrotic and haemorrhagic	Intact endometrium Incomplete surface epithelium. Few villi and glands
28–34	Non-ligated: 5 Ligated: 2	Horn absent (1) Distorted (4) Distorted	Intact surface epithelium Few villi and glands
63–98	Non-ligated: 5 Ligated: 4	Horn absent (4) Normal (1) Horn absent	Intact surface epithelium. Few glands and villi

organs suffering no thermal damage. Animals remained well, even when an entire uterine horn was destroyed and replaced by a fibrous strand. At post-mortem in this group there was no evidence of peritonitis, bowel or bladder damage and adhesion formation was minimal. These animals were possibly able to reabsorb the necrotic uterine tissue over many weeks and this process appeared to be well tolerated. The absence of a horn was first noted at 32 days post-treatment. A similar phenomenon was described when canine bladder was completely destroyed at temperatures ranging from 59 to 69°C and replaced by a fibrous nodule (Linke et al 1972).

This study confirms that the endometrium regenerates if any undamaged epithelial cells or glands remain intact. In both menstruating women and rabbit endometrium subjected to mechanical or chemical trauma, the regrowth of the surface epithelium is derived from the proliferation of two areas: the exposed ends of basal glands and the persistent and intact lining of cornual and cervical regions bordering the denuded areas. This growth is initiated in response to tissue loss and is not hormonally dependent (Ferenczy 1976). Even when there is extensive endometrial and myometrial damage, for instance after cryosurgery, the epithelial surface has regenerated within 7–10 days and after a month the endometrium and its components appear the same as an untreated horn except for patches of fibrosis within the myometrium (Schenker & Polishuk 1972).

These results show that in this animal model if there is inadequate endometrial destruction glandular regrowth occurs. However, because of the extremely thin nature of rabbit myometrium

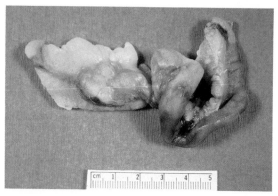

Fig. 8.5 At 32 days the rabbit uterine horn which was treated with overlapping lesions has been replaced by a fibrous strand. The untreated left horn has a normal appearance.

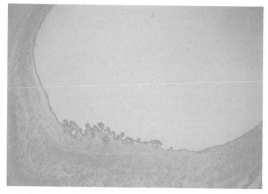

Fig. 8.6 Histological section of a uterine horn treated with overlapping lesions 30 days after treatment. There is abnormal regrowth of villi but re-epithelialisation of the endometrial surface is complete. (Haematoxylin & Eosin, magnification ×8.)

(approximately 1–3 mm) the depth of destruction needed was a fine balance between either too much, causing entire horn loss, or too little, leaving undamaged areas which subsequently regenerated to replace all endometrial components.

Rabbit endometrium was successfully destroyed using this low-power method, and with a suitably designed fibre tip similar biological effects should be produced in the human uterus. The aim of this work was to assess the suitability of using a similar method to treat menorrhagia. Our proposed technique would be to place a suitable fibre tip (diameter 3 mm) into the uterine cavity without cervical dilatation under ultrasound control. Three to four sites would be treated within the uterus to produce large diffuse endometrial lesions at temperatures around 60°C. This procedure could potentially be repeated at intervals until the menopause occurred. If treatment failed it would not affect a subsequent hysterectomy, which remains the treatment for intractable menorrhagia. This low-power technique is shown to be effective, simple and safe and early clinical studies have begun.

PHOTODYNAMIC THERAPY

Photodynamic therapy involves the pretreatment of target tissues with photosensitizing agents which enable light within the visible or infrared region up to about 1000 nm to produce a severe cytotoxic effect. It has been observed that certain tissues, particularly tumours, selectively retain the photosensitizer while adjacent tissue areas contain very little, although this selectivity has often been overemphasized (Bown 1990). Light at a specific wavelength corresponding to an absorption peak of the photosensitizer is then used to activate this drug to produce local necrosis in the required area and leave adjacent tissue undamaged. Laser light is not an absolute requirement for photodynamic therapy but is just a convenient way of producing high-intensity light at exactly the right wavelength. At present, the most suitable laser sources are argon pumped-dye lasers or copper vapour pumped-dye, as the wavelength of the output beam can be tuned to match the absorption peak of the photosensitizer being used.

In tissue the photosensitizer is activated by absorbing light of an appropriate wavelength (Fig.8.7). The activated photosensitizer molecules can react with tissue oxygen to produce singlet oxygen, which is thought to be the cytotoxic agent (Dougherty et al 1983). This is a threshold effect and a certain quantity of singlet oxygen must be produced before a cell is killed. The photosensitizer molecules then return to the ground state and can be activated, again. Activated molecules can also either fluoresce (emit light), returning directly to the ground state, or they can be destroyed by the same activating light (photodegradation). This means that the total quantity of photosensitizer in a tissue is steadily reduced as the tissue is exposed to light.

The use of newer photosensitizers has several advantages over the haematoporphyrin derivatives on which most photodynamic therapy work has been based over the last 10 years, in terms of chemical purity and stability, and some like the phthalocyanines have their major absorption peak in the red part of the spectrum where there is better tissue penetration.

The authors have studied the distribution of two photosensitizers within the endometrium to explore the possibility that photodynamic therapy might be a potentially highly selective and safe treatment for menorrhagia. In rat bladder, highly selective mucosal destruction can be achieved without damage to the underlying musculature or loss of bladder function by

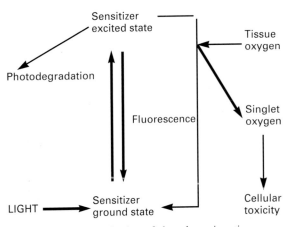

Fig. 8.7 Outline mechanism of photodynamic action.

manipulating the concentration of the photosensitizer and the timing of treatment after sensitization (Pope & Bown 1991). In many cases, like the bladder, there seems to be more selectivity between different normal tissue layers than between a tumour and the normal tissue from which the tumour arose.

In the human uterus, the thick myometrium would allow for adequate endometrial destruction with a large safety margin even if there was some damage to muscle. Adequate tissue penetration is required for complete endometrial destruction and the newer sensitizers have their major absorption bands at longer wavelengths (in the red and near-infrared region of the spectrum) which can produce a maximum depth of necrosis of approximately 5 mm.

Experimental work with photodynamic therapy

The distributions of aluminium disulphonated phthalocyanine (A1S$_2$Pc) and aminolaevulinic acid (ALA) were studied in the rabbit uterus. A1S$_2$Pc is a photosensitizer, whereas ALA is a natural precursor of haem, and in the presence of excess ALA there is an accumulation of protoporphyrin IX (PpIX), a natural photosensitizer and the last intermediate product before haem. Normal rabbits were given either an intravenous dose of ALA or A1S$_2$Pc and then killed at intervals between 30 minutes and 1 week. The uterus was removed at these times and the distribution of PpIX and A1S$_2$Pc studied using quantitative fluorescence microscopy with a charge-coupled device imaging system. This technique produces high-quality colour images which can be digitally analysed to determine relative photosensitizer fluorescence intensities in various parts of the tissue sections (Fig. 8.8) (Barr et al 1988, Pope et al 1991).

The fluorescence levels in the endometrium, stroma and myometrium were individually assessed at each time interval. The endometrium showed a peak fluorescence at 2 and 3 hours with ALA and A1S$_2$Pc, respectively. The stroma and myometrium had fluorescence levels little more than background levels. By 24 hours for ALA and 48 hours for A1S$_2$Pc all uterine layers had

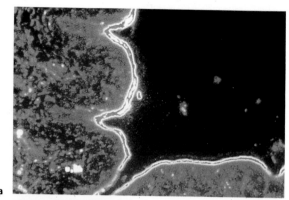

a

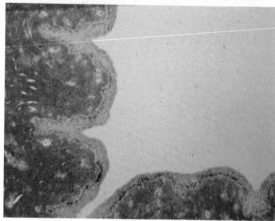

b

Fig. 8.8 **a** Stained section using Van Gieson's technique corresponding to part b showing normal rat uterus (magnification ×60). **b** Fluorescence image 2 hours after sensitization with ALA taken with the charge-coupled device camera from the same section area as part a. This shows high fluorescence in the endometrium with little more than background levels of fluorescence within the stroma and myometrium. The upper colour bar scale indicates fluorescence intensity. (final magnification ×60.)

only background levels of fluorescence. When using ALA and A1S$_2$Pc the endometrium showed fluorescence levels five times higher and 3–4 times higher, respectively, than the stroma and myometrium.

The authors have since applied these parameters to an animal model and produced reliable necrosis of the endometrium without significant myometrial damage and are presently studying the long-term effects on endometrial regeneration. Should this be an effective means of preventing endometrial regrowth, this technique might prove to be a highly selective treatment for women suffering from menorrhagia.

THE FUTURE

For women whose menorrhagia remains resistant to medical treatment, a surgical procedure is often the only option. Methods of local endometrial destruction are now widely used and allow women to be treated and return home usually within 24 hours. However, these techniques are not without their own risk and the aim is to develop techniques with minimal morbidity which could potentially be easily repeatable and performed on an out-patient basis, e.g. a low-power laser hyperthermia technique or photodynamic therapy.

The use of new photosensitizers for photodynamic therapy has the potential to produce extremely accurate endometrial and glandular destruction without the prolonged cutaneous photosensitivity of the haematoporphyrin derivatives. This is because they are either cleared more rapidly from the skin (like ALA), or have a localized absorption peak at a longer wavelength than the porphyrins, away from the main wavelengths in sunlight and thus produce less of a skin reaction (like the phthalocyanines) (Tralau et al 1989).

Adenomyosis is not improved by local endometrial techniques and it is exciting to consider that by manipulating photosensitizer concentrations and pretreatment intervals that glandular destruction could be maximized. From our early studies on the distribution of sensitizers, the myometrium appears to have negligible uptake while glands even when isolated from the main endometrial components show high fluorescence levels and thus a high uptake of photosensitizer. However, much careful research will be required before it is clear what role photodynamic therapy may have to play in treating diseases of the uterus.

REFERENCES

Baumann R, Magos A L, Kay J D, Turnbull A 1990 Absorption of glycine irrigating solution during transcervical resection of endometrium. British Medical Journal 300: 304–305

Barr H, Tralau C J, MacRobert A J, Morrison I, Phillips D, Bown S G 1988 Fluorescence photometric techniques for determination of microscopic tissue distribution of phthalocyanine photosensitizers for photodynamic therapy. Lasers in Medical Science 3: 81–86

Bown S G 1990 Photodynamic therapy to scientists and clinicians — one world or two? Journal of Photochemistry and Photobiology 6: 1–12

Dougherty T J, Boyle D G, Weishaupt K R et al. Photoradiation therapy — clinical and drug advances. In: Porphyrin Photosensitization, ed Kessel D and Dougherty T J 1983 pp 3–13. New York: Plenum Press.

Ferenczy A. Studies on the cytodynamics of human endometrial regeneration. I. Scanning electron microscopy. America Journal of Obstetrics and Gynecology 124: 64–74

Gannon M J, Holt E M, Fairbank J et al 1991 A randomised trial comparing endometrial resection and abdominal hysterectomy for the treatment of menorrhagia. British Medical Journal 303: 1362–1364

Goldrath M H 1983 Uterine tamponade for the control of acute uterine bleeding. American Journal of Obstetrics and Gynecology 147: 869–872

Goldrath M H, Fuller T A, Segal S 1981 Laser photovaporization of endometrium for the treatment of menorrhagia. American Journal of Obstetrics and Gynecology 140: 14–19

Hallberg L, Hoedahh A, Nilsson L, Rybo G 1966 Menstrual blood loss — a population study. Acta Obstetrica et Gynecologica Scandinavica 45: 320–351

Hand J W, Ter-Haar G 1981 Heating techniques in hyperthermia. British Journal of Radiology 54: 443–446

Jacobs A, Butler E B 1965 Menstrual blood loss in iron deficiency anaemia. Lancet ii: 407–409

Irwin A 1991 New gynaecology technique "risky". Pulse July: 23

Judd M D, Hill P D, Potter L A, Bown S G, McColl I 1991 Destruction of the rabbit endometrium using a low-powered neodymium–YAG laser. Lasers in Medical Science 6: 133–140

King A J, Williams D I, Nicol C S 1943 Hyperthermia in the treatment of resistant gonococcal and non specific urethritis. British Journal of Veneral Diseases 19: 141–154

Linke C, Elbadawi A, Netto V et al 1972. Effect of marked hyperthermia upon the canine bladder. Journal of Urology 107: 599–602

Loffer F D 1987 Hysteroscopic endometrial ablation with the Nd–YAG laser using a non-touch technique. Obstetrics and Gynecology 69: 679–682

Lomano J M 1986 Photocoagulation of the endometrium with the Nd–YAG laser for the treatment of menorrhagia. Reproductive Medicine 31: 148–50

Macdonald R M 1944 Toxic hepatitis in fever therapy. Canadian Medical Association Journal 51: 445–449

Magos A L, Baumann R, Turnbull A C 1989 Transcervical resection of endometrium in women with menorrhagia. British Medical Journal 298: 1209–1212

Masters A, Bown S G 1990 Interstitial laser hyperthermia in the treatment of tumours. Lasers in Medical Science 5: 129–135

Matthewson K, Coleridge-Smith P, O'Sullivan J P, Northfield T C, Bown S G 1987 Biological effects of intrahepatic Nd:YAG photocoagulation in rats. Gastroenterology 93: 550–557

Matthewson K, Barton T, Lewin M R, O'Sullivan J P, Northfield T C, Bown S G 1988 Low power interstitial Nd–YAG laser photocoagulation in normal and neoplastic rat colon. Gut 29: 27–34

Matthewson K, Barr H, Traulau C, Bown S G 1989 Low power interstitial Nd–YAG laser photocoagulation: studies in a transplanted fibrosarcoma. British Journal of Surgery 76: 378–381

Morrison L M M, Davis J, Sumner D 1989 Absorption of irrigating fluid during laser photocoagulation of the endometrium in the treatment of menorrhagia. British Journal of Obstetrics and Gynaecology 96: 346–352

Neuwirth R S, Amin H K 1976 Excision of submucous fibroids with hysteroscopic control. American Journal of Obstetrics and Gynecology 126: 95–97

Phipps J H, Lewis B V, Roberts T, Prior M V, Hand J W, Elder M, Field S B 1990 Treatment of functional menorrhagia by radiofrequency-induced thermal endometrial ablation. Lancet 335: 374–376

Pittroff R, Darwish D H, Shabib G 1991 Near fatal uterine perforation during transcervical endometrial resection. Lancet 338: 197–198

Pope A J, Bown S G 1991 Photodynamic therapy. British Journal of Urology 68: 1–9

Pope A J, MacRobert A J, Phillips D, Bown S G 1991 The detection of phthalocyanine fluorescence in normal rat bladder wall using sensitive digital imaging microscopy. British Journal of Cancer 64: 875–879

Schenker J G, Polishuk W Z 1972 Regeneration of rabbit endometrium after cryosurgery. Obstetrics and Gynecology 40: 638–645

Steger A C, Matthewson K, Bown S G, Clark C G 1987a Interstitial hyperthermia: a new technique for intrahepatic neoplasms. Gut 28: A1350

Steger A C, Barr H, Hawes R, Bown S G, Clark C G 1987b Experimental studies on interstitial hyperthermia for treating pancreatic cancer. Gut 28: A1382

Steger A C, Lees W R, Walmsley K, Bown S G 1989 Interstitial laser hyperthermia: a new approach to local destruction of tumours. British Medical Journal 299: 362–365

Sturdee D, Hoggart B 1991 Problems with endometrial resection. Lancet 337: 1474

Tralau C J, Young A R, Walker N P J et al 1989 Mouse skin photosensitivity with dihaematoporphyrin ether (DHE) and aluminium sulphonated phthalocyanine (ALSPc): a comparative study. Photochemistry and Photobiology 49: 305–312

West J H, Robinson D A 1989 Endometrial resection and fluid absorption. Lancet ii: 1387–1388

9. Endometrial resection

C. J. G. Sutton   R. Macdonald   A. L. Magos   J. A. M. Broadbent

PART 1
INSTRUMENTATION
C. J. G. Sutton   R. Macdonald

RESECTOSCOPES

History

It is really quite extraordinary that it took gynae-cologists so long to adapt the technique of trans-urethral resection of the prostate to transcervical resection of the endometrium. Many of us have been working in adjacent operating theatres to our urological colleagues and have watched the operation that is surely destined to be performed by many of us with a sort of detached fascination but few of us had the foresight and perspicacity to translate the modus operandi to endoscopic removal of the endometrium.

It is difficult to find out who first invented the resectoscope. In 1885 the aptly christened Hurry Fenwick designed a 'galvanic ecraseur', in essence a wire snare heated white hot, to cut through the projecting parts of the middle lobe of the prostate, thereby reducing the time and the morbidity of the open operation (Fenwick 1895). In New York, Stevens and Bugbee (1913), and, in France, Luys (1913), used the early operating cystoscopes and rudimentary spark gap diathermy machines to produce a channel through the obstructing bladder neck — a technique called 'foraging' which was often carried out under local anaes-thesia. Loop and punch instruments were available in the 1930s and gradually the mere formation of a 'forage' was extended to removal of the adenoma down to the surgical capsule. By the end of the

Second World War the transurethral technique had become the standard procedure for removal of the benign prostate in the leading urological clinics in North America (Blandy 1978).

It took almost 40 years for the technique to be transposed to gynaecology and the credit for the concept of endometrial ablation by laser must go to Milton Goldrath and his team from Detroit (Goldrath et al 1981). The first reported use of the electrodiathermy resectoscope was by Robert Neuwirth, who used it to remove symptomatic submucous fibroids (Neuwirth 1978), and later DeCherney used it for endometrial ablation in a series of patients with intractable bleeding who, for a variety of reasons, were unsuitable for major surgery (DeCherney & Polan 1983).

The hysteroscope

To perform endometrial resection a rigid hystero-scope is used with a Hopkins rod lens system and a fibreoptic or liquid cable to transmit light from an external power source. For the amazing view afforded by the modern hysteroscope, an enor-mous debt is owed to the inventor of this light transmission system, Professor Harold H. Hopkins FRS of the University of Reading. The telescope, which is 3–4 mm in diameter, provides a 0–30° angle of view and is enclosed in a sheath 4–5 mm in diameter which is encircled by a stopcock at the proximal end. Some resectoscopes have a locking system that is inconveniently placed so that whilst rotating the resectoscope the sheath works itself loose from the resectoscope, resulting in an irritating escape of irrigating fluid — usually over the surgeon. Other resectoscopes utilize a 'snap-in, snap-out' connecting mechanism that eliminates rotary locking. The angle of vision varies widely with the different manufacturers. Generally speaking, an acute angle of vision has been adopted for diagnostic hysteroscopy, the better to see the cornual areas and lateral uterine walls. Resectoscopes run the whole gamut of angles of view from 0° (Olympus and Storz), 12° (Circon ACMI), 25° (Wolf) and 30° (Storz and Circon ACMI). The choice is a matter of individual preference, and before choosing a resectoscope it behoves a surgeon to try the different angles of vision and opt for the one that feels most comfortable.

The resectoscope

The hysteroscopic resectoscope in common use utilizes a continuous-flow outer sheath to allow optimum visibility; the key to any operative hysteroscopy procedure. Low-viscosity fluid, usually sorbitol or glycine, is circulated under rapid flow to rinse the uterus of blood and tissue debris that would otherwise obscure the operator's vision. It is absolutely imperative that isolated inflow and outflow channels run the whole length of the resectoscope so that the irrigant flows around the front of the telescope to maintain clear vision at all times (Fig. 9.1). Instruments have been seen where the two ports are opposite each other, and even when the hysteroscope is inserted the line of least resistance is followed and most of the fluid exits the system the moment after entering it, a system which is absolutely useless for the type of procedures considered here.

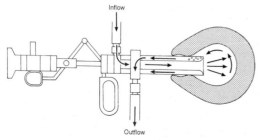

Fig. 9.1 Irrigant flow through the resectoscope and within the uterine cavity. The resectoscope has isolated inflow and outflow channels throughout its length. Clear inflow fluid therefore does not mix with blood and tissue debris. Drainage perforations situated outside the visual field on the outer sheath of the resectoscope.

The position of the outflow ports are extremely important. When the outflow holes are provided only on one surface, as with the Storz and Wolf models, the surgeon has to keep rotating the resectoscope, especially when working on the anterior wall, to keep the field of view clear of bubbles. Both Olympus and Circon ACMI make sheaths with outflow ports that encircle the sheath on the top and bottom surfaces, respectively. This design allows the bubbles that inevitably form during the procedure to be automatically removed and to rise to the top of the uterine cavity, making it unnecessary to have to perform shaking movements of the end of the resectoscope to clear bubbles from the operator's view (Brooks 1990).

The working lengths of the instruments vary from 18 to 35 cm and the outer sheath diameter varies from 6.3 mm (19 French (Fr)) to 9 mm (27 Fr). The metallic components are made from surgical-grade stainless steel and the insulation, when used, is usually Teflon. All available resectoscopes can be soaked in sterilizing solutions, and those made by Olympus and Wolf can also be autoclaved. This may be an important factor for nursing colleagues, who are becoming increasingly concerned by the occupational health hazards associated with sterilizing solutions. The similarities and differences of the commonly available resectoscopes are listed in Table 9.1 and illustrated in Figures 9.2–9.6.

Cutting loops

In order to determine the optimal diameter of the cutting loop it is necessary to obtain a compromise between effectiveness and safety. There can be little doubt that the 24 Fr cutting loop is the safest to use. There is less risk of perforation and, by limiting the depth of tissue excision, the large vessels deeper in the myometrium tend to be spared and profuse haemorrhage obscuring vision is unusual. Unfortunately, technology has not advanced sufficiently for loops of this diameter to achieve sufficient strength, and wire fracture is a frequent and irritating problem. The larger loop, borrowed directly from urologists, is extremely strong but the depth of tissue destruction achieved if the loop is allowed to sink to its

Table 9.1 Comparison of commonly avalable resectoscopes

Manufacturer	Agent in UK	Model	Outer sheath diameter	Working length	Angle of vision	Continuous flow	Position of outflow holes at distal end of outflow sheath	Auto-clavable	Types of electrodes available	Price (set)	Other options
Olympus	Keymed	A4000–A4002 A4003–A4008	8 mm (24 Fr)	19 cm	0°	Yes	Circumferential	Yes	Roller bar Cutting loop Angled cutting loop	£3000	Total video capability and OTV–S2 camera
Olympus	Keymed	A2011A–A2012A A2129–A2130 A2754 A2203 A2183 A2129 A219	9 mm (27 Fr)	19 cm	12° or 30°	Yes	Top and bottom	Yes	Roller Bar Cutting loop Angled cutting loop	£3000	Total video capability and OTV–S2 camera
Storz	Rimmer Bros	27040 SL	8.66 mm (26 Fr)	19.5 cm	30°	Yes	Top	No	Rollerball and bar Knife electrode Cutting loop or wire	£2412	Optical biopsy forceps, injection canula, video capability, extra electrodes and Schmidt insert tube
Richard Wolf	Wolf	8654.433	9 mm (27 Fr)	19 cm	25°	Yes	Top	Yes	Rollerball Forward cutting loop knife, 90° wire (hook) button	£2614	Video capability
Circon ACMI	Cory Bros	GYI-525	8.33 mm 25 (Fr) 9 mm	18 cm	12° or 30°	Yes	Top and bottom	No	Roller bar/ball Various cutting loops	£4422	Bridge to convert continuous-flow resectoscope sheath to operating hysteroscope
Circon ACMI	Cory Bros	GYI-527	9 mm 27 (Fr)	18 cm	12° or 30°	Yes	Top and bottom	No	Roller bar/ball Various cutting loops	£4422	Bridge to convert continuous-flow resectoscope sheath to operating hysteroscope

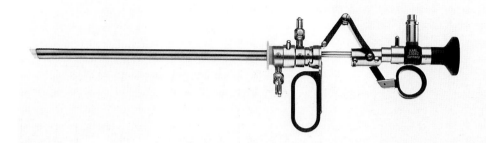

Fig. 9.2 Storz 27 Fr resectoscope based on a similar design to the urological transurethral resectoscope.

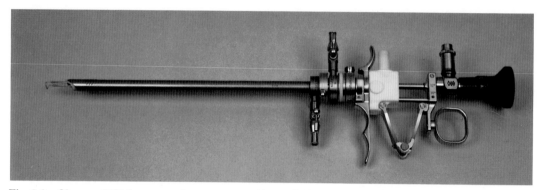

Fig. 9.3 Olympus 25 Fr hysteroscopic resectoscope. Also available in 27 Fr gauge.

full extent can cause serious problems, particularly in the hands of the inexperienced resectoscopist.

The ideal compromise at the moment would appear to be a 24 Fr loop, which is sufficiently

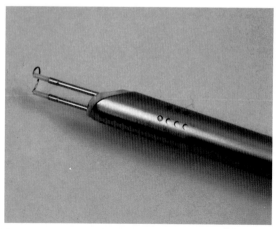

Fig. 9.4 Close up of Figure 9.3. Note the outflow holes encircling the tip to allow easier removal of bubbles.

strong and yet safe, because it excises tissue strips which are of sufficient depth to be effective. The authors have used a loop of this size in one of their hospitals for the past 1.5 years without any perforations and only one patient sustaining haemorrhage sufficient to require balloon tamponade and an overnight stay in hospital. The results have been identical to those the authors have achieved with the large loop (87% success rate), but with this size of loop the authors have had two perforations and seven cases of heavy bleeding, one of them so heavy that an emergency hysterectomy had to be performed.

In addition to the size, attention should also be paid to the configuration of the loop. As stated previously, most manufacturers of resectoscopes have directly translated the design of urological equipment to gynaecology with little consideration for the different requirements of the procedure. A circular loop configuration inevitably leaves ridges between adjacent cuts and requires the operator to make a second pass to obliterate

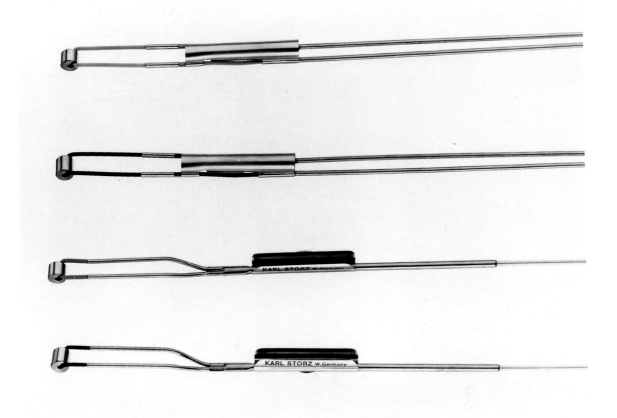

Fig. 9.5 Series of roller bars for Storz resectoscope.

these ridges. This is of no real consequence in transurethral resection of the prostate because multiple cuts are required to remove all the prostatic tissue but the need to make repeated furrows in transcervical resection of the endometrium invites the inexperienced operator to go dangerously deep, resulting in perforation or profuse haemorrhage. On the other hand, failure to remove the ridges leaves the bases of the endometrial glands in situ, inviting regrowth of the endometrium, resulting in a poor clinical outcome.

A square (or almost square) loop configuration allows the furrows to approximate more closely the ideal geometrical shape needed for complete endometrial ablation. Such a loop has been devised by the Olympus Corporation, but is not in commercial production at the time of writing.

Undoubtedly, the hardest part of an endometrial resection is the complete removal of endometrial tissue from the cornual area around the ostia of the fallopian tubes. This is the thinnest part of the uterus and requires great caution to avoid perforation, but access is difficult and it can be hard to ensure complete removal of the endometrium. Recurrent bleeding from active endometrium in this area can result in the formation of a haematometra presenting as cyclical pain without external bleeding because the myometrium has often scarred over distally, preventing the egress of menstrual blood. The one great advantage of the neodymium:yttrium aluminium garnet (Nd:YAG) laser is its superior effectiveness and access in this area, but regrettably it is extremely tedious and time-consuming when used on the four walls.

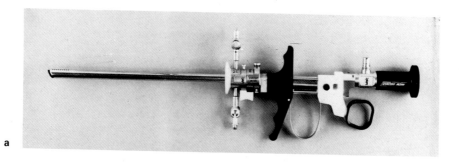

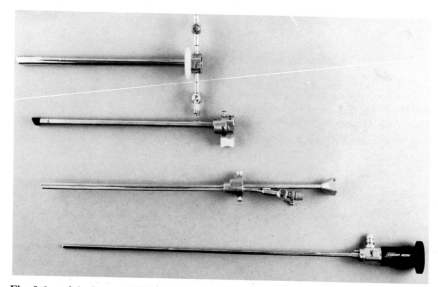

Fig. 9.6 a & b Circon ACMI combined resectoscope with channel for laser fibre or biopsy forceps. Note the all-round outflow ports for bubble-free vision and the 'snap-on' connecting mechanism that avoids unlocking during operative manouevres.

The rollerball held initial promise but owing to difficulties in keeping the ball moving in this confined space it is easy to produce an area of thermal necrosis which undergoes coagulative liquefaction and then 'blows out' due to the hydrostatic pressure inside the uterus. If one is using the resectoscope it is probably best to use a loop slanting 45° forwards and to start the procedure by resecting the cornual endometrium, paying careful attention to the depth of penetration, which may only be 4 mm at this point, then join the two ostia by a series of furrows in the fundus before changing to a 90° loop to complete the resection of the side walls.

The rollerball or bar (Fig. 9.5) is extremely useful to stem the flow of blood from some of the severed vessels at the end of the procedure, especially when used in conjunction with spray diathermy. The rollerball provides a large contact area (approximately 4 mm^2), which allows the spread of electric energy over a large area. It is therefore almost impossible to obtain sufficient power density to actually cut through the uterine wall (Vancaille 1989), but it is vital to keep the ball moving otherwise the extensive tissue destruction results in weakness of the myometrium which can then give way under the pressure of the irrigating fluid.

A drawback to the rollerball as a primary method of tissue destruction is that, like the laser, it does not provide a specimen for histology and therefore requires a preceding diagnostic dilatation and curettage, and hysteroscopy. In addition, many of the papers describing rollerball treatment have used adjunctive therapy in the form of depot preparations of medroxy-progesterone acetate, which will produce oligo- or amenorrhoea in up to 50% of patients, and since this can take as long as 2 years to clear from the system the results are bound to be biased (Townsend et al 1990).

Instrument manufacturers

Before choosing an instrument, advice should be obtained from colleagues who have a long experience in this technique. Any complaints about poor service and the length of time taken to carry out repairs by the supplier should be noted. Some manufacturers do not seem to be prepared to provide an acceptable back-up service and recently there has been a growing practice of being unable or unwilling to loan an instrument whilst repairs are taking place. To avoid problems make sure that the supplier has an efficient and reliable representative in the area who visits the hospital frequently and gets to know you and your operating department personnel.

Inevitably, several different instruments will be tried before a large amount of money is invested in new equipment. Newcomers to this technique should rely on the advice of the more experienced and never attempt the procedure on a patient before having performed several tens of diagnostic hysteroscopies and had some live 'hands on' training with an experienced resectoscopist. Different instruments can be tried out on a hysterectomy specimen, or the instruments used without electrodiathermy on patients who are having diagnostic hysteroscopies. Surgeons must, however, resist the temptation to try instruments on patients unless they are confident of their ability with the technique of transcervical resection of the endometrium.

ELECTROSURGICAL INSTRUMENTATION

The tissue effects involved in both endometrial resection and rollerball ablation are induced by electricity. Radio frequency current is required and to generate this a standard high-frequency diathermy unit is entirely sufficient. Such units are readily available in most operating theatres and are routinely employed whenever diathermy is required during laparotomy or for transurethral resection of the prostate.

It is, however, important to realize that the ultimate tissue effect of this type of electrical energy is mediated through the production of localized heat (Pearce et al 1983). This is also the mode of action of both Nd:YAG laser- and radio frequency-induced endometrial ablation. Similar thermodestruction principles therefore apply. Focused tissue heating to high temperature (100–1000°C) leads to mechanical injury and produces an incision through complete tissue destruction by cell vaporization and localized combustion; less focused heating to lower temperatures (45–100°C) has a coagulative effect due to dessication and protein denaturation. When using electrosurgical instrumentation the former effect is best achieved with the pure cut mode and the latter with the coagulation mode.

Tissue heating is therefore fundamental and its extent is a function of current density and the time for which the electrical energy is applied. Tissue conductivity, density, specific heat and initial temperature are also important and the relative contribution of each of these factors is summarized in the following modification of the bioheat equation (Pearce et al 1986):

$$T = \frac{1}{\sigma \rho c} \times J^2 t$$

where T is the final tissue temperature (K), σ is the electrical conductivity (S/m), ρ is the tissue density (kg/m^3), c is the tissue specific heat (J/kg.K), J is the magnitude of the current density (Am^2) applied, t is the duration of activation (seconds) and T_0 is the initial temperature (K).

Precise and predictable tissue effects can be achieved with appropriate manipulation of current density. This is mainly done by varying either the waveform and power output from the electrosurgical unit or by altering the electrode size. These mechanisms will be discussed in more detail later in the chapter.

The development of diathermy

Strictly speaking, the term 'diathermy', which was introduced by Nagelschmidt in 1907 (Greek: 'dia', through; 'therme', heat), should be confined to the use of short-wave diathermy (10–100 MHz) for physiotherapy, the aim being to promote healing of soft tissue injury through heating of the deep tissues by induction, which causes vasodilatation and increased metabolic rate. Surgical diathermy is therefore a misnomer as it is the alternating current and not heat which passes through the patient. Electrosurgery is a more apt term as electrically induced tissue heating is confined to a localized area of high current density around the active electrode.

Cushing and Bovie (1928) are usually credited with popularizing electrosurgery. Diode or valve circuits became available in the 1920s and enabled generators with rectified waveform outputs to be manufactured. These units made localized tissue cutting possible. Previously available spark gap generators did have a tissue cutting capability and were successfully employed by Doyen in France (1909) and Clark in the USA (1911) to remove skin blemishes. Both power and waveform controls were poor and cutting was imprecise. Spark gap generators, however, gave good tissue coagulation and for many years this type of circuit was employed whenever coagulation was required. More accurate tissue cutting and the facility to rapidly change from the cut to the coagulation mode, or to an intermediate blend, however, required better waveform control and had to wait for the innovation of transistors and solid state circuits.

Modern electrosurgical generators

Modern electrosurgical generators are sophisticated devices which employ integrated 'micro-chip' circuitry to synthesize output (Fig. 9.7). The basic frequency, of 475–750 kHz is generated in a primary oscillator circuit. When the cut mode is required this reference signal is simply amplified to produce a continuous output. When coagulation or blend modes are required the reference signal is modulated through an electronic gate by a burst oscillator, and an interrupted waveform is produced. The frequency of

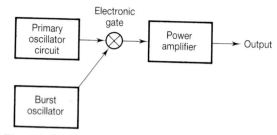

Fig. 9.7 Basic components of s solid state electrosurgical unit. The basic frequency, generated in the primary oscillator circuit, is either relayed directly to the amplification stage to produce a pure cut output or modified through an electronic gate by a burst oscillator to produce a coagulation or bleed output.

this secondary pulse output is usually within the range of 22–33 kHz. Unlike spark gap and valve generators, solid state devices have separate waveform synthesis and power amplification stages. Complex waveform synthesis, therefore, takes place in a low-power circuit before this pulsed signal is amplified to meet output requirement.

The Valleylab Force 2 and Eschmann 411-RS generators are shown in Figure 9.8 and are illustrative of the most recent products from these manufacturers. They offer certain theoretical advantages, particularly with respect to speed and cleanness of cut, but previous models from these and other manufacturers are entirely suitable for endometrial resection or rollerball coagulation. The basic output requirements are pure cut, coagulation and intermediate blend modes with the facility to alter power. Top-range generators give the surgeon a wide and daunting choice. Some units provide two cut modes, high-voltage and low-voltage coagulation (fulguration and dessication, respectively), and up to three blend modes. Although there are theoretical differences between these extra output options, a great deal of experimental work is required to establish how much tissue effects are influenced.

The power supply for the above units in the UK is simply from a 240 V 50 Hz mains socket and the basic output frequency is 475–750 kHz with maximum peak-to-peak voltage and output power of 3800–7000 V and 300–400 W, respectively.

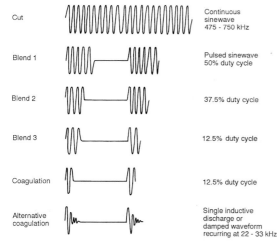

Fig. 9.11 Output waveforms (x axis, time; y axis, voltage). The duty cycle is expressed as a percentage of each secondary pulsed cycle recurring at 22–33 kHz.

a frequency of 22–33 kHz rather than 50–100 Hz. This inductive discharge can be used alone for pure coagulation or in combination with an interrupted sinewave to produce a blended current which will have both cutting and coagulative effects.

Effective cutting requires a continuous train of short-duration, high-current-density discharges. These discharges or sparks are highly localized both in space and time, and by their nature produce intense heat which vaporizes surrounding cells. When the cutting process is underway the electrode–tissue interface is separated by steam. Electrical contact only exists when an arc is established and between arcs the steam barrier acts as an insulator. This is fundamental to the arcing cycle (Fig. 9.12). A magnetic field forms around the cutting electrode. This causes ionization of molecules within the steam and, once a sufficient quantity of ions is present, the barrier, which can no longer function as an insulator, is traversed by a spark. Heat radiating from the spark causes further tissue vaporization and thereby replenishes the steam barrier, which once again will function as an insulator. In theory, a 500 kHz electrosurgical generator can produce arcing 1 million times per second (one arc per half cycle); however, it is likely that only a proportion of half cycles produce an arc (Pearce 1986).

The tissue–electrode gap is therefore both physical and electrical, and failure to maintain this gap will stop the cutting process. For example, the gap will close if the surgeon moves the cutting loop too quickly. This, in fact, is the reason why certain electrosurgical generators seem faster than others; these units can simply maintain the spark gap at a higher electrode speed.

Problems sometimes occur initiating the arcing cycle. Urologists empirically try to speed up this process by activating the electrode prior to tissue contact. The first arc should then occur across a glycine–tissue interface. If the electrode is activated after tissue contact, the cut mode causes dessication and coagulation by resistive heating of surrounding tissue. This dessicated rim of tissue is a poor conductor and therefore will act as an insulative barrier across which arcing can occur. Establishing the arcing cycle in this way is slow and cutting is inefficient, particularly if the spark gap breaks down repeatedly. To get round this problem the more recent Valleylab units have a rapid start or power surge facility: each time the cutting process is initiated there is a transient output surge. Establishment and maintenance of the arcing cycle is therefore more efficient.

A more recent development in electrosurgical waveform is the square wave (Eschmann). The square wave produces a rapid rise to peak voltage and then flattens off to a plateau. Compared with the continuous sinewave, this waveform produces more power at a lower voltage and generates a more controlled and localized spark. Theoretically,

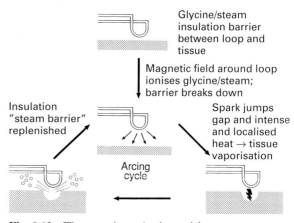

Fig. 9.12 Tissue cutting or 'arcing cycle'.

these technological advances should provide a more precise and predictable tissue cut.

Electrode size

The electrically induced temperature change is proportional to the square of the current density at the active electrode–tissue interface (bioheat equation). Therefore, at a steady output, reducing the electrode size will exponentially increase the current density. Varying the electrode size is analogous to focusing or defocusing a laser beam and a suitably focused current should cut with precision comparable to a laser instrument.

Unfortunately, there are other variables which affect the relationship between the electrode size and current density. At a given power output, the electrode size can only be reduced so much before increasing impedance to current flow causes excessive electrode heating. If the cut mode is applied with an overpowered needle electrode an arc will form, but tissue cutting will be less precise due to the coagulative effect of the hot electrode. Precise cutting can be achieved with small electrodes, but the output must first be appropriately lowered to avoid excessive electrode heating (Hausner 1989).

Hazards and safety

Electrosurgical burns

Irreversible tissue damage will occur whenever the current density is sufficient to raise the tissue temperature to 55°C (Moritz 1947, Pearce 1983). Conduction through tissue within the body is diffuse, and only in exceptional circumstances is current channelling of sufficient density to produce a burn. On the other hand, electrical burns may arise on body surfaces if the area of electrical contact is small enough. There are three potential sites where the current may concentrate and lead to a burn:

1. Under the active electrode
2. Under the dispersive electrode
3. Due to current division where the current returns to the electrosurgical generator via an earth at a site other than under the dispersive electrode.

The first site is of course intended, the latter two are not and many safety features have been introduced to minimize their occurrence.

Return electrode monitor (REM). Poor pad–patient contact leads to current channelling under the dispersive electrodes. If the concentration is sufficient the underlying skin will be exposed to resistive heating. The REM has been developed by Valleylab to ensure adequate pad contact.

The REM pad consists of two functional halves. For the purpose of completing the patient circuit they act as one, but within the pad they are electrically isolated. When connected in series to an interrogation current passing through independent wires in the dispersive electrode cable, a local circuit forms between each half of the pad, which is completed by conduction through the underlying skin. Resistance in this circuit is monitored and if it falls outside a certain range (between 5 and 135 Ω) the electrosurgical unit automatically shuts down. Poor pad–patient contact will increase resistance within the REM circuit and shutdown will occur before significant heating takes place. Alternatively, damage to the dispersive electrode cable may short circuit the REM and lead to low-resistance shutdown.

Circuit sentry. This is a primitive predecessor of the REM system which was developed in the 1970s to prevent current division. Current division is mainly a problem of earthed patient circuits and this is more likely to cause a burn if the dispersive electrode is disconnected. The circuit sentry ensures that this electrode is connected to the electrosurgical unit. As with the REM system, two wires run through the dispersive electrode cable. When the pad is properly attached to the cable these wires form an electrical circuit which inhibits an alarm. If the generator is used when the pad is not connected the alarm goes off. It is important to note that the alarm is still inhibited when a pad with a properly connected cable is not in contact with the patient. This sentry system is unnecessary for earth isolated patient circuits as they will simply not work if the pad is not connected.

Earth-isolated patient circuits. Burns due to current division are now rare owing to the introduction of earth-isolated patient circuits

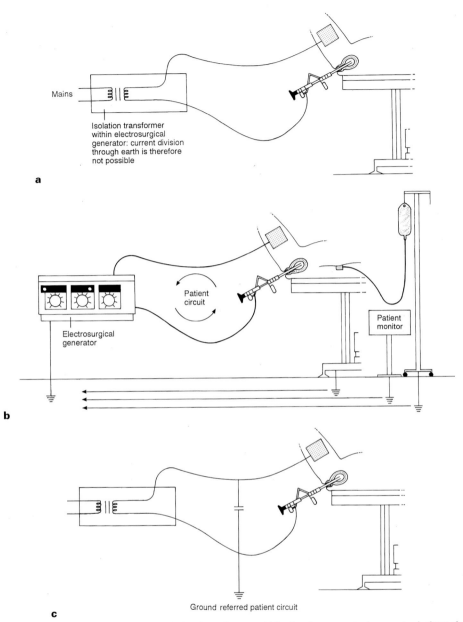

Fig. 9.13 a Earth-isolated patient circuit. An isolation transformer within the electrosurgical generator isolates the patient circuit from earth. **b** Earthed patient circuit. The current may divide in the patient circuit and, instead of the dispersive electrode completing the circuit, the current may return to the electrosurgical generator via any earthed object in electrical contact with the patient. British Standard 5724 (1979) has effectively abolished this type of circuit. **c** Ground-referred patient circuit. The patient circuit is isolated at mains frequencies (50 Hz), but the dispersive electrode is earthed with respect to radio frequency current. As complete isolation of patient circuits is not possible when high-frequency (or radio frequency) current is employed, there is a risk of current division. This risk is minimized if the dispersive electrode circuit within the electrosurgical unit is earthed via a capacitor with low resistance to radio frequency current. This encourages radio frequency current within the patient circuit to flow through the dispersive plate rather than to earth via an alternative pathway.

(Fig. 9.13a). British Standard 5724 (1979) states that patient circuits should be isolated at mains frequencies (50 Hz). If the patient circuit is earthed, current may return to the electrosurgical generator via the dispersive electrode or through any contact point the patient has with earth (Fig.

9.13b). There are many possibilities, earthing may occur through the surgical table, via leg stirrups, a drip stand or any unearthed monitor in electrical contact with the patient. Earthing through an electrocardiograph or other patient monitor is now unlikely because British Standard 5724 (1979) also requires all electrical equipment in the theatre to be earth isolated.

Earth-isolated circuits do not, however, prevent all causes of site burns. Complete isolation is not possible with radio frequency current. As the frequency increases the impedance falls and the possibility for both resistive and capacitative current division increases. A circuit which is isolated at low frequencies therefore may not be isolated at higher frequencies.

To get round this problem a ground-referred balanced output (Fig. 9.13c) has been introduced (Valleylab Force 4, 750 kHz). The patient circuit is earth isolated for mains frequencies (50 Hz), but is ground referred at radio frequencies to minimize the risk of radio frequency current division. The balanced output control mechanism monitors the integrity of the patient circuit and the system will only work if the dispersive plate is connected. Current flow through the output electrode is continually matched with current flow through the dispersive electrode. Any discrepancy, usually due to current division, leads to the immediate automatic shut down of the generator.

ACKNOWLEDGEMENTS

The authors would like to acknowledge gratefully the help given by Sister Diana Miles, Operating Theatre Superintendent, Mount Alvernia Hospital, for checking the details of the currently available resectoscopes.

Technical advice on the electrosurgical section was gratefully received from Michael Brett, IEng, FIEIE, Valley Lab, UK and from Gary Cobb, Eschmann, UK.

REFERENCES

Blandy J P 1978 Transurethral resection, 2nd edn. Pitman Medical, London
Brooks P G 1990 Resectoscopes for the gynaecologist. Contemporary Obstetrics/Gynaecology June: 51–56
Clark W L 1911 Oscillatory destruction in the treatment of accessible growths and minor surgical conditions. Journal of Advanced Therapy 29: 169–183
Cushing H and Bovie W T 1928 Electrosurgery as an aid to removing intracranial tumors. Surgery, Gynecology and Obstetrics 47: 751–784
DeCherney A H, Polan M L 1983 Hysteroscopic management of intrauterine lesion and intractable uterine bleeding. Obstetrics and Gynecology 61: 392–397
Doyen E 1909 Sur la destruction des tumeurs cancereuse accessible. Archives d' Electricité Médicale et de Physiotherapie du Cancer 17: 791–795
Fenwick E H 1895 Urinary surgery, 2nd edn. John Wright, Bristol
Goldrath M H, Fuller T A, Segal S 1981 Laser photovaporization of endometrium for the treatment of menorrhagia. American Journal of Obstetrics and Gynecology 140: 14–19
Hausner K 1989 Electrosurgery — macro vs micro. In: Laser vs electrosurgery, practical considerations for gynaecology. Elmed Incorporated Publications, p 7–9
Luys G 1913 Traitement de l'hypertrophie de la prostate par la voie endoureterale. Clinique 44: 693
Nagelschmidt F 1907 Verhandlungen der Deutschen Naturforschaft für Aer 79: 58
Neuwirth R S 1978 A new technique for and additional experience with hysteroscopic resection of sub-mucous fibroids. American Journal of Obstetrics and Gynecology 131: 91–94
Moritz A R 1947 Studies of thermal injury III. The pathology and pathogenesis of cutaneous burns — an experimental study. American Journal of Pathology 23(6): 915–933
Pearce J A 1986 Electrosurgery. Chapman and Hall, London
Pearce J A, Geddes J, Van Vleet J F et al 1983 Skin burns from electrosurgical electrodes. Medical Instrumentation 17: 225–31
Richard R M, Townsend D E 1989 A new technique for ablating the endometrium. Contemporary Obstetrics/Gynaecology April: 90–94
Stephens A R 1913 Value of cauterisation by high frequency current in certain cases of prostatic obstruction. New York Medical Journal 98: 170
Townsend D E, Richart R M, Paskowitz R A, Woolfork R E 1990 "Rollerball" coagulation of the endometrium. Obstetrics and Gynecology 76: 310–313
Vancaille T 1989 Electrocoagulation of the endometrium with the ball-end resectoscope. Obstetrics and Gynecology 74: 425–427

PART 2
TECHNIQUE
A. L. Magos

As with all forms of surgery, the basic principles of a particular operation are generally accepted, but most surgeons imprint their personality by performing minor variations on a theme. It should not be surprising, therefore, that there is more than one way to perform an endometrial resection. What follows is largely a description of the author's personal technique, which was inspired by Jacques Hamou from Paris, and adapted, altered and developed by experience over the years. The author does not claim that it is the only way to perform endometrial resection, or that it is superior to the technique used by others, but it has proved the best for the author.

PREOPERATIVE ASSESSMENT

Although this has been discussed in Chapter 3, the author would like to emphasize the importance of preoperative assessment by ultrasound, hysteroscopy and endometrial sampling if one is not to come across unexpected pathology from time to time. For instance, the author has operated on patients with a slightly bulky uterus who were found at surgery to have a large submucous fibroid filling the entire uterine cavity, thereby turning what was planned to be a fast and straight forward endometrial resection into a prolonged and complicated hysteroscopic myomectomy. Or patients whose endometrium looked sufficiently abnormal for resection to be abandoned to await the histological assessment of the biopsy which should have been taken before. Forewarned is to be forearmed.

There are several advantages to a thorough preoperative work-up. Ultrasound will provide data about overall uterine size, endometrial thickness, the site and size of fibroids, and any ovarian pathology. Information concerning fibroids and the ovaries are particularly useful as hysteroscopy only allows the examination of the uterine cavity and gives no details about the rest of the pelvis. Hysteroscopy will confirm any uterine cavity abnormalities and allow the procedure to be 'planned'. Finally, endometrial biopsy will show up any premalignant changes which would be contraindications for hysteroscopic surgery.

ENDOMETRIAL PREPARATION

There are two schools of thought with regard to the use of agents to thin the endometrium to facilitate surgery. There are those who see no advantage in subjecting their patients to what are rather noxious drugs in the weeks before resection, and instead prefer to operate on their patients as soon after menstruation as possible when the endometrium is naturally at its thinnest. Logistically this can be difficult in a busy clinical service, and partly for this reason the author prefers to pretreat all his patients and is thus able to operate optimally at any phase of the menstrual cycle. The author uses danazol at a dose of 200 mg 3 times daily for 6 weeks prior to surgery, which has been shown to reduce the endometrial thickness to an average of 1.2 mm compared with untreated average values of 3 mm in the proliferative and 7 mm in the secretory phase of the cycle (Reid & Sharp 1988); other agents such as progestogens and, particularly, gonadotrophin-releasing hormone (GnRH) agonists can also be used (Brooks et al 1991).

The advantage of endometrial preparation for endometrial resection is immediately apparent when one considers the dimensions of the resectoscope loop; a 26 French (Fr) resectoscope is fitted with a 24 Fr diameter cutting loop, which means that it will cut to a depth of approximately 4 mm. Ensuring that the endometrial thickness is less than this value by 1–2 mm means that the basement membrane can be reliably undercut with a single stroke and each area of the cavity does not have to be treated more than once. Surgery is therefore both easier and faster.

There are other benefits to the use of agents such as danazol. The endometrium becomes not only thinner but also less fluffy, so the suction holes on the outer sheath of the resectoscope do not get blocked by endometrial debris. There is also evidence that pretreatment reduces the volume of uterine irrigant that is absorbed during surgery (Magos et al 1991), and perhaps blood loss afterwards.

ANTIBIOTICS

There are several reasons why the author routinely gives a single dose of prophylactic antibiotics prior to surgery, currently metronidazole and cefotaxime. Operating via the vagina means that one is working in a contaminated environment. The uterine irrigant, 1.5% glycine solution in the author's case, while being sterile is not intended for intravenous use, and yet that is exactly what happens during surgery when vessels are transected during resection of the endometrium. There is also spillage of the solution into the peritoneal cavity via the fallopian tubes. The potential for infection therefore seems high, but it must be said that there are many who do not administer antibacterial agents without any apparent risk to their patients. The matter can only be resolved by a large, randomized, placebo-controlled study.

CHOICE OF RESECTOSCOPE

As is evident from Part 1, several sizes and types of resectoscope are available for endometrial resection. Having tried the Hallez-type myoma resectoscope initially, which was considered to be unnecessarily narrow with a flimsy cutting loop, the author prefers to use a standard urological resectoscope fitted with a 26 Fr continuous-flow sheath, 24 Fr cutting loop, passive handle mechanism and a 4 mm 30° telescope (Table 9.2). This combination gives the surgeon just the right depth of cut after endometrial preparation, optimal control over fluid dynamics, and additional safety as the cutting loop rests inside the inflow sheath at rest, thereby minimizing the risk of accidental trauma to the uterus.

Table 9.2 Basic equipment and settings for endometrial resection

1. Resectoscope	26 Fr gauge continuous-flow sheath 24 Fr cutting loop Passive handle mechanism 4 mm 30° fore-oblique telescope

2. Irrigation system	Sterile 1.5% glycine solution
	Hamou Hysteromat set at:
	    100–125 mmHg insufflation pressure
	    –50 mmHg suction pressure
	    300 ml/min maximum flow rate

3. Electrosurgical generator	Valleylab Force 2 set at: 100–125 Watts cutting power Blend 1–3 50 W coagulating power

Whatever the choice of resectoscope, there is no doubt that operating off a high-resolution colour monitor with the help of a small chip video camera attached to the eyepiece is becoming the standard *modus operandi*. The advantages are considerable in terms of operator comfort (just ask any urologist who has been performing endoscopic prostatectomies under direct vision for a number of years if he has any back problems!), particularly with patients with an acutely anteverted uterus in whom the conventional alternative would be to, literally, operate off the floor. Video monitoring is also the best way to teach and supervise juniors under training. As an additional benefit, patients who have not been given a general anaesthetic have the opportunity to follow the resection procedure 'live', something which a surprisingly large proportion of patients in fact do.

ANAESTHESIA

Endometrial resection is potentially not only a day case procedure, but one which can be performed without general anaesthesia using a combination of local anaesthesia, intravenous sedation (or more correctly 'anxiolysis'), and supplementary intravenous analgesia (Magos et al 1989). As will be seen later in the chapter, about two-thirds of women choose to be asleep during surgery, but some prefer to be conscious. The basic principles in using local anaesthetic are two-fold. First of all, the uterine cavity is relatively insensitive to noxious stimuli such as cutting and heating, two of the modalities used in resection, although it is more sensitive to distension. Secondly, what is commonly labelled as 'sedoanalgesia' (sedation with analgesia) has been shown in many other branches of medicine to be a highly effective technique for certain invasive procedures with advantages over general anaesthesia in terms of medical manpower, turn-around time and patient recovery.

The technique itself is relatively straightforward. Patients receive a premedication cocktail of temazepam 20 mg orally and diclofenac 100 mg per rectum (or mefenamic acid 0.5–1 g orally) 1 hour before surgery. In the anaesthetic room (or operating theatre or endoscopy suite), monitoring of the heart rate, electrocardiogram, oxygen saturation and blood pressure is commenced as detailed in Chapter 6. The patients are then given a small intravenous dose of an opiate analgesic such as fentanyl, and 5 minutes later an anxiolytic such as midazolam. The author routinely gives facial oxygen as both agents are potent respiratory depressants.

When comfortable and relaxed, the patients are placed in the lithotomy position and prepared for surgery in the usual manner. Before the cervix is dilated, 10 ml of 1% lignocaine containing 1:200 000 adrenaline is injected into the paracervical nerve plexus (2.5 ml at 3, 5, 7 and 9 o'clock behind the cervix, respectively), and a similar volume into the substance of the cervix (Fig. 9.14). The resectoscope is assembled and connected to the irrigation system, light source, etc., while the anaesthetic takes effect, the only difference being that a narrow injection cannula fitted with a Luer lock is inserted in place of the cutting loop.

After a few minutes the uterus is sounded and the cervix dilated, and the resectoscope is gently steered into the distended uterine cavity. After ensuring that there is no contraindication to surgery, a further 20ml of the lignocaine/adrenaline mixture is injected at 10–15 points into the myometrium to a depth of 1cm, the latter being judged by a burr mark at the distal tip of the cannula. Most of the injections are made around the uterine fundus and cornua as these are the areas which are the least anaesthetized by the paracervical block. Surgery can then continue as under general anaesthesia, additional small doses of fentanyl or midazolam being administered if further analgesia or anxiolysis is required (Fig. 9.15 and 9.16).

Endometrial resection under local anaesthesia usually works well, and most patients feel nothing at all during surgery. There are some women who do find the procedure uncomfortable, and in these cases relatively large doses of fentanyl are ultimately given. It is extremely rare, however, to have to convert to general anaesthesia. As described in the next section, the author now routinely offers his patients this choice of anaesthesia and about one-third choose to avoid being put to sleep. Endometrial resec-

tion under local anaesthesia can also offer the option of surgery for patients too unfit for general anaesthesia (Lockwood et al 1990).

It must be emphasized that endometrial resection under local anaesthesia and sedation is not an 'office' procedure. There has to be a dedicated member of the medical staff, not necessarily an anaesthetist, who is responsible for the sedation and monitoring of the patient. Close and continuous monitoring of respiratory function and other vital signs is mandatory, and facilities for resuscitation, intubation and, of course, laparotomy have to be immediately available. Lastly, the operator should be someone experienced who can complete the required surgery quickly, efficiently and safely.

IRRIGATION SYSTEM

Details concerning irrigation fluids and systems which can be used for hysteroscopic surgery have been given in Chapter 5. Along with most practitioners in the rest of Europe and an increasing number of Americans, the author prefers to use a non-viscous fluid as it is easier to use and control. As there is a long tradition for

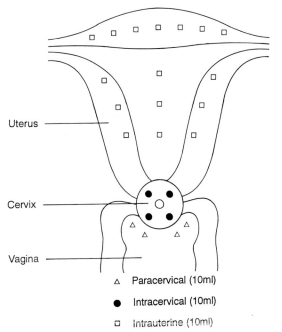

Fig. 9.14 Local anaesthetic injections for endometrial resection.

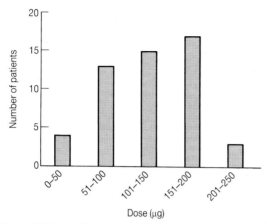

Fig. 9.15 Doses of intravenous fentanyl used during endometrial resection under local anaesthesia.

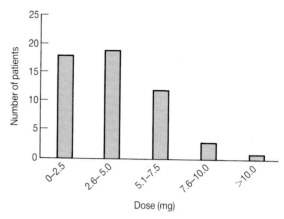

Fig. 9.16 Doses of intravenous midazolam used during endometrial resection under local anaesthesia.

the use of sterile 1.5% glycine solutions in the UK by urologists, it was quite natural for gynaecologists to utilize the same fluid for endometrial resection, which after all is nothing more than the gynaecologist's version of a transurethral prostatectomy.

As for the irrigation system, the author currently uses a dedicated irrigation/suction unit, the Hamou Hysteromat (manufactured by Storz, Tuttlingen, Germany). This gives convenient control over uterine distension and irrigation, prevents overinflation of the uterus, and makes monitoring of fluid absorption relatively simple. The pump settings vary to some extent from patient to patient, but typical figures are a distension pressure of 100–125 mmHg, suction pressure of –50 mmHg, and flow rates of up to 300 ml/min. The system is adjusted so that (1) the minimum distension pressure is used which gives an adequate view of the uterine fundus and cornual areas (to reduce fluid absorption), and (2) the minimum suction pressure is used which keeps the uterine cavity clear of debris (to reduce the volume of fluid infused into the uterus). When faced with problems of insufficient distension or a cloudy view, it is important to realize that it is the irrigation pressure which controls the former and the suction pressure which regulates the latter.

The Hysteromat is expensive, and equal if less convenient results can be achieved simply with a combination of gravity (which is cheap!) and

standard theatre suction. A less costly alternative system is the Quinones pump (also manufactured by Storz), provided a safety valve is built into the irrigation circuit to prevent air being pumped into the uterine cavity when the irrigation bottle is emptied. All these various methods of irrigation involve continuous-pressure/variable flow of the irrigant; what must not be used is any system which is based on continuous-flow/variable pressure as very high intrauterine pressures can develop with the consequent risk of severe fluid overload.

ELECTROSURGICAL GENERATOR SETTINGS

We use a Force 2 electrosurgical generator (manufactured by Valleylab UK) at settings of 100–125 W at blend 1–3 for cutting and 50 W for coagulation of bleeding points at the end of surgery. The precise power used does not seem to matter particularly, provided the endometrium/ myometrium is cut with ease and there is little or no drag on the loop during resection. The advantages of blending the cutting current are probably more theoretical than real: it may reduce fluid absorption and bleeding by sealing small blood vessels, and by coagulating under the loop unresected islands of endometrium may be destroyed thereby reducing the chance of endometrial regeneration after surgery. The disadvantage, particularly with the higher blend numbers, is charring of the myometrium and adhesion of the resected chippings onto the loop, which in combination make the landmarks of the myometrial fibres less distinct and surgery slower. As a compromise, the author generally carries out resections at a power setting of 100 W on blend 1.

TECHNIQUE OF ENDOMETRIAL RESECTION

Endometrial resection shares many similarities with other hysteroscopic techniques of endometrial ablation. The patient is placed in lithotomy poles, and washed and draped in the usual fashion as for dilatation and curettage. There is no reason to catheterize the patient. The author prefers a slight head tilt despite the theoretically increased risk of air embolism should the irrigation circuit be faulty and air allowed to enter the uterine cavity (Wood & Roberts 1990); the reasoning behind a Trendelenburg tilt is also no more than conjecture, but should the uterus be perforated during resection then the chance of bowel trauma may be reduced as loops of bowel are no longer in direct contact with the uterus.

Following bimanual examination of the uterus, the cavity is sounded and the cervix dilated sufficiently to admit the resectoscope comfortably and allow for in and out movement. If a 26 Fr gauge resectoscope is used, which has an outer diameter of just under 9 mm, than dilatation to Hegar size 10 is adequate and will ensure that loss of irrigant between the sheath and the cervix is minimal. The fully assembled resectoscope can then be introduced into the endocervical canal, the irrigation system turned on, and the instrument guided into the uterine cavity under direct vision; there seems no logic behind using an obturator to insert the resectoscope blindly.

Once inside the uterus, the cavity is inspected, local anaesthesia injected if required as described earlier, and the resection started. Resection is performed systematically and follows a set sequence in all patients to ensure that areas are not left untreated (Fig. 9.17). Thus, the fundus is treated first, this being both the most difficult area to resect with the greatest risk of uterine perforation if one is not careful, and the part of the uterus which becomes obscured most quickly by the resected chippings. For this the author now utilizes a 10° forward-angled cutting loop, which is simply a standard cutting loop physically bent forward (Fig. 9.18); rather than bending the loops backwards and forwards, one or two loops are kept at the desired angle for resecting the fundus and cornual areas, and the author simply changes to a standard backward-angled loop for the rest of the cavity.

Using the forward-angled loop, the endometrium is undercut between the two cornua in a series of small chips, taking care never to push the loop more deeply into the myometrium than is necessary. Particular care has to be taken over the two tubal ostia where the myometrium is at its thinnest, and it is best to take a series of shallow shavings until all the endometrium has been resected here rather than make one large cut and risk perforation. Although this all sounds somewhat complicated and dangerous, resection of the fundus is not difficult to learn and is also safe provided the above guide lines are followed; for instance, the author has never yet perforated the uterus when resecting this part of the cavity. There are surgeons, however, who prefer to coagulate the fundus and cornual regions using a rollerball and then switch to the loop for the rest of the procedure.

Once the fundus has been treated, the standard cutting loop can be used to resect the walls of the uterus. It is best to treat the posterior wall first as the endometrial debris collects there and gradually obscures this part of the cavity. Although the chips can be removed from the cavity strip-by-strip, this is slower, there is fluid leakage via the cervix, and each inflation/deflation cycle is associated with uterine bleeding which further obscures the hysteroscopic view. The author prefers instead to operate without interruption and leave the resected pieces in the uterine cavity until the end of the procedure, keeping them at the fundus. This is more manageable if the chippings are relatively small, so the author relies entirely on the travel of the cutting loop as determined by the handle mechanism, about 2.5 cm, and does not move the resectoscope itself to increase the length of the cut.

Using this technique, the resection is started at 9 o'clock and the endometrium excised system-

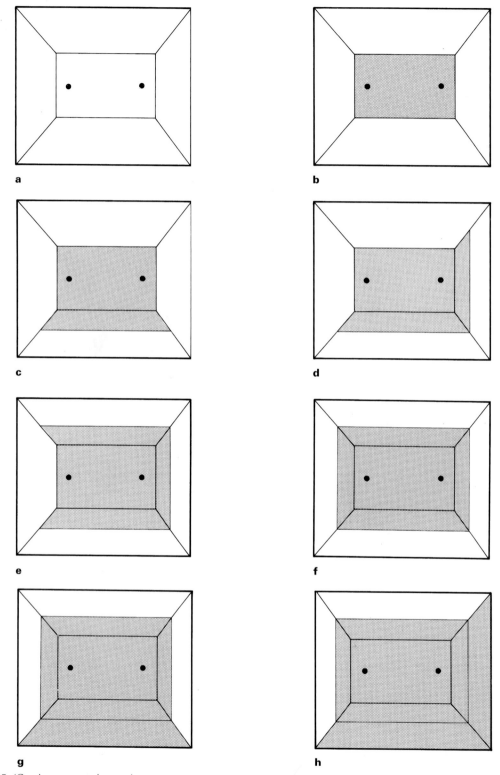

Fig. 9.17 (Caption on opposite page)

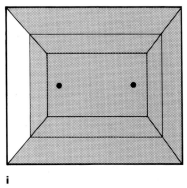

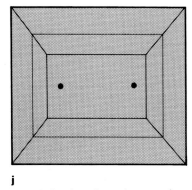

i   j

Fig. 9.17 Schematic representation of the uterine cavity showing the fundus, two tubal ostia and anterior, posterior and two lateral walls to demonstrate the sequence of endometrial resection (shaded area).

atically in an anticlockwise fashion, clearing the top third of the cavity first, then the middle third, and finally, if a total endometrial resection is to be performed, the lower third down to the cervical canal. The depth of cut is determined by the thickness of the endometrium, the aim being to undercut the endometrium by 2–3 mm, which is sufficient to remove all but the deepest extensions of the endometrium but not too deep to cut into larger vessels. If the endometrium has been prepared with an agent such as danazol, it is unusual to need more than one cut to achieve the desired depth of treatment.

Any submucous fibroids present no great problem to the resectoscope provided they are not gross (less than 3 cm in diameter), as, after all, myomectomy was the first gynaecological procedure performed with the instrument as long ago as 1978 (Neuwirth 1978). Larger fibroids can also be treated provided the principles set out in Chapter 12 are followed. Overall, about a quarter of the author's patients undergo a combined procedure of endometrial resection and myomectomy.

When resection appears to be complete, the resectoscope is withdrawn from the uterus and

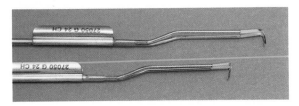

Fig. 9.18 The forward- and backward-angled cutting loops.

the bulk of the endometrial chips are removed with polyp forceps or a flushing curette. The author has tried other instruments such as an Ehrlich aspirator, which is used by urologists after prostatectomy, but it does not work as it is impossible to flush the uterine cavity sufficiently because of its relatively small volume compared to the bladder. Neither has the author found a suction curette as used for termination of pregnancy any more successful. Irrespective of the method, it is virtually impossible and probably unnecessary to remove all the debris as the particles are small and should be passed via the dilated cervix over the next few days. What is removed is sent to the pathologist for histological examination, and this the author believes to be one of the major advantages of endometrial resection compared to the other ablative techniques which destroy the endometrium in situ.

Once the uterus has been emptied, the resectoscope is introduced back into the uterine cavity to check for any untreated areas or major bleeding points (Fig. 9.19–9.22). The former are simply resected, and this demonstrates the beauty of all visual techniques, while the latter are coagulated using the loop or a rollerball. Because of the relatively high intrauterine pressure created by the irrigation system, bleeding during resection is unusual; bleeding points will become more obvious if the distension pressure is reduced, but it is doubtful if it is worth spending time coagulating individual vessels or areas unless the haemorrhage is considerable.

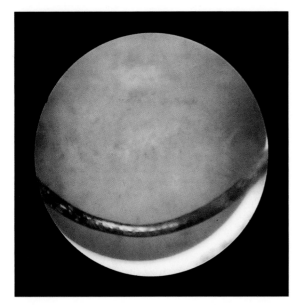

Fig. 9.19 The uterine cavity at the start of endometrial resection.

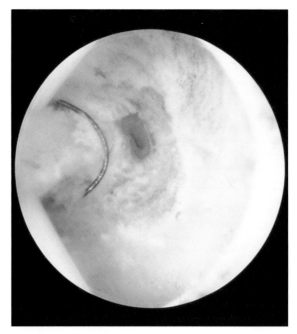

Fig. 9.20 Resecting around the left tubal ostium. (Courtesy of Dr. Jacques Hamou).

Finally, if the aim of surgery is amenorrhoea, we resect the upper half of the endocervical canal to ensure that the lower margins of the endometrium are excised. Resection has to be relatively shallow, especially laterally where the descending branch of the uterine artery is located, but the author has never as yet had any problems with bleeding. As with the uterine fundus, rollerball electrocoagulation of the endocervix is another alternative, but here secondary haemorrhage may occur following sloughing. Resecting the endocervix does not seem to cause

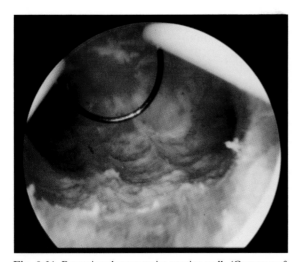

Fig. 9.21 Resecting that posterior uterine wall. (Courtesy of Dr Jacques Hamou).

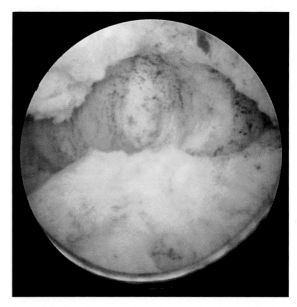

Fig. 9.22 The uterine cavity at the end of endometrial resection.

cervical stenosis, probably because the canal is actually widened by this procedure.

TOTAL AND PARTIAL ENDOMETRIAL RESECTION

As is apparent from the foregoing description, the difference between total and partial endometrial resection lies in the extent of surgery towards the cervix rather than the depth of cut. In *total resection*, the entire uterine cavity is treated, together with, at least in the author's practice, the upper part of the endocervix. Conversely, *partial resection* is not synonymous with 'partial thickness' resection of the endometrium over the cavity, but 'full thickness' resection of the top two-thirds, leaving a rim of untreated endometrium of approximately 1 cm in width in the region of the uterine isthmus.

There are those who routinely restrict their surgery to partial resection for fear of inducing cervical stenosis and subsequently a haematometra if functioning endometrium has been left in the uterine cavity. This concern is, however, unfounded. As can be seen from the next part of this chapter relating to results and complications, cervical stenosis is in fact extremely rare despite the extensive nature of a total resection and, if haematometra do develop, they tend to be fundal rather than isthmic. Unless the patient prefers to continue menstruating following surgery, there seems no rationale for not treating the entire cavity, which is exactly what is carried out with the other ablative techniques described in this book. Indeed, there is a strong case for total resection in that the menstrual results both in terms of amenorrhoea and hypomenorrhoea are far superior after the more extensive procedure. The author now rarely performs partial resection intentionally.

PRINCIPLES OF RESECTOSCOPIC SURGERY

There are four basic principles to using the resectoscope safely and effectively which often cause problems in the early part of the learning curve (Table 9.3). Firstly, it must be remembered that it is not the cutting loop per se which

Table 9.3 Basic principles of resecting safely and effectively

1. It is the electrical current that cuts, not the loop
2. Only cut when moving the loop towards the resectoscope sheath
3. Continue cutting until the loop is totally within the sheath
4. Apply sufficient pressure between the loop and uterus when cutting

cuts the endometrium but the current passing through it from the electrosurgical generator; the loop must therefore be activated to make a cut. Secondly, cutting must only take place when moving the loop towards the resectoscope sheath, as an active loop pushed away from the sheath can easily perforate the uterus. Thirdly, the loop should be brought fully into the inner sheath before the generator is turned off in order to make a clean cut, otherwise a part of the resected tissue will remain attached to the uterus. Finally, in most cases the mobility of the uterus is such that a considerable pressure has to be applied between the cutting loop and the uterus during resection to avoid merely skimming the surface of the cavity; this is achieved by angling the whole instrument more and more the closer the loop gets to the sheath, the cervix acting as the fulcrum for this movement. Beginners tend to be too 'gentle' for fear of gouging out a large chunk of tissue and perforating the uterus, and forget that the physical characteristics of the cutting loop are such that it is virtually impossible to make a cut greater than 4 mm in depth provided the other rules outlined above are adhered to.

MONITORING DURING SURGERY

Close monitoring of the patient during surgery is just as mandatory for endometrial resection as for the other ablative techniques. Endometrial resection may seem to be a minor procedure in terms of surgical time, lack of external scars, and hospitalization of the patient, but is still major surgery in terms of potential risks. The safety aspects of endometrial ablation must always be at the forefront, and careful monitoring is an important component of this. This aspect of surgery has been the subject of other chapters of this book, but two particular risks of endometrial resection which the surgeon and other staff should always be on the look-out for ought to be emphasized: uterine perforation and fluid overload. Under normal circumstances and in trained hands neither should happen, but these are undoubtably potential problems for the beginner in particular. These and other complications are covered in detail in the next part of this chapter but, briefly, it is advisable to stop and look if a perforation is suspected, and to stop if there is concern about fluid overload.

DIFFICULTIES DURING SURGERY

Every operative procedure has its own unique set of problems which can only be mastered by experience. The commoner difficulties peculiar to endometrial resection are listed in Table 9.4 together with the likely causes and the appropriate solutions. Although it is easy to say from the comfort of one's armchair, most are a matter of technique and common-sense.

Perhaps the most frequent problem, particularly when not using a pump for uterine distension, is poor access to the uterine fundus and tubal ostia. It is imperative that, irrespective of whether one resects or uses a rollerball, the anterior and posterior walls of the uterus should be sufficiently separated by the irrigation fluid to be able to visualize the entire uterine cavity without guessing. Poor distension is often compounded by bleeding because of the low pressure within the uterus, and the scene is then set for incomplete resection or, worse, uterine perforation. The commonest solution is to increase the distension pressure, and it is indeed remarkable how non-compliant some uteri are, particularly those which are enlarged by fibroids.

The converse problem is the presence of small particles of endometrial debris inside the uterus giving a hazy view through the endoscope. This can be very annoying and is especially common when the endometrium has not been hormonally thinned. The solution is to increase the suction pressure, but often the resectoscope has to be

Table 9.4   Practical problems and their solutions during endometrial resection

Problem	Cause	Solution
Poor uterine distension	Low distension pressure Uterine perforation Cervical incompetence	Increase distension pressure Stop and check abdomen Cervical suture or tenacula around cervix
Slow clearance of debris/blood	Insufficient suction pressure Blocked outflow hole in sheath	Increase suction pressure Clean sheath
Inefficient cutting	Cutting power too low Cutting loop not in sheath at rest Cutting loop broken	Increase cutting power or reduce blend Gently bend loop into correct position Replace cutting loop
Poor view of endometrium and uterine cavity	See Poor uterine distension See Slow clearance of debris/blood Resected chips restrict view Bubbles on the anterior wall Fibroids	 Remove chips before continuing with surgery Increase suction pressure Hysteroscopic total or partial myomectomy
Rapid fluid absorption	Distension pressure too high Uterine perforation	Reduce distension pressure Stop and check cavity
Bleeding during surgery	Low distension pressure Insufficient coagulation during cutting Resection too deep Fibroids	Increase distension pressure Increase coagulation blend Coagulate vessel(s) and resect more shallowly Coagulate vessels round pseudocapsule
Haemorrhage after surgery	Resection too deep Infection Resected debris in cavity	Uterine tamponade with balloon catheter Antibiotics Evacuate and give antibiotics

removed from the uterus and the small outflow holes in the outer sheath, which easily get blocked up due to their small size, cleaned of tissue.

Another irritating difficulty is when the resected tissue is not cut cleanly off but floats around the uterine cavity rather like a large polyp. This is most often due to the electro-surgical generator not being activated contin-uously to the end of the cut, that is, until the cutting loop has been fully drawn into the inner sheath. If this is not the case then it is worthwhile ensuring that the loop has not been deformed in such a way that it no longer rests inside the resectoscope sheath. Bending of the loop tends to occur with increasing usage and also if cuts are attempted without cutting diathermy.

The small resected chips can be troublesome until one learns how to keep them all at the fundus. If this seems an insurmountable prob-lem, then the answer is either to empty the uterus before continuing with the resection or, alterna-tively, to change to cutting full-length strips which are removed immediately.

Although it has been mentioned before, rapid absorption of fluid should alert one to the possibility that the uterus has been perforated. This needs to be excluded before surgery can continue, but a check should also be made that the irrigant is not being pumped into the uterus at too high a pressure.

CONCLUSIONS

Endometrial resection is undoubtably a skill which has to be learnt. It is a technique which can be applied to a broad range of menorrhagic women, from those with dysfunctional bleeding and a small uterus, to those with a sizeable uterus enlarged with fibroids. This versatility together with advantages in terms of cost, operative time and histology makes it a skill worth learning.

REFERENCES

Brooks P G, Serden S P, Davos I 1991 Hormonal inhibition of the endometrium for resectoscopic endometrial ablation. American Journal of Obstetrics and Gynecology 161: 1601–1608

Lockwood M, Magos A L, Baumann R, Turnbull A C 1990 Endometrial resection when hysterectomy is undesirable, dangerous or impossible. British Journal of Obstetrics and Gynaecology 97: 656–658

Magos A L, Baumann R, Cheung K, Turnbull A C 1989 Intra-uterine surgery under intravenous sedation: an out-patient alternative to hysterectomy. Lancet ii: 925–926

Magos A L, Baumann R, Lockwood G M, Turnbull A C 1991 Experience with the first 250 endometrial resections for menorrhagia. Lancet 337: 1074–1078

Neuwirth R S 1978 A new technique for and additional experience with hysteroscopic resection of submucous fibroid

Reid P C, Sharp F 1988 Hysteroscopic Nd:YAG endometrial ablation: an in vitro and in vivo laser-tissue interaction study. Abstract from the IIIrd European Congress on Hysteroscopy and Endoscopic Surgery, Amsterdam, p 70

Wood S M, Roberts F L 1990 Air embolism during transcervical resection of endometrium. British Medical Journal 300: 945

PART 3
RESULTS AND COMPLICATIONS
J.A.M. Broadbent A.L. Magos

Although increasingly widely practised by gynae-cologists in both Europe and the USA, published information concerning the results of endometrial resection for menorrhagia is restricted to only six detailed published series (Magos et al 1989, Hill & Maher 1990, Maher & Hill 1990, Derman et al 1991, Magos et al 1991, Pyper & Haeri 1991) and a few short communications. (Boto et al 1989, Chappatte 1989); of these, Derman et al concentrate primarily on hysteroscopic myom-ectomy rather than endometrial ablation and do not give specific details about the effects of the latter on menstruation. In addition, as the proce-dure is relatively new, information concerning long-term follow-up is limited to just over 3 years with respect to what is becoming the standard procedure, total endometrial resection.

Nonetheless, it is gradually becoming clear which patients are most suitable for this form of intervention, what sort of results are to be expected when surgery is performed by experi-enced operators and, not least, what are the risks of surgery, both intra- and postoperative.

PATIENT SELECTION

The success of any surgical intervention depends on a number of factors, of which appropriate patient selection is an important part. Although discussed in Chapter 3, the authors wish to highlight their treatment criteria for this form of surgery, which is based on their experience of over 300 procedures (Table 9.5). Endometrial resection is not a panacea for all menstrual ills, and the indications as well as the limitations of surgery are gradually becoming manifest. Some contra-indications to surgery are absolute and unlikely to change through the years (e.g. premalignant endometrial histology), whereas others are relative and are operator- and equipment-dependent (e.g. treatment of a large fibroid uterus).

The criteria outlined in Table 9.5 should enable the identification of those women suffering from menstrual abnormalities who are most likely to benefit from this procedure; conversely, the incidence of treatment failure and operative complications is likely to rise if patient selection is less critical. It has been estimated in one study that up to 58% of patients currently being treated by hysterectomy would be suitable for endometrial resection, including women with moderately sized uterine myomata (Rutherford et al 1991). This is not an inconsiderable advantage compared with other ablative procedures which are generally restricted to the treatment of women with dysfunctional menorrhagia.

Not only must the surgeon choose the right patient for surgery, but he must also ensure that the surgery is right for the patient. Careful counselling with respect to the risks of the procedure,

Table 9.5 Operative criteria for endometrial resection

1. Menstrual problems justifying hysterectomy
2. Symptoms resistant to medical therapy
3. Uterine size smaller than the equivalent of a 12 week pregnancy (or uterine cavity <10 cm in length)
4. Submucous fibroids <5 cm in diameter
5. Benign endometrial histology
6. Completed family
7. No other gynaecological problems indicating alternative surgery (e.g. prolapse, endometriosis, cervical intraepithelial neoplasia)
8. Careful counselling (e.g. amenorrhoea cannot be guaranteed, fertility implications, unknown long-term risks)

the likelihood of menstrual improvement, including postoperative amenorrhoea, and, arguably the most important, discussion regarding the long-term 'unknowns', such as the possible risks of uterine malignancy in years to come (which may not be a real risk at all) are integral to the patient selection process. To give an example, there is little point in insisting that a patient undergoes an ablative procedure if what she wants is a guarantee that she will never menstruate again following her surgery; none of the currently available ablative techniques can promise this, only hysterectomy.

OPERATIVE RESULTS

It is unusual not to be able to complete the intended hysteroscopic procedure. Rarely, it is impossible to dilate the cervix sufficiently to be able to introduce a 26 French (Fr) resectoscope, and in these cases a smaller instrument is the only alternative. Other reasons for incomplete treatment include inaccessibility to parts of the cavity because of fibroids, difficulties because of a grossly thickened, untreated endometrium, and operative complications such as uterine perforation, fluid overload or haemorrhage. Uterine perforation and excessive absorption of uterine irrigant may in fact be linked, and a sudden increase in the amount of uterine irrigant absorbed should alert the surgeon to the possibility of uterine perforation. Surgery should stop *immediately*, both to make the diagnosis and prevent any further extrauterine trauma. In the authors' experience, however, all these problems are unusual and less than 5% of those patients who request the most extensive form of resection, total removal of the endometrium, finish up with partial resection (Magos et al 1991).

DURATION OF SURGERY

According to Maher & Hill (1990), operating times range from 30 to 90 minutes with the actual resection requiring 15–45 minutes. In the authors' experience, the average operating time is 33.6 minutes (Fig.9.23), uncorrected for teaching (Magos et al 1991). As with hysterectomy, the duration of surgery not only depends on the operators' experience but also the presence of

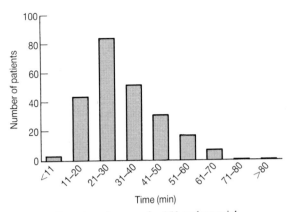

Fig. 9.23 Duration of surgery for 250 endometrial resections.

pathology. It would appear that hysteroscopic experience is by far the greatest determinant of duration of surgery; for instance for one of the authors (A.L.M.) the first 25 procedures took an average of 54.2 minutes compared with an average of 24.5 minutes for procedures 226–250 (Fig.9.24). The presence of fibroids and the lack of preoperative endometrial preparation also prolong operating time (39.0 versus 32.0 minutes and 36.9 versus 31.9 minutes, respectively) (Magos et al 1991). The majority consensus certainly seems to be that treatment given to thin the endometrium prior to surgery facilitates resection (Brooks et al 1989).

FLUID BALANCE

As discussed in detail in Chapter 5 and later in this part, the assessment of fluid balance is

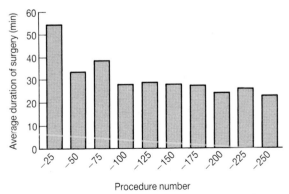

Fig. 9.24 The 'learning curve' for endometrial resection.

paramount to patient safety, the consequences of excessive fluid absorption being not only serious but potentially fatal. Fluid dynamics during surgery depend on a number of factors, but provided the correct infusion system is used (one controlled by pressure and not flow) and surgery is completed as quickly as possible, then absorption of large volumes of irrigant is unusual. As can be seen in Table 9.6, the average volume of 1.5% glycine solution absorbed in our experience is under 500 ml; only 8% of women absorbed more than 1 litre, and 3% more than 2 litres (Fig. 9.25). In otherwise healthy patients it is now our usual practice to stop surgery when the total volume of fluid absorbed during surgery exceeds 2 litres.

BLOOD LOSS DURING SURGERY

It is difficult to accurately assess operative blood loss as any bleeding gets diluted by the uterine

Table 9.6 Operative details of 250 endometrial resections

Number of procedures	250	
Endometrial preparation	189	(75.6%)
Mean uterine size (weeks of pregnancy)	6.6	(range 4–12)
Mean uterine cavity length (cm)	8.0	(range 4–14)
Fibroid uterus	60	(24.0%)
Anaesthesia		
General anaesthetic	156	(62.4%)
Sedation + local anaesthetic	94	(37.6%)
Hysteroscopic procedure		
Total TCRE	227	(90.8%)
Partial TCRE	22	(8.8%)
Planned	11	
Unplanned (total TCRE not possible)	11	
Failed	1	
Simultaneous hysteroscopic myomectomy	56	(22.4%)
Operative time (minutes)	33.6	(SD 14.2)
Fluid balance		
Mean fluid in (ml)	4632	(range 1100–20 900)
Mean fluid out (ml)	4154	(range 950–20 800)
Mean overall fluid balance (ml)	479	(range –250 to +4350)
Mean estimated blood loss (ml)	93.1	(range 10–500)

From Magos et al (1991) with permission. TCRE, transcervical resection of the endometrium; SD, standard deviation.

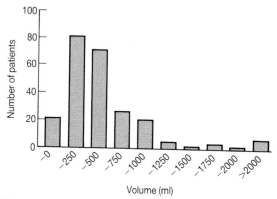

Fig. 9.25 Fluid balance during 250 endometrial resections.

irrigant. Provided the intrauterine pressure during surgery is in the range 80–120 mmHg, the impression is that bleeding is minimal. One report which included objective measurement of intraoperative bleeding quoted an average figure of only 33 ml (range 2–190 ml) (West & Robinson 1989). Bleeding can be troublesome when dealing with a fibroid uterus or if intra-uterine pressure is too low, but generally most of the bleeding associated with endometrial resection takes place after and not during surgery.

HISTOLOGY OF RESECTED ENDOMETRIUM

One of the advantages of resection over other methods of endometrial ablation which involve destruction of the endometrium *in situ* is the ability to examine the resected tissue histologically. The potential importance of this has recently been highlighted by a case report describing the finding of an unsuspected adenocarcinoma in a woman of 38 years which was missed by preresection hysteroscopy and curettage (Dwyer & Stirrat 1991).

As it is difficult and time-consuming to remove all the endometrial/myometrial chippings from the uterine cavity, measurement of the volume or weight of tissue resected tends to be an under-estimate. Typical figures in the authors' practice are 6.67 g (range 0.98–45 g) of tissue removed, the larger figures being associated when myomectomy is performed simultaneously (Magos et al 1991). Typically, after endometrial preparation with agents such as danazol, the endometrium is reported as being 'basal', 'inactive' or 'atrophic'.

Recent studies have suggested that luteinizing-hormone-releasing hormone (LH-RH) agonists are the most consistent at thinning the endometrium, followed by danazol and then progestogens (Brooks et al 1991).

As discussed in Chapter 14, the histological interpretation of the endometrial/myometrial chippings may not always be straightforward. Firstly, there is the problem of diathermy artefacts and thermal necrosis, particularly if resection is performed slowly with a blended current (Duffy et al 1991). Secondly, the angle at which the endometrial chipping are resected makes it not only difficult to assess the percentage of myometrium present in the surgical specimen, but also to determine the presence of adenomyosis. For this reason, and to act as a kind of quality control for the thoroughness of surgery, the authors now routinely biopsy the anterior and posterior walls of the uterine cavity at the end of the surgery; a finding of endometrial glands or stroma in these specimens suggests either the presence of adenomyosis or partial thickness resection. Although these two may be impossible to distinguish on an individual basis, a frequent reporting of endometrium in these biopsies would suggest a tendency for incomplete resection and thus a need to change one's technique.

CONCURRENT OPERATIVE PROCEDURES

Whilst hysterectomy may be the surgical procedure of choice for menorrhagia occurring with other gynaecological pathology (e.g. uterine prolapse), some patients can still avoid major surgery if endometrial resection is combined with other minimally invasive techniques. For instance, we have used operative laparoscopy to treat women with pelvic pain secondary to endometriosis or ovarian cysts.

POSTOPERATIVE RECOVERY

As with other 'minimally invasive techniques', endometrial resection is an ideal day case procedure provided the patient is otherwise well and is accompanied by a responsible adult (Table 9.7). This is particularly so if surgery is per-

Table 9.7 Postoperative recovery[a]

Postoperative hospital stay (days)	0.79	(0–13)
Duration of bleeding (days)	12.1	(1–42)
Duration of discharge (days)	12.0	(0–120)
Return to normal domestic activities (weeks)	1.30	(0–4)
Return to work (weeks)	2.12	(0–6)

From Magos et al (1991) with permission.
[a]Values are means (range in parentheses).

formed under local anaesthesia, when post-operative recovery is exceptionally quick (Fig. 9.26) and is associated with minimal nausea and pain (Fig. 9.27); indeed, about one-third of our patients voluntarily opt to have their surgery without general anaesthesia. Whatever the mode of anaesthesia, however, hospitalization is still short (Fig. 9.28), and recovery in terms of return to normal domestic activities and work generally

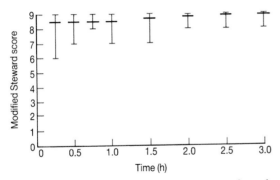

Fig. 9.26 Recovery after endometrial resection performed under local anaesthesia and intravenous sedation as assessed by a modified Steward score (score of 9 is equivalent to total recovery).

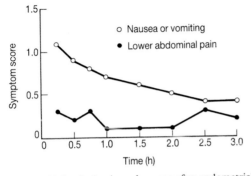

Fig. 9.27 Abdominal pain and nausea after endometrial resection performed under local anaesthesia scored on a scale of 0–3 (0, no symptoms; 1, mild symptoms; 2, moderate symptoms; 3, severe symptoms).

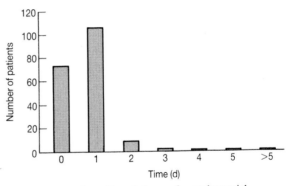

Fig. 9.28 Duration of hospital stay after endometrial resection.

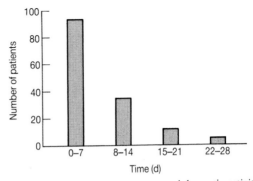

Fig. 9.29 Time taken to return to normal domestic activities after endometrial resection.

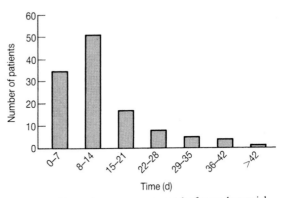

Fig. 9.30 Time taken to return to work after endometrial resection.

fast (Figs. 9.29 and 9.30) (Maher & Hill 1990, Magos et al 1991). Reasons for a prolonged hospital stay are usually related to operative complications or concurrent medical conditions.

Surgery is typically followed by bleeding and vaginal discharge which can last from days to weeks (Figs. 9.31 and 9.32). The bleeding is rarely

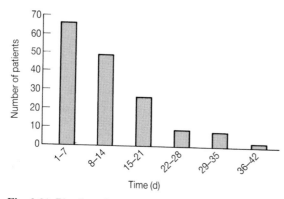

Fig. 9.31 Bleeding after endometrial resection.

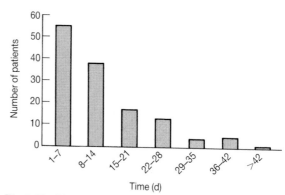

Fig. 9.32   Vaginal discharge after endometrial resection.

Table 9.8   Factors which may influence the results of endometrial ablation

Patient characteristics	Younger patients and those with fibroids/enlarged uteri may have worse results
Surgical experience	Better results with experience
Technique	Rates of amenorrhoea and hypomenorrhoea less likely with partial ablation
Postoperative hormonal suppression	Better results expected early on but benefit may not be permanent
Definitions	Inconsistent meaning of 'hypomenorrhoea' and similar terms can influence the way results are presented
Duration of follow-up	Failures more likely with increasing time

heavy after the first 12–24 hours, and none of our patients has so far had a secondary haemorrhage.

EFFECT ON MENSTRUATION

The short- to medium-term effects on menstruation of endometrial resection have not yet been widely published. The series with the longest follow-up of several years, that of Derman et al (1991), does not distinguish between endometrial resection and hysteroscopic myomectomy and so is difficult to interpret. Further problems include those listed in Table 9.8 which makes objective comparison of not only the data concerning endometrial resection but comparison with the other ablative techniques a complex matter. These difficulties should always be borne in mind.

The results of some of the larger published and

Table 9.9   Menstruation and further surgery after endometrial resections

Series	Maher & Hill (1990)	Magos et al (1991)	Pyper & Haeri (1991)	Shaxted (unpublished)	Holt (unpublished)
Number of patients	100[a]	250	80	274	350
Menstrual result (%)					
Amenorrhoea	21	27–42[b]	6–8[b]	59[c]	42[c]
Improved	95	92	81	91	97
Not improved	3	8	19	9	3
Further surgery					
TCRE	3 (3%)	16 (7%)	15 (19%)	NA	8 (2%)
Hysterectomy	0 (0%)	10 (4%)	4 (5%)	NA	11 (3%)

TCRE, transcervical resection of the endometrium; NA, not available.
[a] Two patients lost to follow-up.
[b] Amenorrhoea rate after total TCRE dependent on time after surgery.
[c] Some given depo-provera after surgery.

explained by the factors noted in Table 9.9. For instance, the low incidence of amenorrhoea reported by Maher & Hill (1990) must be related to these authors' reluctance to resect into the endocervical canal due to the risk of uncontrollable haemorrhage and possible cervical stenosis (a complication not encountered by others); they now use rollerball electrocoagulation to this area and expect to achieve a higher incidence of amenorrhoea.

However, what is without doubt is that irrespective of the technique and other factors, up to 97% of patients treated by endometrial resection experience an improvement in their menstruation such that relatively few require further surgery. What is also clear from both our results and those of others is that endometrial resection can be repeated safely and effectively in those cases who failed with the initial procedure; indeed, Pyper & Haeri (1991) report one patient who underwent a total of three resections before she was cured of her menorrhagia. At least in the short term, the chance of a successful menstrual result from repeat surgery is over 81% (Magos et al 1991).

The authors' results over a 2.5 year period are shown in more detail in Figs. 9.33–9.40. It can be seen that over 80–90% of patients report an

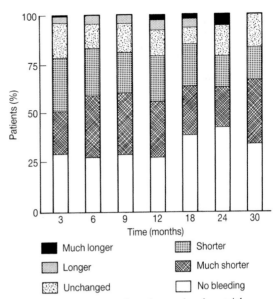

Fig. 9.34 Menstrual duration after total endometrial resection.

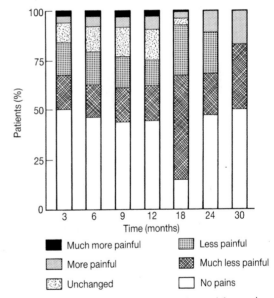

Fig. 9.35 Menstrual pain after total endometrial resection.

improvement in their periods, which either cease completely or become much lighter or lighter (Fig. 9.33). About two-thirds of the women who continue to menstruate find that their periods become shorter or much shorter (Fig. 9.34). Not only that, but menstrual pains are generally reduced or absent after endometrial resection (Fig. 9.35). The end

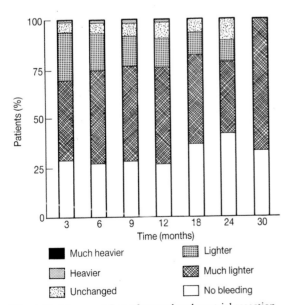

Fig. 9.33 Menstrual flow after total endometrial resection.

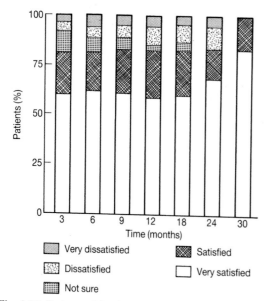

Fig. 9.36 Patient satisfaction after total endometrial resection.

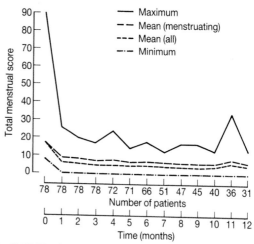

Fig. 9.37 Total menstrual scores after total endometrial resection scored daily on a scale of 0–3 (0, no bleeding; 1, light bleeding; 2, moderate bleeding; 3, heavy bleeding).

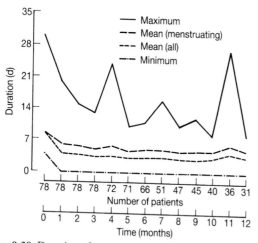

Fig. 9.38 Duration of menstruation after total endometrial resection.

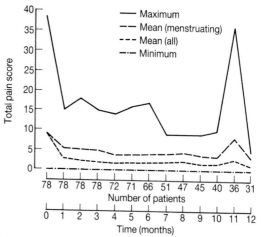

Fig. 9.39 Total menstrual pain scores after total endometrial resection scored daily on a scale of 0–3 (0, no bleeding; 1, mild pain; 2, moderate pain; 3, severe pain).

result is a high rate of patient satisfaction (Fig. 9.36). These retrospective reports were confirmed by a subgroup of women who kept a menstrual calender for up to 1 year (Figs. 9.37–9.39), as well as by objective measures of menstrual blood loss (see Ch. 15). As an indication of the longer-term results of surgery, very few women who achieved a good menstrual result 3 months after surgery subsequently relapsed (Fig. 9.40).

THE UTERINE CAVITY AFTER ENDOMETRIAL RESECTION

The effect that resecting the endometrium has on the uterine cavity is of some interest to the gynaecologist and can be assessed by ultrasound scanning and hysteroscopy. Ultrasonographically, the volume of the uterine cavity can be seen to shrink from an average of 3 to 1 ml, whereas the total volume of the uterus remains unchanged

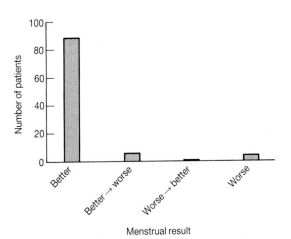

Fig. 9.40 Menstruation 3 and 12 months after total endometrial resection.

(Baumann & Magos, *unpublished observations*). Hysteroscopic examination of the uterine cavity reveals marked fundal fibrosis, with a narrow cavity which is occasionally totally obliterated.

Histological examination of tissue biopsies from the uterine wall typically shows myometrium, a single-cell lining or inflammatory cells. Surprisingly, about 25% of women who become amenorrhoeic after surgery are found to have microscopic deposits of endometrium, an important finding with respect to later hormone replacement therapy for the menopause. This finding is in keeping with the original description of Asherman's syndrome where inactive endometrium was found despite ovulation (Asherman 1948).

COMPLICATIONS OF ENDOMETRIAL RESECTION

Whenever a disorder is treated with surgical intervention, the potential benefits must be balanced against the potential hazards of the procedure itself, and this applies to endometrial resection just as to the other forms of endometrial ablation. However, one should not look at the complications of surgery in isolation but in relation to the procedure it is replacing, that is, hysterectomy. Hysterectomy is major surgery, and carries a relatively low but definite mortality rate of 6:10 000 when the indication is for benign disease (Wingo et al 1985). The morbidity rate

after hysterectomy is, however, much higher, figures of 24.5:100 and 42.8:100 for vaginal and abdominal hysterectomies respectively having been reported in one large audit (Dicker et al 1982). There is also increasing evidence that hysterectomy can be followed by long-term problems such as urinary and intestinal dysfunction (Taylor et al 1989), premature ovarian failure (Siddle et al 1987), cardiovascular disease (Centerwall 1981) and, possibly, osteoporosis. It is important to be aware of these problems when assessing the safety of hysteroscopic surgery.

The potential complications of endometrial resection, as far as the authors are aware of them at present, are listed in Table 9.10, and their incidence in some large series are summarized in Table 9.11.

Uterine perforation

Uterine perforation is potentially one of the most serious complications of endometrial resection as it can be associated with fluid overload as well as trauma to the gastrointestinal and genitourinary tracts and major blood vessels, leading to peritonitis, fistulae or torrential haemorrhage. Uterine perforation was documented in the authors' initial series using the resectoscope (Magos et al 1989), but is not unique to transcervical resection of the endometrium as Goldrath had similar problems with laser ablation during his early learning phase (Goldrath et al 1981). The reported incidence of uterine perforation with the resectoscope is between 1 and 3.7% (Maher & Hill 1990, Sturdee & Hoggart 1991, Magos et al 1991, Pyper & Haeri 1991). The

Table 9.10 Potential complications of endometrial resection

Intraoperative	Postoperative	
	Short term	Long term
Uterine perforation	Infection	Recurrence of Symptoms
Fluid overload	Haematometra	Pregnancy
Primary haemorrhage	Secondary haemorrhage	Uterine malignancy
Gas embolism	Cyclical pain	
	Treatment failure	

Table 9.11   Complications of endometrial resection in different series

Complication	Maher & Hill (1990)	Magos et al (1991)	Pyper & Haeri (1991)	Shaxted (unpublished)	Holt (unpublished)
Number of patients	100[a]	250	80	274	350
Uterine perforation (%)	1	2	4	2.5	1
Fluid overload (> 2 litres) (%)	NA	3	0	NA	1
Haemorrhage (%)	5	0.4	2.5	NA	1
Infection (%)	2	0	NA	NA	4
Haematometra (%)	2	1	NA	1	2
Pregnancy (%)	1	1	0	1.5	8
				0.6	1

NA, not available.
[a]Two patients lost to follow-up.

authors' own figure of 1.6% correlates well with the 1.5% rate reported by Macdonald & Phipps (1992) following a large anonymous postal questionnaire where 2796 resection procedures were surveyed.

It is becoming evident that uterine perforation is very much related to the experience of the operator; in our series of 250 cases, no perforations occurred in the last 193 procedures, and Macdonald & Phipps (1992) reported that 52% occurred during the first five cases of each individual's experience, 33% during the first case. The danger area is also the most difficult area to treat with resection, namely the cornual areas of the fundus. Although by no means totally safe, rollerball electrocoagulation of this part of the cavity is technically easier and probably safer for the less experienced.

Perforation may be obvious if the peritoneum or bowel is visualized, but it can be difficult to make the diagnosis. Sudden absorption of uterine irrigant by the patient should always arouse one's suspicion, and if this happens a careful search should be made for a perforation before continuing with surgery. Alternatively, the patient's abdomen may become increasingly distended, and similar checks are then required.

The significance of this complication depends on the method of perforation. If perforation occurs as a result of instrumenting the uterus, e.g. when dilating the cervix, or inserting the resectoscope, or with the use of polyp forceps/flushing curette when extracting the endometrial chippings, then damage to the intra-abdominal viscera and vasculature is unlikely and inspection via the laparoscope is sufficient. If the perforation site is bleeding then haemostasis can be achieved by laparoscopic suturing or diathermy, thereby avoiding laparotomy. If, however, perforation occurs whilst using the resecting loop then structures adjacent to the uterus (bowel, bladder, large vessels and ureters) are likely to be traumatized, and in the authors' opinion immediate laparotomy is mandatory.

Learning points

1. *Do not resect deeply in cornual areas*
2. *Always resect towards the sheath and never away*
3. *Do not cut too deep*
4. *Carefully inspect cavity if sudden absorption of fluid by the patient occurs.*

Fluid overload

Of all the complications of operative hysteroscopy, most attention has been focused on the risks of fluid overload as a result of absorption of the uterine irrigating fluid from intravasation into the uterine veins or peritoneal absorption following transtubal leakage. As discussed in Chapter 5, the use of non-electrolytic solutions such as 1.5% glycine for electrosurgery and the relatively non-compliant nature of the myometrium requiring high pressures to achieve uterine distension predispose to the absorption of large quantities of irrigating fluid, producing what is known to urologists as the transurethral resection (TUR) syndrome. As congestive cardiac failure, hypertension, hyponatraemia, neurological symptoms, haemolysis, coma and even death can develop as a result of fluid overload, careful monitoring of fluid balance is vital.

The biochemical sequelae of fluid absorption during endometrial resection when 1.5% glycine solution is used as the uterine irrigant has been well documented (Baumann et al 1990, Boto et al 1990, Magos et al 1990). There is a major dilutional effect (Figs. 9.41–9.43) and, of most clinical relevance, a fall in plasma sodium concentrations which is proportional to the volume of irrigant absorbed (Fig. 9.44). Large changes in electrolytes can develop during surgery, particularly if the uterus has been perforated (Fig. 9.45). *Close* intraoperative fluid monitoring is therefore essential.

In view of the potential seriousness of fluid overload the authors now have strict guidelines concerning fluid balance, which have eradicated this complication as surgery is stopped before any danger can occur to the

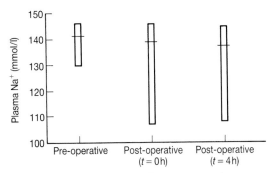

Fig. 9.43 Changes in plasma sodium concentration (expressed as mean and range) after endometrial resection using 1.5% glycine solution for uterine distension (n = 56).

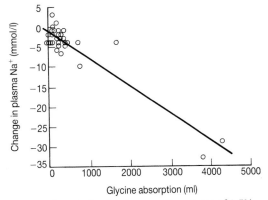

Fig. 9.44 The relationship between the volume of 1.5% glycine solution absorbed and changes in plasma sodium concentration.

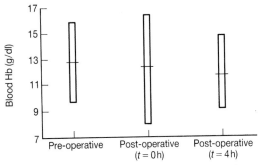

Fig. 9.41 Changes in blood haemoglobin concentration (expressed as mean and range) after endometrial resection using 1.5% glycine solution for uterine distension (n = 56).

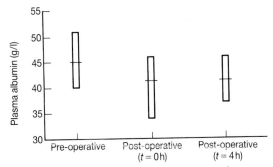

Fig. 9.42 Changes in plasma albumin concentration (expressed as mean and range) after endometrial resection using 1.5% glycine solution for uterine distension (n = 56).

patient (Table 9.12). Fluid balance measurements are made at intervals, such as when a bag/bottle of the irrigant is drained completely, when the collecting bottle becomes full and, finally, at the end of surgery. Whether more sophisticated methods of continuous assessment of fluid absorption, such as the use of intravascular sodium electrodes or tagged irrigant (e.g. with 1% ethanol) will further improve safety remains to be seen.

Finally, it is possible to identify 'high-risk' patients for fluid overload. Women who have a large fibroid uterus, who have not been sterilized and in whom the endometrium has not been prepared for surgery pharmacologically are at most risk from fluid absorption, partly because surgery takes longer under these circumstances. Beginners would therefore do well to pick 'low-risk' women for their early procedures.

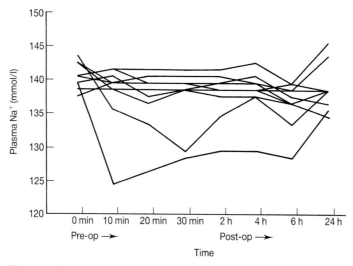

Fig. 9.45 Changes in plasma sodium concentrations during and after endometrial resection using 1.5% glycine solution for uterine distension.

Learning points

1. *Be familiar with the factors which influence fluid balance*
2. *Monitor intraoperative fluid balance closely*
3. *Adhere strictly to fluid balance guidelines*
4. *Suspect uterine perforation when sudden excessive fluid absorption occurs.*

Haemorrhage

Although the uterus is a vascular organ, haemorrhage is a rare complication of endometrial resection provided the myometrium is not cut too deeply, that is, more than 3–4 mm into the subendometrial layer. It is indeed somewhat remarkable how 'bloodless' endometrial resection is, even if combined with hysteroscopic myomectomy. There are three reasons for this: firstly, the subendometrial vessels are of small calibre and unlikely to be the cause of major haemorrhage, the larger branches of the uterine artery being deep to the resection; secondly, use of a blended cutting current seals small vessels during resection; and, thirdly, the intrauterine pressure generated by the irrigant opposes any tendency to bleed into the uterine cavity. The importance of the last is clearly demonstrated when the uterus is deflated during or at the end of surgery when a degree of bleeding is immediate.

If myometrial bleeding points do occur, they can usually be easily controlled by electrocoagulation. If there is a general ooze at the end of surgery, particularly when myomectomy has also been performed, insertion of a 30 ml Foley catheter balloon for 6–8 hours to produce uterine tamponade is generally sufficient to control the bleeding. Silastic balloons have also been specially designed for this purpose (Derman et al 1991). Prior endometrial preparation with gonadotrophin-releasing hormone (GnRH) agonists and danazol, by reducing uterine vascularity, may also lower the risk of excessive bleeding, but this remains to be proven.

Another area of potential danger is in the endocervical canal, as too deep lateral resection

Table 9.12 Guidelines for the management of fluid absorption during hysteroscopic surgery using electrolyte-free aqueous solutions (e.g. 1.5% glycine)

Volume absorbed (ml)	Effect	Action
<1000	Well tolerated by healthy patients	Continue surgery
1000–2000	Mild hyponatraemia likely	Complete surgery as quickly as possible
>2000	Severe hyponatraemia and other disturbances likely	Stop surgery

may damage the descending branch of the uterine artery; for this reason, some workers advocate stopping the resection at the level of the uterine isthmus, and others suggest electro-coagulation in the cervical canal using a rollerball (Maher & Hill 1990). The authors, however, routinely resect the upper half of the endocervical canal as part of total endometrial resection and have never yet had any problems with either primary or secondary haemorrhage.

> **Learning points**
>
> 1. *Do not resect too deeply*
> 2. *Use a rollerball if not experienced*
> 3. *Danger areas include cornual and isthmic regions.*

Gas embolism

Wood & Roberts (1990) reported a case of suspected air embolism during endometrial resection, describing cardiovascular and oxygen saturation changes consistent with this diagnosis. Air embolism can occur whenever an open vein is exposed to air in the presence of an air pressure that is greater than the venous pressure. This situation arises when the operating site is raised above the level of the heart and is particularly risky when the patient is breathing sponta-neously. They suggest that anaesthetic tech-niques using positive-pressure ventilation may be preferred and that patients should not be nursed in a head-down position during surgery. The counter argument against this position is that a Trendelenburg tilt will encourage bowel to fall away from the pelvis and thus reduce the risk of direct bowel trauma should the uterus be perforated during surgery.

Equipment used during endometrial ablation may result in gas embolism, and irrigation pumps using air at pressure to deliver the uterine irrigant should always employ an air-trapping valve system. Baggish & Daniell (1989), for instance, described two fatalities due to air embolism during laser endometrial ablation when gas-cooled sapphire tips were used to deliver the laser energy into the uterine cavity. Although a rare event, the possibility of gas embolism should always be remembered and steps taken to reduce the likelihood of this potentially fatal condition happening.

> **Learning points**
>
> 1. *Avoid air entering the uterine cavity during surgery*
> 2. *Never use an air pressure pump without a safety gas valve.*

Infection

The true incidence of postoperative infection after endometrial resection is not known, mainly because infection tends to be diagnosed on clinical grounds following discharge from hospital rather than on positive culture of swabs. Suggestive symptoms of intrauterine or pelvic sepsis include fever, pain, offensive vaginal dis-charge, persistent uterine bleeding, uterine tenderness and other non-specific prodromal symptoms. Antibiotics are then dispensed, symp-toms resolve, and the diagnosis thus appears to be confirmed. Maher & Hill (1990) reported a 2% incidence in their series, and the authors have certainly had several patients treated by their general practitioners but without confirmatory microbiological evidence. Nonetheless, the authors are concerned sufficiently about this risk to routinely use preoperative prophylactic anti-biotics. This is an aspect of hysteroscopic surgery which needs to be addressed in more detail.

> **Learning points**
>
> 1. *Use antibiotic prophylaxis (not proven)*
> 2. *Confirm uterine infection by bacteriology culture.*

Mortality

The greatest hazard to the patient from endo-metrial resection is not the surgery but the surgeon. There have been reports of fatalities associated with resection of the endometrium either because of severe fluid overload which was not recognized or treated early enough, or uterine perforation leading to catastrophic intra-abdominal haemorrhage. Although precise details are rarely available, the common denominator seems to be inexperience or a frank lack of basic knowledge and skills. Hysteroscopic surgery is not for the novice. Confidence with diagnostic hysteroscopy is a mandatory prerequisite and, conversely, laparoscopic expertise is no substitute as the two techniques are so different. Adequate and supervised training in operative hysteroscopy, including knowledge of the indications and contra-indications, limitations and complications, is essential to ensure the proper management and safety of patients. Although endometrial resection and other ablative techniques are considered to be 'minimally invasive', they can be 'maximally invasive' in the wrong hands.

Learning points

1. *Be familiar with diagnostic hysteroscopy before attempting operative surgery*
2. *Attend workshops and other teaching sessions*
3. *Perform the early cases under supervision*
4. *Restrict yourself to the treatment of women with normal uterine cavities at the beginning.*

Haematometra

The theoretical risk of stenosis at the cervical isthmus causing haematometra is the reason that Hamou advocates partial endometrial resection and why he leaves a rim of endometrium 1 cm in width at the lower pole of the uterine cavity. In practice, this risk is more theoretical than real; cervical stenosis is extremely rare even when the upper portion of the endocervical canal is resected, and indeed the authors have never yet seen a patient with a haematometra secondary to cervical stenosis. In contrast, both the authors and others have come across patients with haematometra localized in the fundus of the uterus, but this complication is equally likely with partial resection and results from viable endometrium loculated off by postresection fibrosis. Symptoms in these cases include cyclical or constant pain, and sometimes vaginal bleeding. Diagnosis is easily made by

ultrasound, and treatment involves opening and re-resecting the cavity to prevent a recurrence. Whether routine probing of the uterine cavity in the first few weeks after surgery reduces the risk of this complication remains to be proven (Loffer 1988), but such intervention is associated with the risk of infection and even uterine perforation.

Learning points

1. *Haematometra needs to be excluded in cases of postoperative pain by ultrasound*
2. *Incidence is not increased by total as opposed to partial resection*
3. *Treat by repeating the resection to remove remaining endometrium.*

Cyclical pain

A related problem to the development of haematometra is quite severe lower abdominal pain, often cyclical, but in the absence of blood in the uterine cavity and even menstruation. This is a definite complaint by a small number of women, and there are also some who experience reduced bleeding but report increased menstrual pains following surgery (Fig. 9.35). The aetiology in this cases is often uncertain, and it could be argued that laparoscopy should be performed to exclude endometriosis and other causes of pelvic pain although, if the pain arises de novo, there is as yet no evidence that endometrial ablation can induce endometriosis externa. More likely is the possibility that foci of endometriosis interna have been created, with small islands of endometrium being buried within the myometrium. It is notable that one of the symptoms originally described by Asherman as being associated with intrauterine synechiae was pelvic pain, which affected 25% of his patients (Asherman 1950).

As for therapy, simple analgesics should be tried first but these will tend to fail in severe cases. Laparoscopic uterine nerve ablation can be attempted but as yet no data on the efficacy of this mode of management is available. Sadly, some women with intractable pain require hysterectomy.

Pregnancy

Although logic suggests that the chance of conception after endometrial resection must be slight because of the small, scarred uterine cavity that typically results from surgery, probable cornual blockage, and the age-related reduced fertility in this age group, the procedure should not be equated with absolute sterility. Several pregnancies have been reported, both intrauterine and tubal. Uterine pregnancies often abort spontaneously or are terminated, but term pregnancies have also been reported with no apparent fetal or placental complications (C. J. G. Sutton, *personal communication*, Maher & Hill 1990).

For these reasons, patients should be carefully counselled prior to endometrial resection with regard to their contraception following surgery, and offered elective sterilization if appropriate. In the authors' experience, only 1:6 patients at risk of pregnancy following resection request sterilization, the remainder preferring to use barrier methods of contraception or to accept this small but definite risk. A large number of 'at risk' women will have to be monitored for a number of years to better define the chance of pregnancy after this procedure.

Treatment failure and recurrence of symptoms

Clinically, it is important to draw a distinction between failure of treatment with no improvement in symptoms after surgery, and recurrence of symptoms after an initial period of improvement. As is evident from the earlier discussion and Table 9.9, in most hands 80–90% of patients achieve a satisfactory menstrual result after a single procedure. Relapse after successful surgery appears to be relatively uncommon (Fig. 9.40). Although this form of surgery is relatively new and so the follow-up data necessarily limited, most women who benefit from surgery early on continue to do so, a feature which is in accord with the results of laser ablation (Loffer 1988). There are exceptions, and the authors have had one patient who became amenorrhoeic following total endometrial resection only to suddenly develop severe menorrhagia after 2 years. There is no reason why both primary treatment failures and those with secondary recurrence of symptoms cannot be retreated, hysterectomy being reserved for those patients who specifically request it. This new procedure must certainly not be forced on patients against their will.

Uterine malignancy

Two aspects of uterine malignancy need to be discussed, namely, occult endometrial carcinoma and the prospect of long-term cancer risk. One of the advantages of endometrial resection over other ablative techniques is the provision of tissue for histological examination. As already noted, what was a theoretical risk of missing occult early endometrial carcinoma has since been realized (Dwyer & Stirrat 1991).

The other concern is the possibility of buried islands of endometrium undergoing malignant change and, because of the presence of intrauterine adhesions or cervical stenosis, presenting at a later stage than would be expected under normal circumstances. This is as yet a purely theoretical risk and to the authors' knowledge no patient has developed a carcinoma following endometrial ablation. It may be that endometrial ablation will ultimately be associated with a reduced risk of endometrial cancer, the commonest malignancy of the uterine corpus, as so little if any of this tissue remains in situ at the end of surgery. Neither is there is any particular reason why sarcomatous change should occur in the myometrium. The chance of tumours affecting the cervix or ovary will remain, of course, unchanged.

There is one practical implication of the finding that endometrial glands and stroma may be found even in women who become amenorrhoeic after endometrial resection (Magos et al 1991): as pointed out earlier, menopausal hormone replacement therapy should be of the combined kind to prevent the development of endometrial atypia with unopposed oestrogens.

> **Learning points**
>
> 1. *Exclude premalignant or malignant endometrium preoperatively*
> 2. *Use opposed oestrogen replacement therapy where indicated.*

FINANCIAL BENEFITS

Provided endometrial resection remains as safe and successful in the long term as in the short term in controlling menorrhagia, then this procedure becomes a very attractive alternative to hysterectomy. The hospital costs of the two procedures have been compared in the UK by Rutherford & Glass (1990), showing a small reduction in operative costs but a much greater benefit in terms of reduced hospitalization and ward costs. The benefits of course continue once the patient is discharged, faster return to work being associated with a reduction in sickness benefits. A similar cost/benefit ratio is to be expected with the other ablative techniques described in this book.

Use of the resectoscope also has important financial advantages over the other methods of endometrial destruction in terms of capital and running costs. For instance, a resectoscope costs approximately 1/25th the price of a laser unit, while cutting loops (and rollerballs) are not only considerably cheaper than laser fibres, but can be reused several times before they become non-functional.

CONCLUSIONS

Endometrial resection has been shown by several investigators to be a highly effective treatment for menorrhagia. Although this approach to endometrial ablation is more recent than other hysteroscopic techniques using laser and electrocoagulation, results appear to be comparable with advantages in terms of speed of surgery, ease of performing submucous myomectomy, the provision of histological specimens, and relatively low capital and running costs. Clearly, the long-term results have yet to be determined but there is no reason to expect that these will be different to other treatment modalities.

Mention is sometimes made of a recent large retrospective comparison of transurethral resection of the prostate with open prostatectomy showing a small but significantly increased risk of death from cardiovascular causes for up to 8 years following the endoscopic procedure (Roos et al 1989); while endometrial resection shares many similarities with this transurethral resection, the patient population and operative conditions are totally different and it is inappropriate to apply the above findings to hysteroscopic endometrial surgery. Nonetheless, this study serves to illustrate the potential for long-term effects which may not be predictable from short-term experience. Only careful long-term monitoring of patients undergoing these new techniques will truly address the question of safety and efficacy.

ACKNOWLEDGEMENTS

The authors gratefully acknowledge information supplied by Mr Edward Shaxted, Consultant Obstetrician and Gynaecologist at Northampton, UK, and Mr Eddie Holt, Consultant Obstetrician and Gynaecologist at Reading, UK.

REFERENCES

Asherman J G 1948 Amenorrhoea traumatica atretica. Journal of Obstetrics and Gynaecology of the British Empire 55: 23–30

Asherman J G 1950 Traumatic intra-uterine adhesions. Journal of Obstetrics and Gynaecology of the British Empire 57: 892–896

Baggish M S, Daniell J F 1989 Catastrophic injury secondary to the use of coaxial gas-cooled fibers and artifical sapphire tips for intrauterine surgery. Lasers in Surgery and Medicine 9: 581

Baumann R, Magos A L, Kay J D S, Turnbull A C 1990 Absorption of glycine irrigating solution during transcervical resection of the endometrium. British Medical Journal 300: 304–305

Boto T C A, Fowler C G, Djahanbakch O 1989 Transcervical resection of the endometrium in women with menorrhagia. British Medical Journal 298: 1518

Boto T C A, Fowler C G, Cockroft S, Djahanbakch O 1990 Absorption of irrigating fluid during transcervical resection of endometrium. British Medical Journal 300: 748–749

Brooks P G, DeCherney A H, Loffer F, Neuwirth R S 1989 Resectoscopy: mastering the challenges Contemporary Obstetrics/Gynaecology 34: 131–148

Brooks P G, Serden S P, Davos I 1991 Hormonal inhibition of the endometrium for resectoscopic endometrial ablation. American Journal of Obstetrics and Gynaecology 161: 1601–1608

Centerwall B S 1981 Premenopausal hysterectomy and cardiovascular disease. American Journal of Obstetrics and Gynaecology 139: 58–61

Chappatte O 1989 Transcervical resection of endometrium. British Medical Journal 298: 1709

Derman S G, Rehnstrom J, Neuwirth R S 1991 The long-term effectiveness of hysteroscopic treatment of menorrhagia and leiomyomas. Obstetrics and Gynaecology 77: 591–594

Dicker R C, Greenspan J R, Strauss L T et al 1982 Complications of abdominal and vaginal hysterectomy among women of reproductive age in the United States. American Journal of Obstetrics and Gynaecology 144:841–848

Duffy S, Reid P C, Smith J H F, Sharp F 1991. In vitro studies of uterine electrosurgery. Obstetrics and Gynaecology 78: 213–220

Dwyer N A, Stirrat G M 1991 Early endometrial carcinoma: an incidental finding after endometrial resection. Case report. British Journal of Obstetrics and Gynaecology 98: 733–734

Goldrath M H, Fuller T A, Segal S 1981 Laser photovaporisation of endometrium for the treatment of menorrhagia American Journal of Obstetrics and Gynaecology 140: 14–19

Hill D J, Maher P J 1990 Intrauterine surgery using electrocautery. Australian and New Zealand Journal of Obstetrics and Gynaecology 30: 145–146

Loffer F D 1988 Laser ablation of the endometrium. Obstetrics and Gynaecology Clinics of North America 15: 77–89

Macdonald R, Phipps J 1992 Endometrial ablation: a safe procedure. Gynaecology and Endocrinology (in press)

Magos A L 1990 Management of menorrhagia. British Medical Journal 300: 1537–1538

Magos A L, Baumann R, Turnbull A C 1989 Transcervical resection of the endometrium in women with menorrhagia. British Medical Journal 298: 1209–1212

Magos A L, Baumann R, Turnbull A C 1990 Safety of transcervical endometrial resection Lancet i: 44

Magos A L, Baumann R, Lockwood G M, Turnbull A C 1991 Experience with the first 250 endometrial resections for menorrhagia. Lancet 337: 1074–1078

Maher P J, Hill D J 1990 Transcervical endometrial resection for abnormal uterine bleeding-report of 100 cases and review of the literature. Australian and New Zealand Journal of Obstetrics and Gynaecology 30(4): 357–360

Pyper R J D, Haeri A D 1991 A review of 80 endometrial resections for menorrhagia. British Journal of Obstetrics and Gynaecology 98: 1049–1054

Roos N P, Wennberg J E Malenka D J et al 1989 Mortality and reoperation after open and transurethral resection of the prostate for benign prostatic hyperplasia. New England Journal of Medicine 320: 1120–1124

Rutherford A J, Glass M R 1990 Management of menorrhagia. British Medical Journal 301: 290–291

Rutherford A J, Glass M R, Wells M 1991 Patient selection for endometrial resection. British Journal of Obstetrics and Gynaecology 98: 228–230

Siddle N, Sarrel P, Whitehead M I 1987 The effect of hysterectomy on the age of ovarian failure: identification of a subgroup of women with premature loss of ovarian function and literature review. Fertility and Sterility 47: 94–100

Sturdee D, Hoggart B 1991 Problems with endometrial resection. Lancet 337: 1474

Taylor T, Smith A N, Fulton P M 1989 Effect of hysterectomy on bowel function. British Medical Journal 299: 300–301

West J H, Robinson D A 1989 Endometrial resection and fluid absorption. Lancet ii: 1387–1388

Wingo P A, Huezo C M, Rubin G L et al 1985 The mortality risk associated with hysterectomy. American Journal of Obstetrics and Gynaecology 152: 803–808

Wood S M, Roberts F L 1990 Air embolism during transcervical resection of endometrium. British Medical Journal 300: 945

10. Electrocoagulation of the endometrium

T. G. Vancaillie

INTRODUCTION

Electrocoagulation of the endometrium once was extremely popular in Germany (Bardenheuer 1937, Baumann 1948), Austria and the Netherlands. Results published by Baumann in 1948 showed a high degree of success, not withstanding the fact that technology was not as far advanced as it is today. Using a 5–8 mm steel ball electrode on a 20 cm long insulated shaft, surgeons of the 1930s and 1940s coagulated the endometrium in a blind fashion without any form of anaesthesia. This method cannot compare with current standards. However, Baumann (1948) reports on his 10 year experience, involving 387 cases (Table 10.1) with a combined failure and complication rate of only 3.4%! Astonishing to say the least. The question comes to mind why a successful method vanished from textbooks and memories. Political and economic reasons related to the Second World War certainly play a role. However, it can safely be postulated that there are two main reasons why this successful treatment of uterine bleeding was not maintained. First of all the situation which had triggered the development of electro-coagulation of the endometrium, i.e. economic hardship, lack of hospital beds, high risk of anaesthesia etc., vanished during the 1950s. At the same time it became apparent that a related method, menolysis by radiotherapy (X-rays or radium) led to the induction of secondary malignancies. Authors such as Baumann unsuccessfully defended the method of electrocoagulation, pointing out the difference between the latter and radiotherapy. In an era of progressively more invasive surgery, defence was vain. One answer brings the next question: In what aspect have social parameters changed, leading to revival of a once doomed intervention? Economic aspects do play a role, but cannot ipso facto explain the renewed interest in endometrial ablation. Greater involvement of the patient in the decision-making process of medical therapy comes to the forefront.

When these old publications surged, they brought with them one important piece of information. Although apparently a great number of these interventions were performed, there was no report on carcinogenicity. As this is only a histor-

Table 10.1 Complications and failures after electrocoagulation of the endometrium as reported by Baumann (1948)

Indication	Number	Complication		Hysterectomy		Repeat electro-coagulation
		Early	Late	Early	Late	
Metrorrhagia	324	2	1	2	1	2
Myoma	58	3	0	0	2	0
Postmenopause	5	0	0	0	0	0
Total	387 (100%)	5 (1.3%)	1 (0.26%)	2 (0.52%)	3 (0.78%)	2 (0.52%)

ical fact, conclusions cannot be drawn hastily, but at least it is encouraging.

PATIENT SELECTION

Excessive rather than abnormal bleeding remains the main indication for performing endometrial ablation. It is obvious that endometrial carcinoma and some less common situations such as placental polyps are treated by different means. The early authors point out correctly that the greatest success is achieved in perimenopausal dysfunctional bleeding. One should bear in mind, however, that the surgery will reduce the total amount of bleeding but not necessarily rectify the erratic pattern of metrorrhagia. When novices select a first patient, a good rule is that a multiparous woman with a normal sized uterus and heavy but regular bleeding is the ideal candidate. In addition, sterilization should not be an issue, ideally because of previous tubal ligation.

Reduction of menstrual bleeding or total eradication brings alongside effects which one should consider beneficial. First of all dysmenorrhoea is reduced, almost parallel with menstrual flow.

Furthermore, a woman in surgically induced amenorrhoea may be considered sterile. There is also evidence that premenstrual symptoms are reduced (Lefler 1989, Lefler & Lefler 1991) and there may be a beneficial effect on the (re)occurrence of pelvic inflammatory disease. Analysing the potential benefit of ablation, as a method of female sterilization, one should acknowledge that it is the only method (besides hysterectomy) which offers a physiological indicator of success, namely the occurrence of amenorrhoea.

When the surgeon's objective is to target these effects in addition to reduction of menstrual flow, then it is evident that the aim should be complete amenorrhoea. Whether amenorrhoea is the final objective or not is a fundamental question every practitioner should review thoroughly. Because these side-effects have received more than their fair share of attention the reader should be warned that the occurrence of amenorrhoea is unpredictable overall, but predictably absent early on in the physician's personal experience. Therefore, it is recommended to refrain from unattainable promises when counselling patients.

Will endometrial ablation become a method of sterilization? In selected cases, yes. Hysteroscopists will learn with advancing experience to recognize at the time of surgery whether a particular patient will become amenorrhoeic. In a further step, they will be able to apply existing hysteroscopic techniques to ensure amenorrhoea in a particular patient. This implies that more than one approach or technique should be used on a case-per-case basis. Mastering only rollerball ablation of the endometrium is a mistake. Furthermore, knowledge in endocrinology and pharmacology of the lower genital tract is paramount. With regard to sterility, patients should have decided that no further fertility is desired. Quite often year-long problems with menstruation biases a person's decision.

PATIENT COUNSELLING

Expectations

Patients with excessive menstrual flow will be pleased even if amenorrhoea is not obtained. On the other hand, patients with multiple but minimal complaints may well be deceived. Time spent to explain the versatile and unpredictable outcome of the procedure is time well spent. One can summarize the counselling of the patients as follows: the flow of menstruation will be reduced in the majority of cases (>90%); the bleeding pattern is, however, unpredictable. In regard to dysmenorrhoea, a good general statement is that true dysmenorrhoea will be reduced parallel to reduction in blood flow; however, some minor cramps comparable to dysmenorrhoea may occur, even though there is amenorrhoea (and no haematometra). Pelvic pain of different origin (e.g. endometriosis) which the patient mislabels as dysmenorrhoea will not be influenced. A thorough physical examination and possibly a laparoscopy may be required to finalize the diagnosis. Finally with regard to premenstrual syndrome symptoms (Lefler 1989, Lefler & Lefler 1991), it is the author's experience that significant relief is obtained only in cases of amenorrhoea. The symptoms least influenced are the progesterone-linked symptoms such as bloating and breast tenderness. From a psychosomatic point of view it may be argued that the anticipation of menstruation aggravates symptoms, which can be improved by eliminating the menstrual cycle. It is also observed that many women with premenstrual syndrome feel better in anticipation of the surgery. This may reflect the fact that they have taken a firm decision 'to do something about it'.

Complications

Preoperative hormonal endometrial preparations may cause various side-effects, such as hot flushes, which are usually well tolerated by the patient.

A major complication of hysteroscopy is uterine perforation. This is the one complication which should not happen as the endoscopy is introduced under direct visual control. However, cervical dilatation preceding the insertion of the resectoscope does occasionally cause a perforation, which signifies the end of the procedure. Obviously a perforated uterus will not hold the distension medium. Once the resectoscope is introduced in the endometrial cavity, it should not become the instrument of a perforation. Deep trauma to the endometrium is a genuine pitfall, as it does not prevent distension of the cavity but fluid may intravasate into the vascular system even under low-pressure conditions.

Intravasation is a potential danger, which keeps even the most experienced hysteroscopists alert. The minimum pressure to distend the uterine cavity adequately is 35 mmHg whereas capillary and tissue pressures are 15 mmHg or less. There is a positive gradient, and therefore intravasation is always present, even with the most sophisticated control system. The objective of the surgeon and the operating theatre staff is to keep intravasation within acceptable limits. People with normal metabolic functions can cope with a fluid load of 1000 ml with ease. Even larger volumes will be tolerated. Compromised patients, e.g. those undergoing renal dialysis, will not be able to assimilate even a slight increase in vascular volume with encompassing hyponatraemia and hypokalaemia. Many gynaecologists may need a refresher course in electrolyte homeostasis to cope with problems inherent to fluid overload.

As distension media are discussed in a separate chapter, only certain aspects will be emphasized here. First of all Hyskon and related hyperosmolar media cause haemodilution by osmosis, and not by direct fluid overload. These macromolecules do not pass the renal filter and diuretics will therefore not eliminate them. Furthermore, diuretics may cause paradoxical hypovolaemia, because of excessive loss of free water and continued osmotic pressure. Macromolecular media are unsuitable for use with the resectoscope. Hypo-osmotic, non-conductive media such as sorbitol (with or without mannitol) and glycine are currently used widely. It is advisable to obtain electrolyte values several days prior to the surgery. The objective is to detect borderline low values, which can be corrected. Prescribing a potassium-rich diet routinely prior to operative hysteroscopy is also a good idea. When fluid overload occurs, diuresis is initiated by use of, for example, frusemide. Sorbitol, with mannitol admixed, will initiate diuresis by itself. All diuretics used will cause loss of sodium and potassium. Rather than waiting for serum values to drop below normal limits, one can initiate replacement at the time of diagnosis. An example of such treatment is to run an intravenous infusion of Ringer's lactate with added potassium (e.g. 4 mmol per 100 ml) at a rate of 50 ml/h. Every fluid overload of 1000 ml or more requires, at least, monitoring of serum electrolyte values until the excess fluid has been filtered out. One should notice that at the time of diagnosis, usually at the end of the procedure, peripheral serum values may still be normal, due to a latency period in redistribution of fluids. Increased diuresis observed in the patient is welcomed at the time, but this means also that sodium and potassium are being lost at an increasing rate. Understanding the dynamics in electrolyte imbalance is crucial in the immediate postoperative period. A patient may appear well and be discharged 2 hours after the procedure but, on arriving home, she can start to feel miserable and nauseous. Sometimes the patient becomes disoriented. However, more serious complications such as aspiration pneumonia may occur, especially if the patient's state of consciousness is affected.

If only a large-contact electrode (such as the roller) is used during the procedure, fluid overload is unlikely to occur because the tissue is coagulated rather than cut, and therefore vessels tend to be sealed rather than severed. However, large-contact electrodes used improperly may — slowly — burn a path into the uterine wall and open venous sinuses on the way. In conclusion, fluid balance must be monitored at all times under all circumstances. An easy way of doing this is to recuperate the distention fluid through direct aspiration under low negative pressure and using collection containers of the same volume as the infusion bottles.

Electrosurgical complications may occur, although not frequently. Defective insulation and connectors are important sources of misadventures. It is one of the reasons to consider electrodes as disposable items. Through and through burns of the uterine wall with large-contact electrodes will not occur when long, immobile contact with uterine wall is avoided. However, there are areas such as the tubal ostia and hysterotomy sites which are quite thin, resulting in heat conduction to neighbouring organs. In situations where there is direct and continuous contact, such as uterus – bladder or bowel adhesions, this heat conduction may result in necrosis and breakdown of the wall of the bladder or bowel. Therefore, coagulation is performed with caution at the level of the uterotubal junction and uterotomy scars. The real danger of unintended electrical burns with large-contact electrodes is that symptoms will occur several days after the procedure. Patients should be instructed to report haematuria, diarrhoea, fever, pain, etc. Pain requiring medication, other than aspirin or the like, 24 hours after the procedure should be thoroughly investigated. Early publications have mentioned the development of fistulae between the uterus and small bowel (treated by expectant management up to 9 weeks). Under comparable circumstances the large-contact electrodes are far less likely to burn through the uterine wall than loop electrodes, which are designed to do exactly that. This makes the large-contact electrodes the ideal electrodes for the 'novice resectionist'.

Excessive uterine bleeding is an unusual complication, more likely the result of forceful cervical dilatation than from electrocoagulation. When electrocoagulation is performed during heavy bleeding — which is technically possible — the uterine flow will be significantly reduced postoperatively. As a matter of fact, procedures in the 1930s and thereafter were performed to stop — successfully — ongoing metrorrhagia. Postoperative bleeding does not exceed the amount comparable to normal menstrual flow — a vague concept, but very well understood by the patient. Should the bleeding be more copious, the surgeon should suspect a potential problem. Cervical lacerations are cauterized or repaired. If bleeding seems to originate from the uterine cavity, then an intramuscular injection of Methergine (an ergometrine derivative, methylergonorine maltate) 0.2 mg is indicated. Lacerations of the uterine side wall, by electrosurgery or mechanically, may injure branches of the uterine vessels. The latter situation is highly unlikely if only large-contact electrodes are used for intra-uterine surgery.

Sporadic, unpublished reports indicate that pelvic peritonitis and all its consequences occur in the immediate and late postoperative periods. In 1948 Baumann reported on three cases in a series of 387; the symptoms of infection did not occur until 4 or more days after the procedure. Whether this warrants the use of prophylactic antibiotics remains an unanswered question.

Pregnancy, intra- or extrauterine, may be seen as a long-term complication of the procedure. There are no statistically reliable figures. It is estimated that the risk for pregnancy is reduced to about 1%. However, this figure should only be quoted by experienced operators.

ENDOMETRIAL SUPPRESSION

The rationale for endometrial suppression is simply that a suppressed endometrium is less likely to recover from a surgical insult. Preoperative suppression also reduces the bulk of the endometrial tissue and surgery will therefore be easier.

Whether a specific hormonal regimen is superior to another will be difficult to demonstrate.

Ease of use for patient and physician will probably play a major role in determining the choice of hormone therapy.

The regimen used by the author is a single intramuscular administration of Lupron Depot (leuprolide acetate) 7.5 mg during the luteal phase of the cycle. Surgery is scheduled 2–3 weeks after the injection. The total duration of action of Lupron Depot is approximately 6 weeks. A single dose will cover pre- and post-operative suppression of the endometrium.

TECHNIQUE

Positioning of the patient (Fig. 10.1)

The patient is placed in the dorsal lithotomy position. The instrument table and scrub technician are on one side, while the video monitor and fluid containers (in and out) are located on the other. Ideally, a heating blanket is available.

Anaesthesia

Any type of anaesthesia is feasible. When local anaesthesia, i.e. paracervical block, is used, with or without sedation, patients may feel some pain when the surgeon operates in the cornual areas. In addition, heat sensation is not blocked by local anaesthesia. The anaesthesiologist should be made aware of the potential for fluid overload and therefore limit the intravenous infusion.

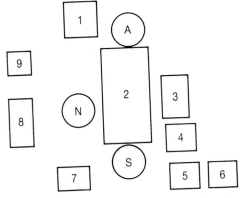

Fig. 10.1 Room set-up: this diagram gives a schematic overview of the special arrangement of the operation room. A = anaesthetist; S = surgeon; N = nurse; 1 = anaesthesia equipment; 2 = theatre table; 3 = video system; 4 = suction curettage equipment; 5 = inflow; 6 = outflow; 7 = Mayo stand; 8 = instrument table; 9 = warmer

Use of vasopressin (Pitressin)

A vasoconstrictor in conjunction with local anaesthesia is beneficial, mainly when the use of the cutting loop in anticipated. The author has extended its use to include all operative hysteroscopic procedures, except for lysis of adhesions.

Additional benefit of vasopressin is that dilatation and curettage can be performed prior to ablation with virtually no bleeding. It also seems that cervical dilatation is easier to achieve when vasopressin is infiltrated into the cervix.

Paracervical block

Even when the patient is operated upon under general anaesthesia, a paracervical block retains some merit. The anaesthetic effect of the block will last well beyond the end of the intervention and therefore reduce the need for postoperative pain medication.

Cervical dilatation

Cervical dilatation is performed with extreme care. If perforation occurs the procedure must stop. More importantly, an incomplete perforation and/or a cervical laceration, which may go unnoticed, will lead to rapid fluid overload, because large venous sinuses are injured.

Preoperative insertion of laminaria is commonplace in some institutions. For several reasons the author does not use this technique. Among them is the fact that, with laminaria, it becomes a little more difficult to distinguish the internal os. Furthermore the cervix needs to be dilated only to a diameter of 10 mm, which is in most instances readily achieved with any type of mechanical dilator.

Curettage

A thorough suction curettage is performed to remove debris and as much of the endometrium as possible. Setting a particular time, e.g. 3 minutes, which is actually monitored, will help to assure that the procedure is done thoroughly. A specimen is sent for histology, except if sampling was performed during previous investigation.

Selecting waveform and power setting (Figs. 10.2–10.5)

There are many variables with regard to the physical characteristics or radio frequency electrical current (Ch. 9). However, when a large-contact electrode is used in contact with tissue, the main tissue effect is coagulation and dessication, because of the immediate spread of energy with a resulting decrease in power density. It is well known from experiments performed early this century that low-power-density electrical energy used over a relative long period of time will cause deeper tissue destruction than an equivalent amount of energy delivered by high-power density. The explanation for this is that increasing coagulation causes an increase in tissue impedance and therefore a decrease in current flow. The ideal current for deep destruction (>5 mm) would be a continuous low-power-density waveform (a 'cutting current' of <20 W for example). The rate of tissue destruction would be very slow and therefore difficult to control for the surgeon. In addition, one has to take into account that once the electrode has coagulated the tissue underneath it and is moved forward, healthy tissue is now located behind a layer of high-impedance, coagulated tissue. It may be beneficial for the sake of understanding the process to separate the initial static phase from the second dynamic phase.

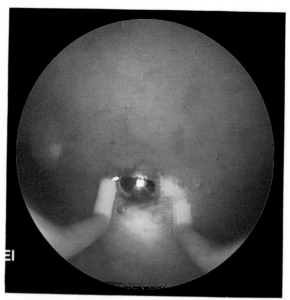

Fig. 10.3 In vivo appearance of the 'initiation phase'. Copyright TEI 1991.

Initiation (Figs. 10.2 and 10.3)

The electrode is gently pressed in contact with the tissue, and the current activated. The volume of tissue to be destroyed is relatively large, and the electrode will therefore require to be held on the same spot for a short period of time before it

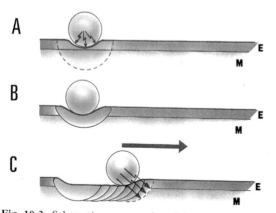

Fig. 10.2 Schematic representation of the bioeffect of electrical current on the endometrium in the **A**, **B** initiation phase and **C** dynamic phase. E, endometrium; M, myometrium.

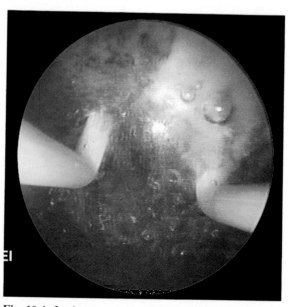

Fig. 10.4 In vivo appearance of the coagulation effects preceding the electrode. Copyright TEI 1991.

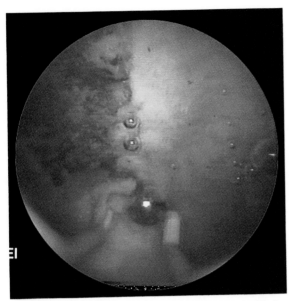

Fig. 10.5 Aspect of the cavity after a single 'stroke' with the electrode. Copyright TEI 1991.

is moved. The time required to obtain blanching around the electrode should, however, still be short (<1 second).

Dynamic phase (Figs 10.2, 10.4 and 10.5)

Once blanching is available all around the electrode, the electrode can be moved, slowly, towards the cervical canal. The speed of progression of the electrode is monitored by observation of a zone of visible tissue destruction preceding the electrode. The power necessary for the electrical current to pass through desiccated tissue and coagulate tissue in front of it is relatively high. The ability for current to transcend a resistance (coagulated tissue) depends on the available voltage. The coagulation current was designed to spark across a gap and is therefore the preferred choice at this stage of the procedure.

To couple depth of destruction with speed of surgery, it seems that a low-wattage coagulation current is a good compromise. Important variations exist among available electrosurgical units. A power output of 40–60 W is, however, a setting which will be workable in most instances.

The surgeon holds the electrode against the uterine wall and presses the coagulation pedal.

Blanching around the electrode should be visible within 1 second. Rapid explosive action is the result of too high a setting, whereas absence of a visible effect indicates that the power setting, after checking whether all connections fit, should be increased. Then the electrode is rolled towards the optic, slowly. At all times coagulation effects should be visible preceding the electrode. A smaller volume of tissue needs to be destroyed, but a shorter period of exposure is allowed, so that in effect an equal amount of energy is absorbed per unit of tissue volume.

The walls of the uterine cavity are coagulated systematically. Whether one starts on the anterior wall or any other is of no importance. However, once adopted, a particular sequence should be religiously adhered to. Obviously, prior to proceeding with electrocoagulation the surgeon explores the uterine cavity for any unexpected pathology. In particular he will look for both tubal ostia and any visible hysterotomy scars.

Fundus, cornua and internal os

The areas most difficult to reach technically are the areas where complications will arise. It requires quite some manoeuvring with the resectoscope to reach areas of the fundus and tubal ostia. Rolling the electrode is often not possible. In that instance the electrode is placed at one point, activated and then retrieved. This cycle is repeated several times until the entire fundus and adjacent cornual areas are coagulated. Care is taken not to force the electrode into the tubal ostia (Figs. 10.6 and 10.7).

The internal cervical os represents the anatomical limit of coagulation. The resectoscope is retrieved within the cervical canal, which will temporarily occlude the outflow. This allows the operator to visualize the narrow part of the internal os. Use of laminaria makes it somewhat more difficult to locate the actual anatomical site. For those who have difficulty in discerning the internal os, there is the possibility of staining the mucosa of the uterus. A drop of methylene blue is diluted in 10–20 ml of physiologic solution and slowly instilled into the uterine cavity prior to dilatation. With an endoscope, 5 mm in diameter or less, the operator can then perform a hystero-

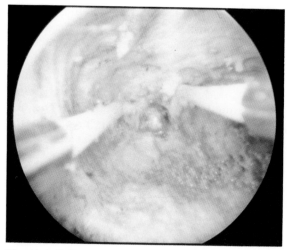

Fig. 10.6 Rollerball coagulation of the fundus by the right tubal ostium. (Courtesy of Dr Jacques Hamou)

scopy and observe the even blue coloration of the endometrium, the dark blue spots of the endosalpinx and the parallel blue lines of the endocervix.

Evaluation of the procedure

At the end of the procedure the surgeon searches for areas which appear untouched. This is extremely difficult, because electrocoagulation modifies significantly the appearance of the endometrial surface. This stresses again the need for making the first run as thorough as possible.

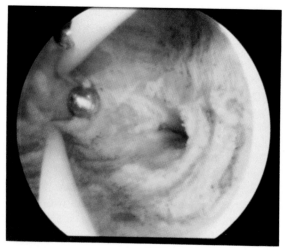

Fig. 10.7 Rollerball coagulation around the left tubal ostium. (Courtesy of Dr Jacques Hamou)

The aspect of the surface allows the operator to evaluate the presence of adenomyosis. As graphically represented in Figure 10.8, the irregular interface between the endometrium and myometrium will cause transverse grooves. Rolling the electrode over such a surface will feel like driving over speed bumps. The reason for the irregularity of the coagulated surface is that endometrium has a lower impedance than myometrium (cell-rich tissue conducts electricity better than fibrous tissue). Therefore, the endometrium is more thoroughly destroyed than the surrounding myometrium, causing these grooves in the wall. Because endometrial glands reach deep into the myometrium, the electrocoagulation of the glandular tissue may be incomplete. Resection of these areas is indicated.

INSTILLATION OF TETRACYCLINE HYDROCHLORIDE

Tetracycline hydrochloride has been used in the past as a caustic for treatment of spontaneous pneumothorax. Each patient who has the drug in intravenous infusion remembers its caustic effect. There is no slow release preparation of the drug. The crystalline form of tetracycline probably remains in situ longer than the parenteral preparation. The author uses the equivalent of 500 mg of crystalline tetracycline suspended in 3 ml of dextran, which is slowly and gently injected into the uterine cavity. Use of a viscous medium such as Hyskon will help avoid spillage of the product into the peritoneal cavity, which would lead to chemical peritonitis. Some of the instillate will escape through the cervical canal into the vagina. This is removed prior to ending the surgery, because it will irritate the vagina slightly.

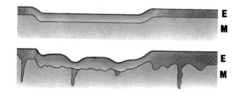

Fig. 10.8 Graphic representation of the difference between absence and presence of adenomyosis after electrocoagulation. E, endometrium; M, myometrium.

FOLLOW-UP

During the immediate postoperative phase, vital signs, vaginal bleeding and diuresis are monitored carefully. It should be stressed that bleeding and infection can occur several days after the procedure. Should one treat a patient who lives far away, one should insist on keeping contact for a period of 10 days or more. The author schedules the first postoperative visit at 6 or more weeks after the procedure. This allows the author to perform a follow-up ultrasonography for measurements of the uterus and detection of a haematometra. No intrauterine manipulation is performed. Pelvic examination demonstrates a firm uterus, slightly smaller than before surgery.

RESULTS

Overall, more than eight in ten patients are quite satisfied with this procedure. The level of satisfaction greatly depends on the expectations of the patient. Adequate preoperative counselling is therefore of primary importance. One should report results in terms of reduction in menstrual flow. However, due to lack of accurate measurement of flow, the number of days per month that a patient experiences vaginal bleeding is an acceptable substitute. Amenorrhoea is total absence of any cyclic vaginal discharge. Spotting is bleeding which lasts less than half a day. Hypomenorrhoea is bleeding lasting less than 2 days.

Patients may not always report accurately what their bleeding pattern is, especially if bleeding occurs sporadically and not on a regular basis. This type of data will always be somewhat inaccurate. In particular, when menstruation is reduced to an amount so small that protection is hardly necessary, the patient may spontaneously report complete amenorrhoea. When the author's initial publication on rollerball ablation was written, minimal spotting was included in the amenorrhoea group. In this chapter, minimal spotting is reported in the column '$<\frac{1}{2}$ day'. This distinction is, as far as the patient is concerned, only of academic importance. However, for the sake of comparing results, precise figures are required. Table 10.2 summarizes the results obtained in 90 patients between June 1986 and June 1991. Series A represents the initial study, series B represents the intermediary period and series C reports the results with the method described in this chapter.

Several comments are required. First of all it is obvious that the results from series B are poorer than those of series A. The reason for this difference is that the author made the mistake of rolling the ball too quickly during the procedure while increasing the wattage of the energy output.

The author now realizes that he gave in to one of the surgeon's natural instincts, namely to increase the speed of moving the electrode, which moreover appeared to be very efficient. Discussions with Roger Odell, electrical engineer, made the author understand that he had to alter the method of applying electrosurgery by using a low wattage — as described — and to use a slower motion.

In series C, the main element of change is the addition of a local instillation of tetracycline hydrochloride suspended in dextran 70. There is no dramatic improvement in outcome, apparently. However, it should be pointed out that more difficult cases, i.e. larger uterine cavities,

Table 10.2 Results of rollerball electrocoagulation of the endometrium[a]

Series	0 days	<1/2 day	<2 days	>2 days	Repeat ablation	Hysterectomy
A (n = 15)	[b]	10 (67%)	1 (6%)	4 (27%)	1	1
B (n = 12)	1 (8%)	4 (33%)	3 (25%)	4 (33%)	1	2
C (n = 63)	17 (27%)	24 (38%)	16 (25%)	6 (10%)	0	0

Series A starts in June 1986, B in October 1988 and C in October 1989.
[a] Average number of days of menstrual bleeding per month.
[b] In series A the results of '0 days' and '<1/2 day' are combined.

were operated upon after October 1988. Too many interfering variables preclude an objective assessment. A prospective study is currently being organized. Although series C is a larger group, no patient has requested a repeat ablation yet and no hysterectomy was performed for failed treatment.

Considering a monthly bleeding of 2 days or less to be an acceptable result, approximately 90% of patients have been cured. Of the others, three have undergone hysterectomy and one has become pregnant. Only two patients have requested a repeat ablation; both became amenorrhoeic. Repeat ablation is not performed on a large scale and therefore somewhat still unexplored.

The method as described in this chapter is not finalized yet. Improving the three aspects of treatment — i.e. hormonal inhibition, thermal destruction, scar stimulation — will eventually lead to an optimal method of endometrial ablation.

REFERENCES

Bardenheuer 1937Elektrokoagulation der Uterusschleimhaut zur Behandlung klimakterischer Blutungen.Zentralblatt Für Gynakologie 209–16

Baumann A 1948Ueber die elektrokoagulation des Endometriums sowie der Zervikalschleimhaut. Geburtshilfe und Frauenheilkunde 8: 221–6

Lefler Jr H 1989Premenstrual syndrome: improvement after laser ablation of the endometrium for menorrhagia. Journal of Reproductive Medicine 34: 905–6

Lefler Jr H, Lefler CF 1992 Ablation of the endometrium: a three year follow-up of improvement in perimenstrual symptoms. Journal Reproductive Medicine 37(2): 147–50

Vancaillie T 1989Electrocoagulation of the endometrium with the ball-end resectoscope. Obstetrics and Gynecology 74: 425–27

11. A comparison of hysteroscopic techniques

F.D. Loffer

Gynaecologists have attempted to destroy the endometrium to decrease menstrual bleeding by a variety of methods. These initially included rigorous curettage, intracavitary radium, cryotherapy, superheated steam, quinacrine, methylcyanoacrylate, oxalic acid, paraformaldehyde and silicone rubber. Only intracavitary radium was successful in destroying the basalis of the endometrium and controlling bleeding. The risk from radiation precluded its continued use. In 1981 a successful endometrial ablation technique using the neodymium:yttrium aluminium garnet (Nd:YAG) laser was described (Goldrath 1981). Later, a unipolar electrical resectoscope technique was used to accomplish the same results (DeCherney & Polan 1983).

Other lasers such as carbon dioxide, argon and potassium titanyl phosphate 532 (KTP 532) lasers, have either not been used or do not appear to be suitable for this procedure. However, several non-hysteroscopic endometrial ablation techniques are currently under investigation including radio frequency-induced endometrial destruction (Phipps et al 1990). A blind technique has the advantage of being less skill dependent than the currently available hysteroscopic procedures.

It is the purpose of this chapter to compare the two clinically proven hysteroscopic endometrial ablation methods which are presently available to gynaecologists: that using the Nd:YAG laser and that using the uterine resectoscope. This comparison will be made on patient selection, pre- and postmedical therapy, equipment differences, hysteroscopic methods, results, complications and future applications. In addition to reviewing the literature the author will draw upon his experience in endometrial ablation with the Nd:YAG laser since 1983 and the uterine resectoscope since 1986.

PATIENT SELECTION

Endometrial ablation was designed for women whose heavy and/or prolonged menstrual bleeding required them to consider a hysterectomy for its control. Both the Nd:YAG laser and resectoscope procedures are able to accomplish this purpose. Neither is, as often called by the lay press, a 'laser' or an 'electrical' hysterectomy, respectively. Since the uterus remains, neither amenorrhoea nor the avoidance of further uterine surgery can be guaranteed.

As discussed in more detail in Chapter 3, there are three types of patients who choose endometrial ablation over hysterectomy: those women who are poor surgical risks for hysterectomy, those who for various personal reasons do not wish to have a hysterectomy and, finally, those who cannot afford the time required for recovery from a hysterectomy. Either technique is suitable for these patients.

There are no specific anaesthesia differences between the techniques. General anaesthesia is not necessary (Magos et al 1989). Both techniques have been undertaken using local, epidural and general anaesthesia. All but acutely ill patients can be treated as out-patients.

Dysmenorrhoea caused by the passage of blood clots will be controlled by either technique. The control of primary dysmenorrhoea and premenstrual syndrome may be another benefit (Lefler 1989).

Submucous fibroids are frequently encountered in women requesting endometrial ablation.

These can be removed at the same time as endometrial ablation using either the Nd:YAG laser or resectoscope. When the Nd:YAG laser is used small fibroids are vaporized at the time of ablation and larger fibroids are cut into pieces and removed. When the resectoscope is used the fibroid is removed using a loop electrode. The ablation may then be done with either a loop resection or roller technique. It is the author's preference to use the resectoscope technique for fibroid removal (Loffer 1990). The author usually removes submucous fibroids prior to endometrial ablation. The reason for this is that the fibroid usually contributes the major component to excessive bleeding. It is removed first in case the procedure would have to be terminated early. Other investigators perform the ablation first since it can be done more easily and quickly than the resection of a large fibroid.

The uterine cavity size is a critical factor in selecting which technique is used. The Nd:YAG laser is not as well suited for the larger uterine cavity as is the resectoscope. Most authors who use the Nd:YAG laser technique prefer the uterus to be no larger than 8 cm with an upper maximum of 10 cm. It is feasible with the resectoscope to operate easily on patients where the cavity is 10 cm with an upper limit of 12–14 cm. This difference exists because of the means by which energy is applied to the endometrial surface. The Nd:YAG laser fibre is 600 μm wide and covers a smaller area of tissue at any given time than the electrical methods. Consequently, there is considerably greater time involved in covering the surface with the Nd:YAG laser and a greater chance of missed or inadequately treated areas. The use of higher power has been advocated to overcome this problem (Indman 1991). However, risks exist if this technique is not properly performed (Perry et al 1990).

PRE- AND POST-TREATMENT MEDICAL THERAPY

Pretreatment to obtain suppression of the endometrial thickness is probably more critical with the Nd:YAG laser technique than with the resectoscope techniques. No authors have advocated ablation of a non-prepared endometrium with the Nd:YAG laser technique but good results have been achieved without preparation using the resectoscope or the Nd:YAG laser after resectoscope ablation.

This difference between techniques is important for two reasons. First, some patients such as those with leukaemia may be bleeding so heavily that there is not time for endometrial preparation. In these cases ablation is undertaken to control the acute bleeding as well as to provide a long-term effect. Secondly, endometrial suppression is costly and often has undesirable side-effects for the patient.

There are two aspects of the non-suppressed endometrium that account for this difference. First the endometrium will be of various degrees of thickness, which makes it difficult for the operator to know whether adequate in-depth penetration has been achieved with laser energy. This problem is less critical with the electrical method since the myometrium can be identified more clearly, allowing the operator to know with somewhat more precision the actual depth of penetration. Secondly, and more importantly, a non-suppressed endometrium will tend to be redder and bleed more easily. The energy of the Nd:YAG laser is absorbed by darker colours and blood. This creates a superficial rather than an in-depth penetration effect.

If endometrial suppression has not been undertaken, a large suction curette can be used to reduce endometrial thickness and to expose the basalis layer (Lefler et al 1991).

Post-treatment endometrial suppression is routinely used by some (Table 11.1) and may be helpful in improving results (Goldrath 1990).

EQUIPMENT DIFFERENCES BETWEEN THE ND:YAG LASER AND THE RESECTOSCOPE

The initial cost of the equipment needed to perform ablation is considerably less with the electrical method than with the laser method. Most institutions have available suitable electrical generators and need only to purchase the gynaecological resectoscope. While the Nd:YAG laser technique uses standard operative hysteroscopic equipment with a laser bridge (Storz

Table 11.1   Published series of endometrial ablation procedures, their ablation method and the use of pre- and postendometrial suppression

Study	Number of patients			Pre-Rx	Post-Rx
	Nd:Yag laser	Resectoscope	Both		
Baggish (1988)	14			D	
Danniell (1986)	18			—	
Davis(1989)	25			—	
DeCherney (1987)		21	—	—	
Derman (1991)		71	P,G,D	P,G	
Garry et al (1991)	859			D,P,G	
Gimpleson (1988)	23				—
Goldfarb (1990)	35			D	D,G
Goldrath (1990)	324			D	D,P,—
Indman (1991)	13			P	—
Lefler (1991)	18				
		20			—
Lomano (1988)	62			—	—
Magos (1991)		234		D	—
McLucas (1990)		12		D,—	
Townsend (1990)		50		D,P, B	P,—
Vancaille (1989)		15		P	—
Van Damme (1992)			200	—	—
Author	100	75		D	—
				D, L	—
Total	1491	498	200		

D, danazol; G, gonadotrophin-releasing hormone (GnRH) analogue; L, luprolide; P, medroxyprogesterone acetate; B, birth control pills; —, nothing.

27021UL), it requires a large capital outlay for the energy source. The contact probes do not, at this time, have a role in endometrial ablation (Zumwalt 1986).

The ability to use an electrolyte-containing distending medium such as Ringer's lactate or normal saline with the Nd:YAG laser technique decreases some of the risk associated with hyponatraemia should excessive absorption occur (Loffer 1992). The safety requirement of using special glasses during Nd:YAG laser surgery is an inconvenience for both the surgeon and the other operating room personnel. No such special precautions are necessary with electrical methods.

METHODS OF ENDOMETRIAL ABLATION

The technical aspects of both techniques have already been discussed in detail elsewhere. Briefly, endometrial ablation techniques can be divided into those which disrupt the endometrial surface and those which leave it intact. Many surgeons find the visual end-point of disruption of the endometrial surface reassuring, indicating that adequate in-depth destruction has occurred. However, it also increases the risk of intra-operative fluid overload and postoperative bleeding because of the vessels that may be opened in the myometrium. It also may increase the risk of uterine perforation with damage to intra-abdominal structures. A combination of both methods can be used.

Disruption of the endometrial surface with the Nd:YAG laser is commonly called a 'dragging' or 'touching' technique. It is created by dragging a bare fibre through the endometrium and into the myometrium (Goldrath 1981). When the resectoscope is used to disrupt the surface a loop electrode is used to cut beneath the surface and resects the endometrium with a portion of the myometrium attached (DeCherney 1987). This is referred to as endometrial resection.

When the endometrial surface is to be left intact during a laser procedure the end of the

Nd:YAG laser fibre is brought as close in a parallel fashion to the surface as feasible without touching it (Loffer 1987). This is called a 'blanching' or 'non-touch' technique. When the resectoscope is used with this technique a roller (bar or barrel) makes contact with the endometrium (Vancaillie 1989). While the endometrium appears to disappear as the roller passes over it, the myometrium is not entered.

Many surgeons using the Nd:YAG laser use a combination technique since blanching (non-touch) is easier to accomplish in the fundus but much more difficult in the lower uterine segment, where a dragging (touching) technique can be more readily accomplished. Those authors who use a combination technique with the resectoscope first resect the endometrium and superficial myometrium and then roll over the surface with a rolling electrode in order to decrease postoperative bleeding. Only one author has advocated first ablation with the resectoscope and then following this with the Nd:YAG laser (Van Damme 1992).

Power settings are difficult to compare since the reaction of tissue varies with the energy source as well as the technique used (Moseley et al 1987, Duffy et al 1991, Indman et al 1991). In a blanching Nd:YAG laser technique, 60–70 W of power is generally used, versus 55–60 W with the dragging technique. In order to achieve adequate cutting of tissue with the resectoscope loop, approximately 100 W in the pure cut mode is the usual power setting. There is not yet a consensus among authors as to appropriate roller electrode power. Suggested power settings have ranged from as little as 35 W to over 100 W (Table 11.2).

PUBLISHED ABLATION SERIES

12 authors have contributed 1491 cases of endometrial ablation with the Nd:YAG laser to the literature (Table 11.1). Included in these figures are the author's published cases (Loffer 1987, 1988), which have been expanded in this report to cover the first 100 patients. There are fewer

Table 11.2 Endometrial techniques, the power and distension media used, and the length of the procedures

Study	Nd:YAG laser (number of patients): surface disrupted		Resectoscope (number of patients): surface disrupted		Power (W)	Media	Time (mean) (minutes)
	Yes	No	Yes	No			
Baggish (1988)	14				25–30	H	40–140 (60)
Daniell (1986)		18			50	NS	—
Davis (1989)	25				50–80	NS	45–120
DeCherney (1987)			21		30–40	H	15–30
Derman (1991)				71	30–40	H	—
Garry (1991)	859				50–80	NS	11–90 (24)
Gimpleson (1988)	23				50–60	NS	30–93 (58)
Goldfarb (1990)	35				50	NS	—
Goldrath (1990)	324				50	DS	30–40+
Indman (1991)		13			100–120	NS	17–65 (31)
Lefler (1991)	18				60–70	RL	(117)
				20	60–100	RL	(66.8)
Lomano (1988)	17				50–60	NS	30–100 (56)
		45			40–60	NS	15–55 (31)
Magos (1991)			234		100–125	G	10–100 (33.6)
McLucas (1990)				12	100	S	20–60
Townsend (1990)				50	50–100	G,S	9–55 (25)
Vancaillie (1989)				15	40–70	H	15–30
VanDamme (1992)					70	G	—
Author	46	54	10	65	55–70	RL	—
					35–100	DW/G	—

DW dextrose and water; DS, dextrose and saline; G, glycine; S, sorbitol; H, Hyskon; NS, normal saline; RL, Ringer's lactate.

published resectoscope ablation series with only seven published reports covering 423 patients. The author has added to those reported in the literature his 75 patients, for a total of 498 patients.

Two authors have had their experience with both the laser and the resectoscope. There is one series of 200 patients which used both the resectoscope and the Nd:YAG laser.

While many surgeons have additional cases that could be contributed to these results we must rely on those who have taken the time to publish their findings.

It is clear the Nd:YAG laser technique as the original ablation procedure has many more published cases but it is of interest that the resectoscope, although comprising a smaller number of cases, has almost an equal number of authors. This would suggest that the resectoscope technique, although newer, may be enjoying wider popularity.

Eight of the 12 surgeons described an Nd:YAG laser technique which disrupted the endometrial surface by making contact of the fibre with the endometrium and myometrium (Table 11.2). Two authors have used only a blanching technique and two have used both techniques. In the author's experience, if the two techniques are compared the results appear to be better with a blanching technique than when a dragging technique is used. One other investigator agrees with this and now advocates non-touch technique (Lomano 1988).

Only two of the eight published series use a resectoscope technique which disrupts the surface with a loop electrode, that is, excises the endometrium. The author has used both techniques (Table 11.2). Others combine these methods with the addition of rolling over the surface with the large-contact electrode after resection. There are, however, no published reports to allow critical evaluation of this approach.

The power used with the Nd:YAG laser ranges between 50 and 120 W, with the majority usage in the range 50–60 W. The resectoscope method has a range of 30–125 W with the higher power less frequently used.

The majority of Nd:YAG laser cases were carried out with an electrolyte-containing solution. Hyskon (dextran) was used only by one author.

The resectoscope cannot use an electrolyte solution and most cases were carried out using low-viscosity fluids. Three surgeons used Hyskon.

Although the range of time between the two techniques was quite variable, the Nd:YAG laser technique generally took longer than the resectoscopic methods.

RESULTS OF ENDOMETRIAL ABLATION

Combining all series, the number of laser cases with adequate follow-up is 1102 (Table 11.3), which can be compared to 418 resectoscope cases (Table 11.4). It is not possible to fully compare the results of endometrial ablation using the Nd:YAG laser with those of the resectoscope. The laser technique has many more reported cases and has had a longer period of usage in which to gain experience and report failures. Differences in hysteroscopic expertise of the surgeon, patient population, technique (total versus partial ablation) and criteria for reporting of results further increase the difficulty in comparing the two methods.

In addition to the author, only one investigative group has published experience with both techniques (Lefler et al 1991). Lefler and coworkers found a higher amenorrhoea rate with the resectoscope as compared to the Nd:YAG laser (60 versus 28%) and a slightly higher failure rate of 10 versus 6% with laser. The authors found a lower amenorrhoea rate with the resectoscope when compared to the Nd:YAG laser (17 versus 19%) and a slightly higher failure rate of 6 versus 5%.

The amenorrhoea rate reported by Leffler et al is less than that given in most series. However, excellent results, defined as amenorrhoea and hypomenorrhoea, are similiar to those of other authors. It should be noted that Leffler et al assign patients to a hypomenorrhoea group if any blood is apparent, even if the patients do not wear pads or report they are 'not having menstrual periods'.

While it is pleasing to both investigators and patients to achieve amenorrhoea, endometrial ablation should be considered successful if a sufficient reduction in bleeding occurs to avoid further surgery. If a satisfactory result is defined as the avoidance of hysterectomy or other sub-

Table 11.3   Results of Nd:YAG laser ablation

Study	Total number of cases	Amenorrhoea	Hypomenorrhoea	Normal menses	Failed	Short F/U [a]
Baggish (1988)	14	10 (71%)	3 (22%)	0	1 (7%)	
Daniell (1986)	18	7 (39%)	6 (33%)	1 (6%)	4 (22%)	0
Davis (1989)	25	2 (8%)	4 (16%)	5 (20%)	14 (56%) [b]	
Garry (1991)	859	288 (60%)	152 (32%)	—	39 (8%) [c]	380
Gimpleson (1988)	23	9 (39%)	6 (26%)	7 (31%)	1 (4%) [d]	
Goldfarb (1990)	35	21 (60%)	—	11 (31%)	3 (9%)	
Goldrath (1990)	324	146 (45%)	146 (45%)	7 (2%)	22 (7%) [e]	3
Indman (1991)	13	9 (69%)	4 (31%)			
Lefler (1991)	18	5 (28%)	4 (22%)	8 (44%)	1 (6%)	
Lomano (1988)	62	31 (50%)	17 (27%)	14 (23%)	0	0
Author	100	18 (19%)	55 (59%)	16 (17%)	5 (5%) [f]	6
Total	1491	546 (50%)	397 (36%)	69 (6%)	90 (8%)	389

[a] Cases are not included in denominator to determine percentage of success.
[b] Four of these patients had a repeat procedure which resulted in one amenorrhoea, hypomenorrhoea, normal menses and another failed.
[c] 23 of these patients had repeat procedures, 16 were successful.
[d] Repeated, with amenorrhoea resulting.
[e] 14 patients repeated with 10 becoming amenorrhoeic.
[f] Two patients had a repeat procedure with one patient now hypomenorrhoeic and one patient still experiencing menometrorrhagia.

sequent uterine surgical procedures (including repeat ablation), then the two techniques are essentially the same with a failure rate of 8% for the Nd:YAG laser and 10% for the resectoscope (Table 11.3 and 11.4).

Neither procedure should promise a patient amenorrhoea since this cannot be guaranteed. However, an effort should be made to decrease the menstrual flow as much as possible, since this will provide the least endometrium for possible regrowth and the potential risk of long-term failure. The Nd:YAG laser results appear to provide a slightly higher degree of decreased menstrual flow. Amenorrhoea occurs in 50 versus 35% of those treated by the resectoscope. However, excellent results (amenorrhoea or hypomenorrhoea) occur almost equally (the Nd:YAG laser at 86% and the resectoscope at 83%), and normal menses occur in 6% of the Nd:YAG laser patients versus 7% of the resectoscope patients. Combining

Table 11.4   Results of resectoscope ablation

Study	Total number of cases	Amenorrhoea	Hypomenorrhoea	Normal menses	Failed	Short F/U [a]
DeCherney (1987)	21	20 (95%)	1 (5%)	—	0	
Derman (1991) [b]	71	—	48 (77%) [b]		14 (23%)	9
Lefler (1991)	20	12 (60%)	4 (20%)	2 (10%)	2 (10%)	
McLucas (1990)	12	8 (67%)	4 (33%)	—	—	
Magos (1991)	234 [c]	75 (37%)	96 (47%)	12 (6%)	20 (10%) [d]	31
Townsend (1990)	50	10 (40%)	10 (40%)	5 (20%)		25
Vancaille (1989)	15	10 (67%)	4 (26%)	0	1 (7%)	
Author	75	10 (17%)	36 (60%)	10 (17%)	4 (6%) [e]	15
Total	498	145 (35%)	203 (48%)	29 (7%)	41 (10%)	80

[a] Cases are not included in denominator to determine percentage of success.
[b] Exact results not specified; 48 patients had successful results and 14 had further abnormal bleeding. Five patients had further surgery: hysterectomy (3) and repeat ablations (2).
[c] Exact results not specified. Results given here are interpretation of findings stated for the 18 months of follow up.
[d] 16 patients had a repeat procedure of which 13 were successful.
[e] One patient had a repeat procedure and became hypomenorrhoeic.

Table 11.5 Complications

Author	Number of cases	Bleed	Fluid overload	Infection	Perforation
Baggish (1988)	14	0	1	0	—
Danniell (1986)	18	0	0	0	0
Davis (1989)	25	0	1	1	—
DeCherney (1987)	21	0	0	0	0
Derman (1991)	71	0	—	—	—
Garry (1991)	859	0	4	4	3[a]
Gimpleson (1988)	23	1	2	—	—
Goldfarb (1990)	35	—	1	—	—
Goldrath (1990)	335	13	5	1	—
Indman (1991)	13	0	0	0	0
Lefler (1991)	38	—	—	—	—
Lomano (1990)	62	—	—	—	—
McLucas (1990)	12	0	0	0	0
Magos (1991)	250	1	7	—	4[b]
Townsend (1990)	50	—	1	—	—
Vancaille (1989)	15	0	0	0	0
Van Damme (1991)	200	1	0	0	2[c]
Author	178	0	0	0	0

0, none reported; —, no specific reference to problem by author; [a] three with scope; [b] three with resection and one with retrieval of chips; [c] one with scope and one with coagulation.

both the laser and the electrical techniques may give better results (Van Damme 1992).

Complications with endometrial ablation are few, with fluid overload being the most commonly reported problem followed by bleeding, uterine perforation and infection (Table 11.5). Fluid overload is an inherent problem of all hysteroscopic surgical procedures (Loffer 1992). Like bleeding, the risk is increased with techniques which disrupt the uterine surface. Reported cases of uterine perforation can occur both during diagnostic hysteroscopy and resection. This complication has been reported with both the laser and resectoscope (Perry et al 1990, Van Damme 1992); however, the author is also aware of serious intra-abdominal injury and death associated with all ablation techniques.

THE FUTURE OF ENDOMETRIAL ABLATION

It is quite possible that simpler techniques than hysteroscopy will be developed for endometrial ablation using other modalities. At the present time the clinician has only the two methods discussed in this chapter to use. As more gynaecologists become experienced in hysteroscopy and more patients become aware of the fact that hysterectomy for heavy menstrual bleeding is generally not required, the number of cases of endometrial ablation will undoubtedly increase. However, the procedure will ultimately fail if surgeons oversell the results of the procedure to their patients or give only a minimal effort to training, knowing that a hysterectomy can be done later. Third party and insurance companies will not reimburse for a procedure which is no more than a stepping stone before the ultimate control by hysterectomy.

The electrical method using the resectoscope would appear to be the more popular technique among surgeons at this time, not only because of its ease and quickness but because of the cost of the equipment. However, the author's experience suggests better results may be more readily achieved using the Nd:YAG laser.

REFERENCES

Baggish M S, Baltoyannis P 1988 New techniques for laser ablation of the endometrium in high-risk patients. American Journal of Obstetrics and Gynecology 159: 287–292

Daniell J, Tosh R, Meisels S 1986 Photodynamic ablation of the endometrium with the Nd:YAG laser hysteroscopically as a treatment of menorrhagia. Colposcopy and Gynecologic Laser Surgery 2: 43–46

Davis J A 1989 Hysteroscopic endometrial ablation with the neodymium–yag laser. British Journal of Obstetrics and Gynecology 96: 928–932

DeCherney A, Polan M L 1983 Hysteroscopic management of intrauterine lesion and intractable uterine bleeding. Obstetrics and Gynecology 61:392–397

DeCherney A H, Diamond M P, Lavy G, Polan M L 1987 Endometrial ablation for intractable uterine bleeding: hysteroscopic resection. Obstetrics and Gynecology 70: 668–669

Derman S G, Rehnstrom J, Neuwirth R S 1991 The long-term effectiveness of hysteroscopic treatment of menorrhagia and leiomyomas. Obstetrics and Gynecology 77: 592–594

Duffy S, Reid P C, Smith J H F, Sharp F 1991 In vitro studies of uterine electro surgery. Obstetrics and Gynecology 78: 213–220

Garry R, Erian J, Grochmal S A 1991 A multi-centre collaborative study into the treatment of menorrhagia by Nd:YAG laser ablation of the endometrium. British Journal of Obstetrics and Gynecology 98: 357–362

Gimpleson R J 1988 Hysteroscopic Nd:YAG laser ablation of the endometrium. Journal of Reproductive Medicine 33: 872–876

Goldfarb H A 1990 A review of 35 endometrial ablation using the Nd:YAG laser for recurrent menometrorrhagia. Obstetrics and Gynecology 76: 833–835

Goldrath M H 1990 Use of danazol in hysteroscopic surgery for menorrhagia. Journal of Reproductive Medicine 35: 91–96

Goldrath M H, Fuller T A, Segal S 1981 Laser photovaporization of endometrium for the treatment of menorrhagia. American Journal of Obstetrics and Gynecology 140: 14–19

Indman P D 1991 High power Nd:YAG laser ablation of the endometrium. Journal of Reproductive Medicine 36: 501–504

Indman P D, Lovoi P A, Brown W W, Lucero R T 1991 Uterine surface temperature changes caused by endometrial treatment with the Nd:YAG laser. Journal of Reproductive Medicine 36: 505–511

Lefler H T 1989 Premenstrual syndrome improvement after laser ablation of the endometrium for menorrhagia. Journal of Reproductive Medicine 34: 905–906

Lefler H T, Sullivan G H, Hulka J K 1991 Modified endometrial ablation: electrocoagulation with vasopression and suction curettage preparation. Obstetrics and Gynecology 77: 949–953

Loffer F D 1987 Hysteroscopic endometrial ablation with the Nd:YAG laser using a non-touch technique. Obstetrics and Gynecology 69: 679–682

Loffer F D 1988 Laser ablation of the endometrium. Obstetrical and Gynecological Clinics of North America 15: 77–89

Loffer F D 1990 Removal of large symptomatic intrauterine growths by the hysteroscopic resectoscope. Obstetrics and Gynecology 76: 836–840

Loffer F D 1992 Complications related to uterine distending media. In: Corfman R S, Diamond M P, DeCherney A H (eds) Complications of endoscopic procedures: intra-abdominal and intra-uterine. Blackwell Scientific, Cambridge, MA

Lomano J M 1986 Photocoagulation of the endometrium with the Nd:YAG laser for the treatment of menorrhagia. A report of ten cases. Journal of Reproductive Medicine 31: 148–150

Lomano J M 1988 Dragging technique versus blanching technique for endometrial ablation with the Nd:YAG laser in the treatment of chronic menorrhagia. American Journal of Obstetrics and Gynecology 159: 152–155

McLucas B 1990 Endometrial ablation with the roller ball electrode. Journal of Reproductive Medicine 35: 1055–1058

Magos A L, Baumann R, Cheung K, Turnbull A C 1989 Intrauterine surgery under intravenous sedation as an alternative to hysterectomy. Lancet ii: 925–926

Magos A L, Baumann R, Lockwood G M, Turnbull A C 1991 Experience with the first 250 endometrial resections for menorrhagia. Lancet 337: 1074–1078

Moseley H, Morris J D, McLeon R W, Davidson M, Hawthorn R J S, Davis J A 1987 Thermal effects of intrauterine Nd:YAG laser therapy for endometrial ablation. Lasers in Medical Science 2: 77–82

Perry C P, Daniell J F, Gimpelson R J 1990 Bowel injury from Nd:YAG endometrial ablation. Journal of Gynecological Surgery 6: 199–203

Phipps J H, Lewis B V, Roberts T, Prior M V, Hand J W, Edler M, Field S B 1990 Treatment of functional menorrhagia by radio frequency-induced thermal endometrial ablation. Lancet 335: 374–376

Townsend D E, Richart R M, Paskowitz R A, Woolfork R E 1990 "Rollerball" coagulation of the endometrium. Obstetrics and Gynecology 76: 310–313

Vancaille T G 1989 Electrocoagulation of the endometrium with the ball-end resectoscope. Obstetrics and Gynecology 74: 425–427

Van Damme J P 1992 One stage endometrial ablation: results in 200 cases. European Journal of Obstetrics and Gynecology and Reproductive Biology 43: 209–214

Zumwalt T, Wesseler T, Jaffee S N 1986 A comparison of artificial sapphire tip with the quartz tip: in invitro endometrial ablation. Colposcopy and Gynecologic Laser Surgery 2: 47–51

12. Radio frequency endometrial ablation

J.H. Phipps   B.V. Lewis

INTRODUCTION

An alternative approach to laser ablation or electroresection in the treatment of dysfunctional uterine bleeding is to use heat to ablate the endometrium without hysteroscopic surgery. The advantages of such an approach are twofold. Firstly, flushing media such as saline neodymium:yttrium-aluminium-garnet ((Nd:YAG laser)) or glycine (resection) are not required, and thus the problems of fluid overload and glycine toxicity are avoided. Secondly, the learning curve required for successful and safe laser endometrial ablation or electroresection is not required. Intravasation of fluids can lead to pulmonary or cerebral oedema (Morrison *et al* 1989), although this is unlikely unless more than 2 litres enters the circulation. Also, if excessive glycine is metabolized, hyperammonaemia may result with severe electrolyte disturbance (Magos *et al* 1990), (Table 12.1). Recently, sorbitol or mannitol has been used,

but although safer in this respect, visual clarity is said to be reduced.

The concept of totally or partially destroying the endometrial cavity by physical or chemical means is not new. In times past, toxic chemicals such as urea, silver nitrate, quinacrine and cyanoacrylate ester ('superglue') have been tried without success. Radium packing was effective, but it remains unclear to what extent the resulting amenorrhoea was due to fibrosis or ovarian irradiation. Moreover, the risk of cancer due to ionizing radiation is significant (Goldrath 1987). Cahan and Brockunier (1971) and Droegemueller *et al* (1971) attempted to 'congelate' (ablate by freezing) the endometrial cavity using a fine probe inside the uterus which was cooled to very low temperatures. Although partly successful, erratic cooling resulted in only partial endometrial destruction in some areas, and full-thickness myometrial destruction and fistula formation in others. Cryosurgery has now been abandoned.

Table 12.1 Potential advantages and disadvantages of hysteroscopic and non-hysteroscopic methods of endometrial ablation

Electroresection/Nd:YAG laser ablation	Radio frequency ablation
Advantages	*Advantages*
Direct view of operative site	Easy to learn
May be used for fibroids	No fluid-related problems
	Perforation unlikely
Disadvantages	*Disadvantages*
Fluid overload	Risk of burns
Glycine toxicity	Useful only for dysfunctional bleeding
Special training required	
Perforation/trauma possible	

Attempts to heat the uterine cavity have been made using either steam or circulating hot fluids contained within a probe or inflatable balloon catheter. These techniques have been unsuccessful for a number of reasons. An intrauterine thermal device would have to achieve a temperature in excess of 60°C in order to achieve a histotoxic temperature at the basalis layer. Thus, any fluid containing protein or blood inside the cavity will be denatured, and hence quickly solidify, causing a progressive insulation of the device with poor thermal penetration into the endometrium. Any system which relies on simple thermal conduction will be inefficient if the uterine blood flow is high, because the greater the flow, the greater the cooling, and hence the lower the heating effect. Thermal penetration is thus erratic. Escape of hot fluid into the peritoneal cavity either directly or as a consequence of catheter rupture may cause severe intra-abdominal burns, and possible intravasation into venous spaces raises the possibility of thrombus formation and embolism. Two patients treated with hot water/steam (Hardt and Genz 1989) suffered serious intestinal burns, and one patient died after 'atmocausis' of the endometrium, presumably due to leakage of hot fluid into the peritoneal cavity.

One method of heating tissue is the use of capacitative heating. When alternating current is passed across biological tissue, an electric field set up around the applicator (the thermal probe in the case of endometrial ablation) leads to a rapid oscillation of charged molecules, ions and dipoles. Local currents are consequently induced, and heating occurs. In physical terms, biological tissues under these circumstances act as 'lossy' capacitors. That is, the flow of current across tissue is not perfectly efficient, and there is a proportion of the current which is not transferred across the capacitor due to alternating charge polarity. That current which does not flow across is 'lost' as heat.

The principle of capacitative heating in which tissue is exposed to an electric field could allow safe and effective heating and destruction of the endometrium, leading to amenorrhoea or reduced menstrual flow.

THEORETICAL ASPECTS

Biology

The Greek physician Parmenedes recognized the potential beneficial effects of heat for a range of medical conditions, and Hippocrates recognized the healing effects of fever, which he felt was a natural response of the body to infection. When the human body temperature rises to 42°C, heat exhaustion occurs, and if that temperature is exceeded for any length of time, death follows. This occurs because of skeletal muscle damage with renal failure and damage to the central nervous system.

At temperatures a few degrees above normal the first changes to occur are denaturation of protein components of the cell wall and cytoskeleton such as spectrin and actin (Gerweck 1977). Human cells can survive until temperatures above 42°C are reached.

Hyperthermia refers to the heating of tissue for the purpose of destruction or inactivation of cells. The only experimental application of hyperthermia in clinical medicine is for the treatment of malignant disease, although whole-body heating has been tried in leukaemia. Temperatures in the range 44–53°C have been used alone or in combination with radiotherapy, although results are very variable. Malignant tumors in both superficial and deep sites have been heated in a number of ways. Such treatment may be given either using non-invasive applicators (superficial hyperthermia) such as bladders irrigated with hot water for tumours, or using applicators surgically placed within the tissues (interstitial hyperthermia) (Streffer 1977).

In vitro, mammalian cells survive for about 1 hour at 43°C and this time is approximately halved for each degree rise (Streffer 1977, Hahn 1982).

Physics

The authors have been investigating a method of generating heat in the endometrium by applying radio frequency electromagnetic energy to the uterine cavity. Radio frequency energy is defined as being within the frequency range 500 kHz to 2–3 gHz (Hand 1987). The frequency of 27.12

MHz was chosen because this is an assigned frequency for medical use, signal generators capable of producing such a signal are available, and the physical characteristics of this form of heating are ideal for application to the endometrium.

An electric field is generated around a probe placed within the uterine cavity, and tissue lying within that field becomes heated. Direct contact is not necessary for a therapeutic (histotoxic) effect. The electric field density falls off geometrically with distance from the radio frequency probe, so that energy penetration beyond 7 mm is minimal (Hand 1987). The amount of tissue damage depends upon the temperature, which in turn is dependent on the power applied and exposure time. These factors are variable.

It is necessary to produce a circuit through which current can flow in order to induce hyperthermia in the uterine cavity. This circuit consists of the intrauterine probe, uterus, abdominal wall and external 'return' ground plane electrode placed around the abdomen to form a resonant series circuit stimulated by the radio frequency energy source. The output of the radio frequency generator is tuned to the electrical characteristics of the individual patient such that maximum power delivery is obtained, in much the same way that a radio set is tuned to a station to give the strongest sound. Tuning is monitored using a meter which measures incident power, which is the total amount of power produced by the radio frequency-generating apparatus, and the standing wave ratio, which is a numerical comparison of voltages of the incident signal and the return signal. At a ratio of 1.0 the voltages are equal, and all of the incident power is absorbed by the tissues as heat (Fig. 12.1).

EQUIPMENT

The radio frequency ablation equipment consists of two components: the generating and monitoring apparatus and the patient application apparatus. The first prototype generator (the Menostat, manufactured by Rocket of London Ltd, UK) was built from standard modules: a radio frequency transmitter, a linear 1 kW amplifier, an antenna tuning unit and the custom-built power, probe temperature and treatment time

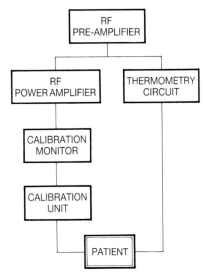

Fig 12.1 Block circuit diagram of the radio frequency endometrial ablation (RaFEA) apparatus.

measuring equipment. This has been superseded by the Mark II wholly purpose-built device (Fig. 12.2). This consists of a radio frequency generator whose output is amplified to a maximum of 400 W, although 150–300 W is typically used clinically. The power is transmitted to the intrauterine probe via a tuning circuit. The return 'arm' of the circuit consists of an insulated ground plane electrode (analogous to the earth pad used in diathermy) which is wrapped around the patient's waist and is connected to the radio frequency generator to complete the circuit.

In an early series of patients, two vesicovaginal fistulae resulted from accidental heating of the anterior vaginal wall in two grossly obese patients (Phipps et al 1990a). This was because there was inadequate retraction of the capacious vagina by the plastic Cusco speculum used. Contact of the vagina with the probe shaft occurred, and bladder damage resulted. In order to prevent this complication, a vaginal thermal guard was designed, consisting of a nylon tube which when inserted into the vagina completely retracts the walls and gives a clear view of the cervix. The bladder and rectum are thereby protected from inadvertent heating (Fig. 12.3).

The sterile thermal probe and vaginal guard are disposable (Fig. 12.4). The tip of the probe is 50, 60 or 70 mm long, according to the size of

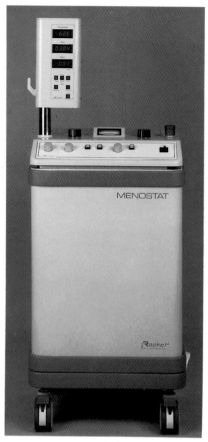

Fig. 12.2 The Menostat radio frequency endometrial ablation (Rocket of London Ltd, UK).

the endometrial cavity. This is accurately measured with a vaginal ultrasonic probe and confirmed with a uterine sound during surgery. Cavity and endocervical canal measurement is important because heating of the latter canal may lead to damage to the bladder base because the myometrium is comparatively thin in this area. The tip of the probe is angulated and is able to rotate during treatment to ensure heat is evenly distributed (Fig. 12.5).

TREATMENT TECHNIQUE

In the initial experimental series, patients were treated in the postmenstrual phase of the cycle when the endometrium is thinnest. Currently, the authors use danazol (600 mg daily for 4–6 weeks) to produce a flat endometrium prior to surgery. The efficacy of progestogens or luteinizing-hormone-releasing hormone (LH-RH) analogues has yet to be assessed.

The patient may be treated under general or regional anaesthesia. The external electrode is placed around the patient's waist, and she is placed in the lithotomy position. No part of the patient should touch earthed metal such as the operating table or metal stirrup frames, because of the risk of skin burns. The cervix is dilated to Hegar size 10, and the length of the cavity is

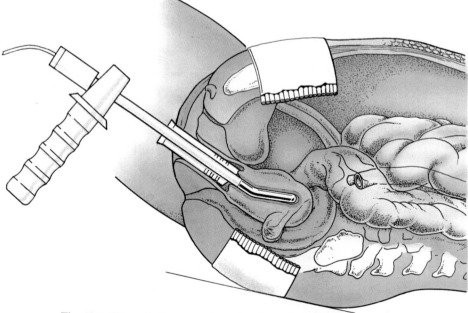

Fig. 12.3   The radio frequency thermal probe vaginal guard in situ.

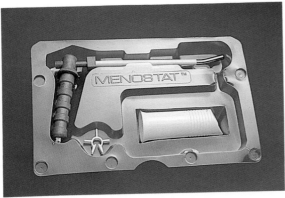

Fig. 12.4 The radio frequency thermal probe, vaginal guard and centralizing clip (Rocket of London Ltd, UK).

measured using a sound, and the length of the cervical canal estimated. The estimated length of the cervical canal is subtracted from the total length, and the corresponding probe size selected. This manoeuvre is necessary so that the cervical canal is not heated.

The thermal guard is inserted into the vagina until the leading edge is in the fornices with the cervix central. No vaginal skin should be visible to protect the bladder and rectum. It is helpful to ensure that the cervix remains central with two stay sutures placed through the anterior and posterior lips of the cervix, and passed through the opening of the guard where they are clipped and held under tension. The probe is then inserted into the cavity of the uterus. If difficulty is encountered in dilating the cervix, if there is any suspicion of perforation or if rotation is not free, the procedure *must* be abandoned.

A safety check is carried out by the surgeon and the anaesthetist before the generator is switched on. There must be no contact between the patient and any metal, and the electrocardiograph and pulse oximeter must be filtered and compatible with the radio frequency equipment. Most older monitoring equipment is unstable in the presence of radio frequency energy, and may cause burns at the site of electrocardiograph electrodes or pulse oximeter sensors if used without adequate filtering and screening because a pathway to earth may form. If monitoring

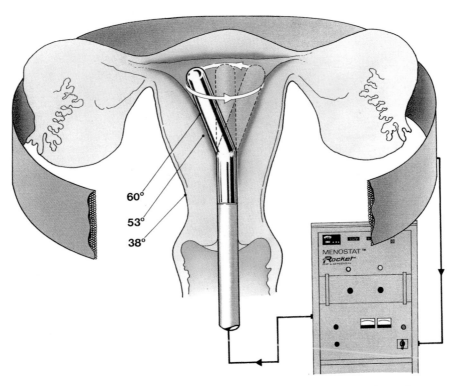

Fig. 12.5 The radio frequency thermal probe in situ showing rotation within the uterine cavity.

equipment is left connected to the patient but switched off, burns may also occur (Table 12.2).

The probe and belt electrode are connected to the radio frequency generator/monitor unit, which is switched on and set to the calibration mode. Tuning is achieved by manipulation of the two calibration controls. After tuning, the machine is switched to the treat mode, and the power increased to an initial power setting specified according to probe length. The probe temperature is measured every 3 minutes with a built-in thermistor in the probe tip, and power levels are varied so that a probe temperature of 62–65°C is maintained. The uterus is treated for a total of 15 minutes, during which time the probe is slowly rotated through 360°. At the end of the procedure, the probe, guard and clip are removed.

EXPERIMENTAL STUDIES

Temperatures achieved during treatment were measured in ten volunteers undergoing abdominal hysterectomy. All studies were carried out with ethical committee approval. Multichannel electronic thermometry was used to measure the temperatures during treatment within the uterine cavity, at various distances from the probe within the myometrium, on the surface of the uterus, surface of the bowel and base of the bladder. These studies demonstrated that, despite an intracavity temperature of around 63°C, the surface of the uterus was only one or two degrees above body temperature, and all other tissues remained at normal body temperature (Fig. 12.6) (Phipps et al 1990b).

The cooling effect of the uterine blood supply was demonstrated when radio frequency endometrial ablation (RaFEA) was performed before and after ligating the uterine arteries on two

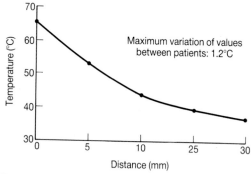

Fig. 12.6 Temperatures at various distances from the radio frequency thermal guard during endometrial ablation (550 W incident power; n=10).

abdominal hysterectomy patients. The temperature rose significantly faster and higher when the uterine vessels were clamped, demonstrating that blood flow has a significant cooling effect (Fig. 12.7).

Systemic venous blood samples were collected before surgery, immediately afterwards, and at 1 and 6 weeks postsurgery. Coagulation profiles, free haemoglobin and bilirubin levels were all normal. Uterine venous blood was sampled from an isolated uterine vein during RaFEA, and examined microscopically. No sample taken showed any of the characteristic red cell crenelation associated with thermal damage (Coakley 1987).

PATIENT SELECTION

Volunteer patients with dysfunctional uterine bleeding were fully informed of the experimental nature of the surgery, and preferred this option to hysterectomy. They had all completed their families, since the effects of endometrial ablation on fertility are unknown. Permanent sterility after the procedure cannot be guaranteed, and so simultaneous laparoscopic sterilization was offered.

Table 12.2 Safety measures

- Patient not in contact with earthed metallic surfaces (finger rings and metallic surgical implants are safe)
- Compatible, filtered electrocardiograph and pulse oximeter in use, switched on
- Power and belt earth electrode cables not in contact with patient
- Blood pressure constantly monitored
- Electrocardiograph pads fresh and correctly applied to clean, dry skin
- Good view of the cervix, maintained centrally within the thermal guard maintained at all times
- Probe temperature must not exceed 66°C

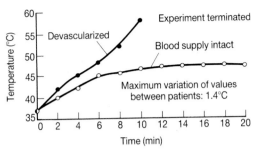

Fig. 12.7 Effect of uterine devascularization on temperature rise during endometrial ablation (450 W incident power; n=2).

Table 12.3   Results of RaFEA

Result	Number of patients
Amenorrhoeic	92
Reduced flow	112
No change	15

Organic disease such as fibroids or polyps is excluded by hysteroscopy and ultrasound scanning. A transcornual diameter of more than 35 mm is unsuitable for treatment, because the thermal probe will be ineffective. An endometrial biopsy is taken to exclude hyperplasia. The uterus must be clinically of normal size and shape, and freely mobile. There must be no suspicion of endometriosis. Patients complaining of cyclical pain or dyspareunia are excluded because of the possibility of adenomyosis. A history suggestive of significantly heavy bleeding is elicited: changing protection every 1.5 hours or more frequently because of saturation or near-saturation.

RESULTS

347 patients have been treated in four UK centres: Watford, Manchester, Glasgow and Rotherham. Of these, 219 were treated at 62–65°C for 15 minutes and have been followed up for between 4 and 14 months. Results are shown in Table 12.3, and indicate that using the definitive treatment regime in patients where the endometrial cavity is normal, either amenorrhoea or significantly reduced flow was achieved in almost 90% of cases. A 'cure' was judged when patients no longer wished further treatment for their heavy bleeding, and considered their periods acceptable.

In 15 patients menstrual loss was recorded over two cycles before and after RaFEA. The radioactive iron-59/whole-body gamma counting method was used, which is more accurate than, and does not suffer the practical disadvantages of, pad-saving studies (see Ch. 16, Part 2). The pretreatment loss was 97–1330 ml, and after RaFEA it was 0–266 ml, with a mean reduction

of 195 ml per cycle (74% reduction in loss, see Fig. 12.8). It is a feature of the technique that several cycles may elapse before the patient achieves her definitive result. Many patients experience several heavy periods after treatment, which subsequently diminish, presumably because of endometrial cavity fibrosis. The longest that any patient has been observed is 18 months. Once either amenorrhoea or a significant reduction in flow is achieved, this appears to be a permanent effect over the observed time period.

The majority of patients are now treated as day cases, and in a series of 140 patients treated only three have required overnight admission for pain relief; all were able to go home the following day. 50% of cases are able to resume work within 10 days, and the majority of the rest within 2 weeks. Approximately 10% of patients need between 2 and 4 weeks of recovery. The principle complaint that prevents return to work seems to be a feeling of general malaise and tiredness. Patients are told that they should refrain from sexual intercourse and take cephradine 250 mg four times a day for a week as prophylaxis against possible infection.

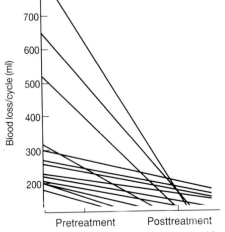

Fig. 12.8 Effect of RaFEA on blood loss measured by radioactive iron-59/ whole-body gamma counting.

Postoperative hysteroscopy at 6 months after surgery has shown a variable appearance within the uterus. In some cases the cavity is completely absent, and passage of the hysteroscope is not possible. In others, the endometrium is replaced by fibrous tissue.

COMPLICATIONS

Most of the patients complained of some abdominal pain after RaFEA, which disappears or becomes a dull ache after 4–6 hours. Two patients required overnight admission for pain control, but were both sent home the following day. All patients report a blood-stained serous vaginal discharge lasting 1–4 weeks. Although prophylactic antibiotics (cephradine 250 mg q.i.d. for 1 week) were prescribed, they are probably not necessary because postoperative infection is not significant.

Of the patients treated in the recent series using the vaginal guard, one patient developed a vesicovaginal fistula, which was subsequently repaired without further complication. The cause of this was a fold of anterior vaginal wall (and therefore bladder) which was trapped by the thermal guard and was in contact with the thermal probe shaft.

Four patients from the series complained of cyclical pain. One of these has settled spontaneously, but the other three continue. Ultrasound scans are unremarkable, but the possibility of small haematometra remains.

Electrocardiograph electrode burns and a pulse oximeter sensor burn have occurred due to the use of non-compatible equipment. It is vital that only approved monitoring equipment is used. Standard electrocardiographs are suitable *provided* a special filter is interposed between the monitor and the patient. Self-powered battery-operated pulse oximeter units are also suitable for use *provided* they have been examined and approved. The purpose-built combined monitoring unit may also be used. Built-in fuses in the latest monitoring equipment (which may also be used for general theatre purposes) mean that, even if a fault develops, burns are prevented by stopping current flow.

Studies have shown that environmental radio frequency electromagnetic energy levels are below the government recommended maximum levels with the equipment operating at power levels in excess of those used clinically. Therefore, hazards to theatre staff and patients due to excessive radio frequency exposure are not a problem. The prevention of complications depends upon the surgeon, the anaesthetist and the theatre staff, who should be familiar with the safety protocol, with the patient under constant vigilance during treatment. Theatre doors should be labelled with appropriate signs stating that radio frequency energy is in use, and entry forbidden by non-authorized staff.

THE FUTURE

Currently, a multicentre trial is underway in four centres in the UK, and it is hoped to expand this to Europe and the USA. The equipment is being continuously modified to improve safety and efficiency.

The authors have successfully treated two patients with severe cardiopulmonary disease — one awaiting pulmonary transplant for terminal bronchiectasis, the other being a postcardiac transplant case. Both women were resistant to medical therapy and were too poor a risk for major surgery. It was considered that possible intravasation of even a few hundred millilitres of fluid would represent a significant risk if hysteroscopic ablation were performed. RaFEA was therefore offered. Both patients were cured of their heavy bleeding. It is possible that RaFEA has a unique role under these circumstances.

The lack of need for specialized operating skills or high-technology operating facilities mean that the technique may be ideal for use in third world countries, particularly in Moslem communities where hysterectomy is culturally undesirable.

In conclusion, RaFEA may offer an alternative to hysteroscopic methods, and has the advantage of simplicity and speed. The estimated cost of the equipment is approximately £35 000, and is therefore considerably cheaper than Nd:YAG laser.

REFERENCES

Cahan W G, Brockunier A 1971 Cryosurgery of the uterine cavity. Obstetrics and Gynecology 38(2): 256–258

Coakley W T 1987 Hyperthermia effects on the cytoskeleton and on cell morphology. Syposia of the Society for Experimental Biology 41: 187–211

Droegemueller W, Greer B, Makowski E 1971 Cryosurgery in patients with dysfunctional uterine bleeding. Obstetrics and Gynecology 38: 256–258

Gerweck L E 1977 Modification of cell lethality at elevated temperatures. Radiation Research 70: 224–235

Goldrath M H 1987 Hysteroscopic laser ablation of the endometrium. In: Sharp F, Jordan J A (eds) Gynaecological laser surgery. Perinatology Press, New York, p 253–255

Hahn G M 1982 Hyperthermia and cancer. Springer-Verlag, New York

Hand J W 1987 Electromagnetic applicators for non-invasive local hyperthermia. In: Field S B, Franconi C (eds) Physics and technology of hyperthermia. Martinus Nijhoff, London, p 126–134

Hardt W, Genz T 1989 Atmocausis vaporisation. Most severe internal burns following intrauterine use of steam. Geburtshilfe und Frauenheilkunde 49(3): 293–295

Magos A L, Lockwood G M, Baumann R, Turnbull A C, Kay J 1990 Absorption of irrigating solution during transcervical resection of endometrium. British Medical Journal 300(6731): 1079

Morrison L M M, Davis J, Sumner D 1989 Absorption of irrigating fluid during laser photocoagulation of the endometrium in the treatment of menorrhagia. British Journal of Obstetrics and Gynaecology 96: 346–352

Phipps J H, Lewis B V, Roberts T, Prior M V, Hand J W, Field S B, Elder M 1990a Treatment of functional menorrhagia with radio frequency endometrial ablation. Lancet 335: 374–376

Phipps J H, Lewis B V, Prior M V, Roberts T 1990b Experimental and clinical studies with radio frequency endometrial ablation. Obstetrics and Gynecology 76(5): 876–882

Streffer C (ed.) 1977 Cancer therapy by hyperthermia and radiation. American Institute of Physics, New York, p 122–124

13. Fibroids

K. Wamsteker S. de Blok A. Gallinat R. P. Lueken

PART 1
RESECTION OF INTRAUTERINE FIBROIDS
K. Wamsteker S. de Blok

INTRODUCTION

Uterine fibroids, also known as leiomyomata, are the most common tumours of the uterus and a frequent indication for hysterectomy. It is estimated that between 20 and 25% of all women over 35 years of age harbour uterine fibroids (Smith 1952).

Although leiomyomata are usually named fibroids, they are of muscle cell origin and do not derive from fibrous tissue. They can be single or multiple and have a dense capsule, quite often with large superficial blood vessels (Fig. 13.1). Normally they decrease in size after the menopause.

Sarcomatous degeneration of fibroids is possible but very rare. The incidence of malignancy in myoma is stated to be less than 0.5% (Novak & Woodruff 1974). Fibroids typically affect women in their fourth or fifth decades, but they can also cause serious bleeding or fertility problems at a younger age.

Uterine fibroids are divided into three groups, according to their localization:

- Submucous — pedunculated or sessile — developing just beneath the endometrium
- interstitial or intramural, localized in the muscular wall
- Subserous — pedunculated or sessile — situated directly under the serosa.

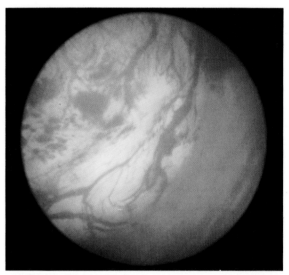

Fig. 13.1 Submucous fibroid with enlarged capsular vessels and submucosal bleeding.

As subserous and interstitial fibroids do not qualify for transcervical hysteroscopic endosurgery, only submucous fibroids will be dealt with here.

SUBMUCOUS FIBROIDS

Submucous fibroids can cause profuse bleeding and are difficult to detect with 'blind' diagnostic procedures. Before the development of hysteroscopic endosurgical techniques they frequently required hysterectomy. The symptomatology of submucous myomata may include:

- Bleeding problems — menorrhagia and metrorrhagia, resulting in anaemia
- Dysmenorrhoea and/or lower abdominal or low back pain
- Infertility
- Fetal loss or premature labour.

Depending on their localization and size, fibroids may also be asymptomatic, detectable only by routine pelvic examination or ultrasonography. Hysteroscopy is a prerequisite for the proper diagnosis and localization of submucous fibroids as they may escape detection with blind diagnostic procedures such as conventional dilatation and curettage.

Pedunculated submucous fibroids are ideal candidates for transcervical hysteroscopic removal. In cases with partial intramural extension, special techniques have to be used and sometimes the complete transcervical removal has to be accomplished in two or more surgical endoscopic procedures. With fibroids which are predominantly localized in the uterine wall, hysteroscopic resection is not advised. Instead, experimental techniques with deep neodymium: yttrium aluminium garnet (Nd:YAG) laser coagulation in these cases are under investigation and appear to yield encouraging results (Donnez et al 1990, K. Wamsteker & S. de Blok, unpublished data).

HYSTEROSCOPIC ENDOSURGICAL TREATMENT

Different techniques have been used to remove submucous fibroids with the aid of hysteroscopic endosurgical procedures. In 1976 Neuwirth & Amin described the first five cases of excision of submucous fibroids with conventional hysteroscopic endosurgery. They used a standard hysteroscope with 32% dextran 70 for distension of the uterine cavity. After excision, the fibroids were removed from the uterine cavity with ovum forceps, in one case after morcellation. One patient required abdominal

hysterotomy. Transection of the pedicle can also be performed with high-frequency electroprobes or the Nd:YAG laser, which still leaves the fibroid to be removed.

A much more elegant technique was introduced by Neuwirth in 1978, using a single-channel 8 mm urological high-frequency electroresectoscope with minor modifications to 'shave' the fibroid from the uterine wall. In 1987 Hallez et al reported the use of a continuous-flow resectoscope for better visualization, using not Hyskon but a 1.5% glycine solution for distension of the uterine cavity. The technique with continuous-flow resectoscopes and low-viscosity distension of the uterine cavity has now been widely accepted as the method of choice for the transcervical resection of submucous fibroids.

INSTRUMENTATION

Conventional mechanical techniques

Conventional techniques require 7 or 8 mm operating hysteroscopes with a working channel and semi-rigid scissors (Fig. 13.2) or high-frequency electroprobes. The scissors should be rigid rather than flexible to be able to cut the dense tissue of the pedicle of a fibroid. Large superficial blood vessels can be coagulated with the high-frequency electroprobe.

For good visualization and the ability to flush the uterine cavity if bleeding occurs a continuous-flow operating sheath is to be preferred (Fig. 13.2). Morcellation and removal of larger fibroids can be very difficult as no equipment adequately adapted to this purpose is available at present. Most authors use an ovum forceps after dilatation of the cervix.

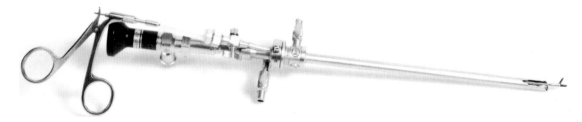

Fig. 13.2 Continuous-flow operating hysteroscope with 4 mm 30° telescope and working channel with semi-rigid scissors.

High-frequency electro-endoresection

For electro-endoresection with high-frequency current a resectoscope has to be used. This can be a resectoscope especially designed for intra-uterine resection or a urological resectoscope. In order to reduce the risk of intravasation and to enable clear visualization only continuous-flow instruments should be used. This type of resectoscope (Fig. 13.3) consists of a telescope, a working element with resection electrodes (Fig. 13.4), an insulated inner sheath and an outer sheath.

The standard resectoscope has a 4 mm tele-scope with a viewing angle of 0, 12 or 30°, to be used according to the preference of the surgeon. The working element includes the connections for the cutting electrode and the cable to the high-frequency generator. It is spring loaded and can be passive or active. In the passive system (Iglesias type) the wire loop electrode is inside the sheath in the resting position and cutting is caused by the power of the spring of the working element. In the active system the wire loop electrode is outside the sheath in the resting position and cutting is performed by actively withdrawing the electrode. The passive resectoscope is safer for intrauterine surgery, as with the active system the wire can touch the fundus of the uterus after insertion and may cause perforation, especially if the footswitch of the high-frequency generator is accidentally activated. This may result in serious bowel complications.

For standard resection of fibroids the 90° U-shaped wire loop electrode should be used (Fig. 13.5A). For the resection of small fundal area fibroids or the resection of the base of a fundal area fibroid, a 45° wire loop (Fig. 13.5B) can sometimes be of benefit, but should be used with great care as the loop can easily penetrate the uterine wall too deeply.

The inner sheath has an insulated end (Fig. 13.4) and serves as the inflow channel while the outer sheath provides for the outflow of the dis-tension medium. An obturator can be used to insert this sheath into the uterine cavity atrau-matically (Fig. 13.3), but some surgeons prefer to do this under direct vision without an obturator.

The outer diameter of the standard continuous-flow resectoscope measures approximately 9 mm (26–27 French(Fr)). Special hysteroresecto-scopes have also been developed with reduction of the outer diameter of the instrument. To this purpose, 3 mm telescopes with a viewing angle of 0° have been used. Using circular electrodes, their diameter has been reduced to 7 mm and, with U-shaped electrodes, which are preferable for myomectomy, to 8 mm (Fig. 13.6). These resectoscopes can be used for smaller fibroids with ease; for larger ones the 9 mm resectoscope is to be preferred.

A standard high-frequency generator provides the cutting and coagulating current, as for endo-metrial resection. For the wire loop electrode, the cutting current should be between 80 and 120

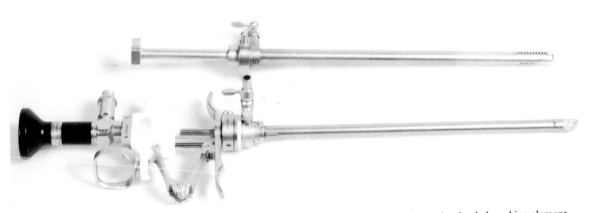

Fig. 13.3 27 French (Fr) continuous-flow resectoscope with 4 mm 12° telescope, passive spring-loaded working element, insulated inner sheath and outer sheath with visual obturator.

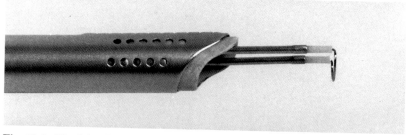

Fig. 13.4 Distal tip of 27 Fr resectoscope with 90° high-frequency wire loop electrode, insulated inner sheath and perforated outer sheath.

W, and 30–50 W for coagulation. A blended current can also be used but the authors prefer to use a pure cutting current for myomectomy.

METHODS

The uterine cavity can be distended with either high- or low-viscosity fluids, just as for conventional endosurgery. The high-viscosity fluid used for uterine distension is 32% dextran 70 in 10% dextrose in water (Hyskon), as originally described by Neuwirth (1978) and subsequently by several other authors for intrauterine resection. This fluid does not mix with blood, an important advantage if using a single-flow resectoscope. A disadvantage is that the instrument and, especially the working element and electrodes can eventually malfunction following caramelization of the dextran. The amount of Hyskon infused into the uterus should be limited to 500 ml. McLucas (1991) reported pulmonary oedema, coagulopathy and anaphylaxis as complications of Hyskon distension during hysteroscopic endosurgery.

For the more recent continuous-flow techniques, low-viscosity fluid is preferable as the uterine cavity can be flushed continuously. The fluids used in resectoscopy are 4% sorbitol, sorbitol/mannitol solution or 1.5% glycine. Although glycine was originally described for this technique by Hallez et al (1987) and is still being used in several countries for urological as well as gynaecological endoresection, the authors do not use this irrigant as they are concerned that in rare cases it may cause hyperammonaemia and encephalitis due to oxalate formation in cases of considerable intravasation.

Whatever liquid is being used, it has to be delivered under pressure. As discussed in earlier chapters, this can be accomplished by hydrostatic pressure (gravity), by means of a pressure cuff with liquid bags, or by an electronically controlled pressure pump. It goes without saying

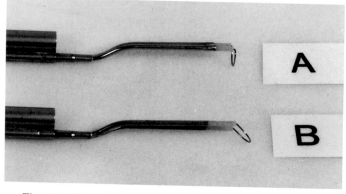

Fig. 13.5 High-frequency wire loop electrodes: A 90° and B 45°.

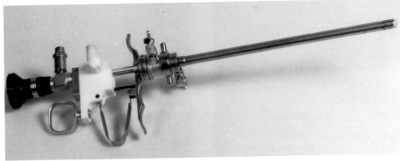

Fig. 13.6 24 Fr continuous-flow resectoscope with a 3 mm 0° telescope and passive spring-loaded working element.

that irrespective of the irrigation system, all the fluid collected through the outflow channel and any leakage from the cervix must be measured continuously and accurately and should be compared with the amount of inflow of fluid. The difference between these two measures should be considered to have been intravasated. The amount of 'missing' fluid must not exceed 1.5–2 litres because of the dangers of pulmonary oedema and electrolyte disturbances.

Finally, when operating on sessile fibroids with considerable intramural extension, laparoscopic control or, alternatively, abdominal ultrasound should be used during the resection to reduce the risk of perforation of the uterus.

OPERATIVE TECHNIQUES

The different techniques for hysteroscopic resection of submucous fibroids can be subdivided into those for pedunculated and those for sessile fibroids.

Pedunculated submucous fibroids

A small pedunculated myoma in the uterine cavity can be resected by cutting the pedicle with the operating hysteroscope and scissors, high-frequency electroprobe or Nd:YAG laser fibre. The pedicle of larger fibroids should not be cut before the fibroid itself has been reduced in size as this will be very difficult to do after transection of the pedicle. The best technique, however, is transcervical endoresection with the resectoscope, which commonly requires regional or general anaesthesia. While the 7 or 8 mm hys-

teroresector (Fig. 13.6) with a 3 mm telescope can be used for small submucous fibroids, the 9 mm resectoscope (Fig. 13.3) with a 4 mm telescope makes for easier and faster resection of the more common larger fibroids.

After dilatation of the internal os, the authors insert the outer sheath with obturator into the uterine cavity. The obturator is then replaced by the inner sheath with the electrosurgical working element, which should be filled with the distension medium before assembling to prevent the introduction of air bubbles. The uterine cavity is flushed until completely clear visualization is obtained. Before starting the resection large superficial vessels and the vessels in the pedicle can be coagulated with the wire loop and coagulating current. The authors prefer to use a pure cutting current for myoma resection as a blended current can cause adherence of the chips to the wire loop.

The fibroid is resected by bringing the wire loop behind the tumour (Fig. 13.7), activating the cutting current and withdrawing the wire loop until the resected chip is completely released from the fibroid. Generally, it is better not to withdraw the loop completely into the sheath, but to partially withdraw the whole resectoscope with the loop a little outside the sheath. The relation of the tumour to the uterine wall can thus be visualized more clearly, avoiding unnoticed resection into the uterine wall or damaging of the internal os.

The base of the pedicle should be resected very cautiously, in order not to damage the surrounding endometrium. In case of bleeding, the base of the pedicle can be coagulated. The removal of the resected pieces of the fibroid, the so-called

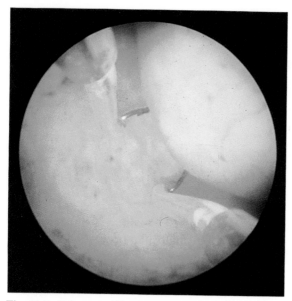

Fig. 13.7 Submucous fibroid with the starting position of the high frequency wire loop electrode before resection.

chips from the uterine cavity can be performed in several ways:

- With the high-frequency wire loop itself or, better, with a dislodging loop:
- Through the outer sheath
- By withdrawing the complete resectoscope
- With an optical forceps
- With a blunt curette
- By means of inversion of the flow of the distension medium after removal of the working element; to this purpose the inflow of the distension medium should be connected to the stopcock of the outer sheath, and thus the liquid will flush chips out through the channel of the inner sheath.

Sessile submucous fibroids

Resection of sessile fibroids requires the use of the resectoscope and, in the authors' practice, simultaneous laparoscopy. The resection of the intracavitary part of the fibroid is identical to the technique for resection of pedunculated fibroids. To resect the intramural part, the cleavage plane between the fibroid and its capsule must be identified: the fibroid tissue is whitish and nodular while the capsule tissue is greyish and smooth.

The fibroid tissue has to be resected from the capsule to be certain of complete removal of the fibroid. Intramural fibroid tissue left in place can be resorbed due to necrosis or can be expelled to the uterine cavity by myometrial contractions, in which case it has to be resected in a second session.

The above technique should only be used for submucous fibroids with less than 50% intramural extension. If the intramural extension of an intrauterine fibroid is more than 50% it should be considered unsuitable for transcervical endoresection treatment, as this quite often will require many repeat procedures. Experimental studies by Donnez et al (1990) and in the authors' centre indicate that in these cases Nd:YAG laser treatment or a combination of Nd:YAG laser treatment and endoresection appears to provide for better endosurgical modalities. The resected chips must always be sent in for histological examination, as sarcomatous degeneration cannot be identified visually.

PRESURGICAL APPRAISAL AND CLASSIFICATION

Before deciding on endosurgical treatment of one or more submucous fibroids a presurgical appraisal has to be performed. A diagnostic hysteroscopy is a prerequisite and the possibilities for successful endosurgical treatment should be ascertained. This includes the determination of the size and nature of the tumour, the number of fibroids, the localization and the amount of intramural extension.

The intramural extension of sessile fibroids can be determined hysteroscopically by observation of the angle of the fibroid with the myometrium at the attachment to the uterine wall. One should realize that the transition of the endometrium, which covers the fibroids to the normal endometrial lining of the uterine cavity, usually smooths away the actual angle (Fig. 13.8).

To be able to compare the results of treatment, the Hysteroscopy Training Centre in Haarlem, The Netherlands, introduced a classification for the intramural extent of submucous fibroids, which has been adopted by the European Society of Hysteroscopy (Table 13.1 and Fig. 13.9). A

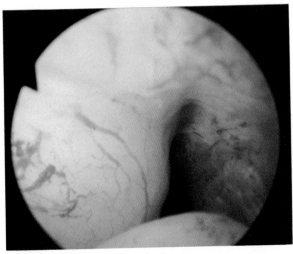

Fig. 13.8 Sessile submucous fibroid with less than 50% intramural extension (type I). Note the covering endometrium smoothing away the actual angle of the fibroid with the uterine wall.

type 0 submucous fibroid is pedunculated and has no intramural extension (Fig. 13.10). In type I cases the intramural extension is < 50% (Fig. 13.8) and in type II fibroid the intramural extension is > 50% (Fig. 13.11). Both type I and II fibroids are sessile.

Table 13.1 European Society of Hysteroscopy classification of submucous fibroids

Type	Degree of intramural extension
0	No intramural extension
I	Intramural extension < 50%
II	Intramural extension ≥ 50%

K. Wamsteker, 1990, Hysteroscopy Training Centre NL, Spaarne Hospital, Haarlem, The Netherlands.

In cases of deep intramural extension or primary intramural localization of fibroids an ultrasonographic investigation has to be performed to map the fibroids to be able to further determine the possibilities for endosurgical treatment and the technique to be used.

PRE-, INTRA- AND POSTOPERATIVE MEDICATION

Endoresection procedures for submucous fibroids should be scheduled in the proliferative

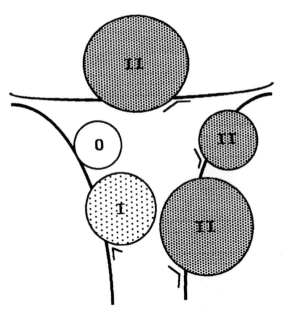

Fig. 13.9 Diagram of the uterine cavity with the three classification types of submucous fibroids: type 0, no intramural extension; type I, intramural extension < 50%; type II, intramural extension 50%.

phase of the menstrual cycle. However, to flatten the endometrium and to facilitate the procedure, preoperative medication with danazol 600 mg for approximately 3 weeks can be prescribed, starting on the first day of the cycle. It can be worthwhile reducing the size of very large fibroids with

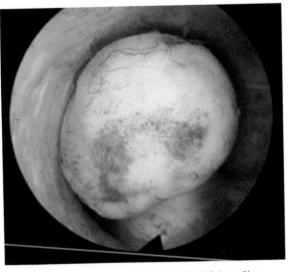

Fig. 13.10 Pedunculated submucous fibroid (type 0) without intramural extension.

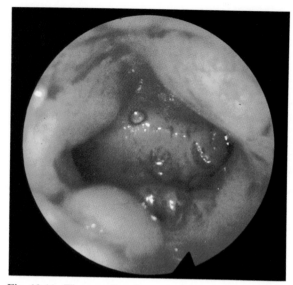

Fig. 13.11 Three sessile submucous fibroids (type II) with > 50% intramural extension.

gonadotrophin-releasing hormone (GnRH) agonist medication for a period of 2 or 3 months. This treatment can considerably reduce the size of the fibroids to facilitate hysteroscopic endoresection.

An intraoperative antibiotic prophylaxis is recommended, especially in infertility patients. The authors give cefuroxime 1500 mg and metronidazole 500 mg at the induction of anaesthesia.

Postoperative bleeding can be prevented by leaving an inflated 16 or 18 Fr balloon catheter in the uterine cavity for 6–18 hours, but this is rarely essential.

With pedunculated submucous fibroids, postoperative medication is not necessary. The authors do not recommend oestrogen medication to enhance re-epithelialization. Endometrial healing appears to be rapid and adequate without exogenous hormones.

If multiple myomectomy has been performed and there is a risk of adhesion formation between opposite uterine walls, a control hysteroscopy is recommended in the first or second cycle after operation to divide any scar tissue between the two planes. Another possibility is to leave an intrauterine contraceptive device in the uterine cavity for one or two cycles.

If the intramural part of the fibroid cannot be completely resected, a GnRH agonist or danazol can be prescribed to enhance resorption of the residual fibroid tissue. In that case a control hysteroscopy should be scheduled 3 months after the operation to determine the necessity for a second procedure.

In all other cases a control hysteroscopy is recommended 2 months after the resection to ascertain the normalization of the uterine cavity and the healing of the endometrium.

RESULTS

The results of resection of submucous fibroids published in the literature confirm the effectiveness of this technique. Excessive bleeding caused by intrauterine fibroids is controlled in more than 90% of the patients, although only a limited number of studies with long-term follow-up is presently available.

Hallez et al (1987) reported on 61 patients with sessile submucous fibroids treated in the period 1984–1986 with endoresection. In 30 of 32 patients with menorrhagia and 38 of 41 patients with metrorrhagia, the bleeding pattern had been restored to normal. In six of seven patients, secondary dysmenorrhoea disappeared. Postoperative hysterograms were normal in 49 of 54 patients. Of 11 infertility patients, seven became pregnant, of whom two had an uncomplicated spontaneous early abortion.

In 1989 Brooks et al published the results of hysteroscopic endoresection of submucous fibroids and polyps in 52 patients with a follow-up of more than 3 months. Resumption of normal menses was achieved in 91% of the patients. The term pregnancy rate in 15 patients with infertility was 33%.

Loffer (1990) published the results of 53 cases of resectoscopic treatment of large symptomatic intrauterine growths. 43 patients had sessile or pedunculated submucous fibroids and ten patients had large endometrial polyps. Long-term results were based on 45 patients with a follow-up of more than 12 months. In 93% of the patients, excessive bleeding was controlled and five patients underwent subsequent hysterectomy (9%). Two patients had repeat endoresection of fibroids and two patients had subsequent non-resectoscopic myomectomy. Seven of 12 infertility patients (58%) delivered live-born infants.

The most extended follow-up has been published by Derman et al (1991), summarizing the results of resectoscopic treatment of submucous fibroids in 94 patients with abnormal uterine bleeding (84%) and infertility (16%) treated in the period 1973–1988. Late postoperative problems occurred in 24.5% of the cases and 15.9% underwent further surgery. After 9 years of follow-up, 83.9% of the patients had not required further surgery. These data suggest that hysteroscopic management of submucous fibroids is effective over the long term, although effectiveness appears to diminish with time. 21 patients subsequently became pregnant, two having a spontaneous abortion and five voluntary termination of pregnancy. In the remaining 14 patients, 13 infants were delivered vaginally and five by caesarean section.

In the authors' centre the first 49 patients with excessive menstrual bleeding and infertility who were treated with transcervical endoresection for submucous fibroids were classified according to the classification for submucous fibroids of the European Society of Hysteroscopy (Table 13.1). Out of 33 patients with menorrhagia, the excessive bleeding was controlled in 30 cases (91%) (Table 13.2). Of 16 patients with infertility as the main indication for surgery, nine (56%) became pregnant after transcervical fibroid resection (Table 13.3), resulting in term delivery in eight cases (50%). In both groups the benefits of the endoresection therapy appear to decrease with the amount of intramural extension.

COMPLICATIONS

Complications of endoresection of submucous fibroids can be divided into complications from the resection itself and complications from the distension medium. During resection the uterine wall can be perforated, which can cause serious intestinal, vascular and other traumatic complications if this occurs unnoticed during activation of the high-frequency generator. For that reason the working element of the resectoscope should be passive and the electrode should never be activated without clear vision.

The most important potential complication is related to the distension fluid, that is, fluid overload resulting in pulmonary oedema and electrolyte disturbances due to intravasation of the fluid. The prevention of this complication has been discussed in Chapter 5 on distension fluids.

In the literature, Hallez et al (1987) reported one case of uterine perforation in 61 resections, which was recognized immediately and repaired by laparotomy. Brooks et al (1989) mentioned one perforation of the uterus during extraction of the resected pieces of a fibroid and one case of febrile endometritis following endoresection in 92 procedures. Neither patient required additional hospitalization.

In 55 endosurgical procedures with the resectoscope, Loffer (1990) reported no major complications, although he mentioned three patients with adverse effects. Two patients had more than 1000 ml of fluid retention with transient hyponatraemia, one of whom retained 4000 ml of dextrose and water with early pulmonary oedema, which should be considered to be a serious complication. Another patient had

Table 13.2 Results of transcervical resection of submucous fibroids (TCRMs): abnormal uterine bleeding

Intramural extension	Type	Number	Number of cases of menstrual bleeding after TCRM	
			Controlled	Not improved
None	0	12	12	— (0%)
< 50%	I	13	12[a]	1 (8%)
≥ 50%	II	8	6	2 (25%)
Total		33 (100%)	30 (91%)	3 (9%)

[a] One patient also had endometrial resection.

Table 13.3   Results of transcervical resection of submucous fibroids (TCRMs): infertility (follow-up >
3 months)

Intramural extension	Type	Number	Number of cases of fertility after TCRM	
			Pregnancy	No pregnancy
None	0	8[a]	5	3[a]
< 50%	I	3[b]	3[c]	0
≥ 50%	II	5	1	4
Total		16	9(56%)	7(44%)

[a] One patient had a separate intramural fibroid.
[b] Two patients had tubal occlusion and had in vitro fertilization.
[c] One patient had immature labour.

a uterine perforation during removal of the intrauterine chips.

Of the 94 women treated by Derman et al (1991), four required intraoperative or postoperative blood transfusion, two of whom underwent laparotomy. In the authors' own material of 108 endoresections for submucous fibroids we had one case of uterine perforation due to a break in the cutting loop, which was noticed immediately, and one patient who developed early pulmonary oedema and hyponatraemia caused by fluid retention of 3.5 litres of 4% sorbitol. The pulmonary oedema was perceived by the anaesthesiologist because of a drop in the oxygen saturation. Treatment consisted of frusemide and positive-pressure ventilation resulting in rapid and complete recovery.

CONCLUSION

Hysteroscopic high-frequency electro-endo-resection is a very elegant and gentle technique and the method of choice for the removal of submucous fibroids. The pedunculated type is the most favourable for this kind of treatment. Before surgery the size, number, localization and intramural extent should be determined by hysteroscopy and/or ultrasonography in order to be able to ascertain the possibilities for endo-surgical treatment and the technique to be used. Sessile fibroids with more than 50% intramural extension can be very difficult to treat with endoresection alone. Laser treatment or com-

binations of laser and endoresection most probably will be preferred in these cases. Conventional hysteroscopic endosurgical methods should only be reserved for very small pedunculated fibroids that can be removed during a diagnostic procedure.

REFERENCES

Brooks P G, Loffer F D, Serden S P 1989 Resectoscopic removal of symptomatic intrauterine lesions. Journal of Reproductive Medicine 34: 435–437
Derman S G, Rehnstrom J, Neuwirth R S 1991 The long-term effectiveness of hysteroscopic treatment of menorrhagia and leiomyomas. Obstetrics and Gynecology 77: 591–594
Donnez J, Gillerot S, Bourgonjon D, Clerckx F, Nisolle M 1990 Neodynium:YAG laser hysteroscopy in large submucous fibroids. Fertility and Sterility 54: 999–1003
Hallez J P, Netter A, Cartier R 1987 Methodical intrauterine resection. American Journal of Obstetrics and Gynecology 156: 1080–1084
Loffer F D 1990 Removal of large symptomatic intrauterine growths by the hysteroscopic resectoscope. Obstetrics and Gynecology 76: 836–840
McLucas B 1991 Hyskon complications in hysteroscopic surgery. Obstetrical and Gynecological Survey 46: 196–200
Neuwirth R S, Amin H K 1976 Excision of submucous fibroids with hysteroscopic control. American Journal of Obstetrics and Gynecology 126: 95–99
Neuwirth R S 1978 A new technique for and additional experience with hysteroscopic resection of submucous fibroids. American Journal of Obstetrics and Gynecology 131: 91–94
Novak E R, Woodruff J D 1974 Novak's gynecologic and obstetric pathology, 7th edn. W B Saunders, Philadelphia, ch 13
Smith C J 1952 Hysterectomy for benign pelvic conditions. American Journal of Obstetrics and Gynecology 64: 1211–1220

PART 2
HYSTEROSCOPIC TREATMENT OF FIBROIDS BY THE USE OF THE NEODYMIUM:YTTRIUM ALUMINIUM GARNET (Nd:YAG) LASER
A. Gallinat   R. P. Lueken

INTRODUCTION

After several early attempts (Mikulicz-Radecki & von Freund 1928, Schroeder 1934), modern surgical hysteroscopy started in the second half of the 1970s. Initially, operations were performed mechanically by the use of forceps and scissors, which allowed for the treatment of small submucous fibroids up to 2 cm in diameter, depending on their localization and the nature of their pedicle (Gallinat 1984). There was, however, no possibility to treat intramural myomata, especially when the biggest part of the fibroid mass was situated in the uterine wall. As summarized by Wamsteker in 1983 '... hysteroscopy in the management of that disorder (fibroids) has not been fully evaluated ...'.

As outlined in the previous part, one major advance in the surgical management of submucous fibroids was the introduction of electroresection by Neuwirth (Neuwirth 1978, 1984). The development of hysteroscopic surgery with the Nd: YAG laser combined with a modified hysteroscope has allowed yet another modality for the management of this common disorder. As a result of these new techniques, most fibroids, independent of size and localization, can be treated hysteroscopically (Neuwirth 1983). Nowadays, there is no need for laparotomy and hysterotomy except for large intramural and subperitoneal fibroids.

INSTRUMENTATION

Hysteroscopes

Different types of hysteroscope are now available: rigid endoscopes have an outer diameter of the metallic sheath ranging from 3.6 to 8 mm. For intrauterine Nd:YAG laser surgery the authors prefer a standard 7 mm hysteroscope. Contact hysteroscopes or microcolpohysteroscopes are of no advantage. Flexible hysteroscopes are used by several authors with good success (Dequesne 1989). However, as there is only a small opening angle from the internal os to the uterine cavity, the authors do not think that there are any real advantages as the steering mechanism for directing and deflecting the tip cannot fully rotate because of the lack of space.

For these reasons the authors favour a rigid 7 mm hysteroscope fitted with an Albarran bridge. An optimal quality of view is obtained using a 4 mm optic with a 30° fore-oblique lens, which is most suitable for the shape of the uterine cavity. This kind of optic enables good visualization of all structures, and the quality of light is perfect. The Albarran bridge makes the quartz glass fibre steerable in certain directions, thereby facilitating contact of the tip with tissue under certain circumstances. However, it is neither possible nor necessary to always achieve a frontal laser application in the small space of the uterine cavity by the use of this steering mechanism.

Lasers

The application of the Nd:YAG laser for hysteroscopy opened up new therapeutic possibilities including myomectomy. In contrast to the resectoscope, a unipolar electrical instrument, lasers are more predictable instruments for tissue destruction. For various reasons the carbon dioxide laser — so familiar in the field of gynaecology — cannot be employed for hysteroscopic surgery. The profuse generation of smoke caused by its vaporization effect would completely obscure vision. As the carbon dioxide laser beam is reflected by mirrors and prisms, coupling problems are encountered in view of the relatively thin hysteroscopes. The use of a liquid distending medium results in the absorption of the carbon dioxide laser beam. The precision of the carbon dioxide laser in the treatment of myomata is counter-productive. Furthermore, for destroying large areas of fibroids the use of the carbon dioxide laser fails on account of its small depth of penetration.

In contrast to the carbon dioxide and other lasers, the Nd:YAG laser has virtually ideal characteristics for hysteroscopic application. Standard instruments can be utilized and the thin quartz fibre that conducts the laser beam can be passed down a normal working channel. Owing to its physical properties with the coagulating effect predominating, only small amounts of smoke are generated (Fig. 13.12), which obscure vision little or only temporarily, so that operative hysteroscopy can be carried out with few problems. The depth of penetration of the Nd:YAG laser — and this physical property in particular makes it highly suitable for intrauterine application — is approximately 5 mm. A liquid irrigation medium can of course be used as detailed in Chapter 7 but, as will be seen later, carbon dioxide gaseous distension is another possibility which does not carry with it the risks of fluid overload.

The argon and potassium titanyl phosphate (KTP) lasers have similar advantages to the Nd:YAG laser. The laser light is also conducted by small quartz glass fibres so they too can be used for surgical hysteroscopy (Donnez 1989). However, these two lasers are not always satisfactory because of their tissue reaction, that is, their depth of penetration of tissue. In this respect, the Nd:YAG laser is preferable for hysteroscopic applications.

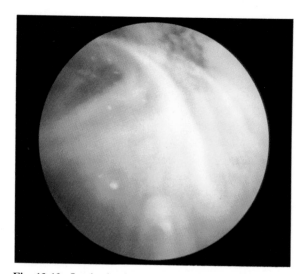

Fig. 13.12 Smoke development under Nd:YAG laser coagulation. View is cleared by the continuous carbon dioxide gas insufflation after a short time.

The limited depth of tissue destruction to about 5 mm enables safe intrauterine laser surgery. The temperature increase beyond this penetration depth is only very slight and does not denature the enzyme system. Basic studies have demonstrated that, even with higher laser output, a temperature rise to less than 50°C was measured 1 cm beneath the area of endometrial surgery, which did not lead to any necrosis (Goldrath 1981, Donnez 1989). The uterine wall, with an average thickness of 1.5cm or more, allows safe laser surgery, deeper structures not being affected.

The authors use the Medilas 40 laser unit (manufactured by MBB, Munich, Germany) or, more recently, the latest Medilas 4060, the Fibertom. For hysteroscopic surgery the exposure time is set to either maximum, that is, 20 seconds when using the Medilas 40, or continuous mode with the new Fibertom. The power output for intrauterine treatment of fibroids is preset to between 30 and 40 W. The authors use a modified quartz glass fibre without a nozzle, the diameter of this fibre being 0.6 mm.

The fibre beside the cladding is coated with a Teflon tube, the outer diameter of which is 1.4 mm (Fig. 13.13). This Teflon coating provides a second channel, which is necessary for a smoke evacuation system, and makes the fibre more rigid, making contact laser surgery easier. The larger diameter also allows better handling, and as a further advantage there is no gas leakage from the stopcocks, which can occur when using the naked thin 0.6 mm fibre.

When the authors started with Nd:YAG laser surgery in 1986 there was still confusion about which kind of fibre to use — with or without sapphire tips. In ignorance of the physical behaviour of carbon dioxide in the human body, especially when using sapphire tips, a so-called coaxial gas cooling system was supplied by the companies. Nearly all complications in Nd:YAG laser hysteroscopy are due to this unnecessarily dangerous system! For endoscopic surgery, sapphire tips are of no use. For hysteroscopic purposes, all kinds of indications can and must be handled with the so-called bare fibre, which makes surgery both easier and safer (Gallinat et al 1989).

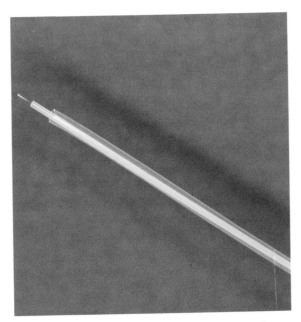

Fig. 13.13 Teflon-coated quartz glass probe that can be passed through the working channel of the 7 mm hysteroscope.

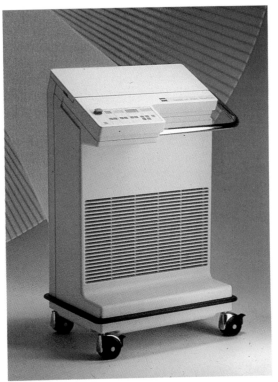

Fig. 13.14 The new Fibertom 4060 (MBB, Munich, Germany).

From the beginning of 1991, the authors have had the chance to work with the new Fibertom (Fig. 13.14). There are many advantages to using this new apparatus. Continuous tip temperature measurement regulates the laser output when changing, for example, from a contact to non-contact technique. The preset tip temperature is always constant, there being no heat congestion. This means that there is no melting or burning of the tip of the fibre. As a result of this new generation of lasers, alteration of the preset power is avoided as the laser application technique is changed. The automatic regulation of the Fibertom and the use of the quartz glass fibres is incomparably easier, and operating times as well as preoperative preparations are reduced dramatically.

DISTENSION MEDIUM

Fluid as well as gaseous distension media can be used when using the Nd:YAG laser. In contrast to resectoscopic surgery where, because of the use of unipolar current, a non-conductive medium without electrolytes must be used, all kinds of fluids can be employed for laser surgery. The use of irrigating fluids can be associated with the well-recognized complications discussed in Chapter 5, such as fluid overload, electrolyte imbalance, hyperglycinaemia and ammonia toxicity (with glycine solution), and anaphylactic reaction (with dextran 70) (Getzen et al 1963, Siegler 1975, Knudtson & Taylor 1976, Donnez 1989). For these reasons the authors almost exclusively perform carbon dioxide hysteroscopy even when performing endometrial ablation or hysteroscopic myomectomy. In comparison to the use of fluids, additional advantages of this dry medium are:

1. Better quality of view
2. Hysteroscopy is performed cleanly and quickly
3. Carbon dioxide is a physiological gas (there are no allergic reactions).

The visibility during carbon dioxide hysteroscopy is not disturbed by particles, blood or mucus. Such matter is pressed against the uterine wall because of the intrauterine gas pressure and cannot float in the distending medium, as occurs when using a liquid (Lindemann et al 1980).

When using carbon dioxide as a distending medium, it is vital to use a special insufflation apparatus such as the Metromat (manufactured by Wolf, Knittlingen, Germany). These special insufflation machines work with a fixed insufflation pressure and a limited carbon dioxide insufflation flow which guarantees the patient's safety (Lindemann 1972, Gallinat 1983). Using such an insufflation machine, the maximum insufflation pressure is about 150 mmHg and the maximal flow rate is limited to below 70 ml of carbon dioxide per minute. In this fixed range, carbon dioxide gas insufflation is safe to use (Gallinat 1978). After 10–20 seconds of carbon dioxide insufflation a good view is obtained as the pneumometra is built up very quickly. Carbon dioxide gas, with a reflection index of 1, also has the best optical qualities of all media.

For a routine diagnostic carbon dioxide hysteroscopy, which lasts about 2 minutes, only 100 ml of carbon dioxide gas is used overall. For intrauterine surgery, which can last 1 hour or longer, far more gas is insufflated but, in contrast to the use of liquid distending media, there are no electrolyte imbalances and of course no fluid overload.

There are, however, some similarities between the use of gas and fluids for uterine distension, such as direct intravasation of the medium, and this is the reason why only purpose-built insufflators should be used during hysteroscopy. The buffer capacity of blood can absorb large quantities of carbon dioxide (Lindemann et al 1976, Hulf et al 1979, Gallinat 1983). Furthermore, carbon dioxide is the gas with the highest diffusion rate, so transport of even larger quantities of carbon dioxide occurs because, after the first passage through the lung, the intravenous carbon dioxide is completely eliminated by the lungs at the first cycle of circulation (Hoeffken et al 1957).

At uncontrolled, high-flow rates tachypnoea, cardiac arrhythmias and even cardiac arrest can occur secondary to severe acidosis (Lindemann et al 1976, Gallinat 1984). When using carbon dioxide as the distension medium it is, therefore, essential to only use special insufflation apparatus. Under these circumstances carbon dioxide is the only medium without side-effects (Buchwald 1965, Lindemann & Gallinat 1976). As an indication of this inherent safety, carbon dioxide for uterotubal pertubation and hysteroscopy was introduced by Rubin in 1925. In 1947, he reported the results from 80 000 carbon dioxide tubal persufflations by 380 different authors and showed no untoward sequelae (Rubin 1947).

Under no circumstances, however, should an additional carbon dioxide tank for cooling or rinsing be used. All complications which have taken place in the last few years, with the introduction of the Nd: YAG laser for hysteroscopic surgery, were due to the so-called coaxial gas cooling system. When using this system for endoscopic procedures, each laser activation by the foot switch passed an additional amount of 500–800 ml of carbon dioxide into the uterine cavity. Ignorance of the physical behaviour of carbon dioxide insufflation can lead to a lethal outcome. Such deaths led to the US Food and Drug Administration unreasonable recommendation not to use the Nd: YAG laser in carbon dioxide hysteroscopy!

SMOKE EVACUATION SYSTEM

The only disadvantage of using carbon dioxide as a distending medium is the smoke production during Nd: YAG laser surgery. While there is only a small amount of smoke production when performing endometrial ablation, especially after optimal preoperative hormonal treatment, large amounts of smoke are produced with the treatment of large tissue masses such as broad-based septae or myomata. For continuous laser surgery, without long working gaps, production of large amounts of smoke necessitates a smoke evacuation system.

The carbon dioxide is usually insufflated via the telescope and flows from the cervix towards the fundus. If the target area is located within the upper part of the uterine cavity, the smoke collects there before condensing in the areas of the cornua. In many cases vision is improved when carbon dioxide insufflation is affected via the laser light guide, in which case the gas issues from the tip of the light guide, dispelling the smoke and keeping the view unobstructed. However, at higher outputs a considerable amount of smoke is still generated, hindering the view.

To avoid breaks in operating, the authors use a smoke evacuator for continuous gas circulation (Fig. 13.15). Essential to the development of such a machine was the fact that the carbon dioxide insufflation should not be allowed to exceed 100 ml/min (Lindemann 1972); in fact, under normal uterotubal conditions the carbon dioxide flow is about 30–40 ml/min. By controlling the inflow pressure, this new machine simultaneously clears the smoke by suction via a microfilter and, at the same time, replaces the carbon dioxide, preventing a collapse of the pneumometra (Fig. 13.16). This means that the gas insufflation from the Metromat takes place within fixed physiological limits while at the same time the intrauterine gas volume is cleared of smoke. The programmed control system is such that there is no interference between the smoke evacuator and carbon dioxide gas insufflation.

As stated earlier, the authors use a Teflon-coated probe for intrauterine Nd: YAG laser surgery. The carbon dioxide is insufflated via this Teflon-coated laser probe. The gas is delivered to the same area that smoke is produced by tissue vaporization (Fig. 13.17). The smoke is blown aside and visibility remains clear. While laser sur-

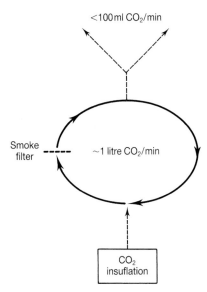

Fig. 13.16 Principle of smoke evacuation. Carbon dioxide insufflation takes place by the special insufflation machine for hysteroscopy. Under Nd:YAG laser treatment carbon dioxide-gas is aspirated from the cavity, carrying with it smoke. At the same time the carbon dioxide cleaner replaces the same amount of carbon dioxide which is aspirated, preventing collapse of pneumometra.

gery continues, the distending carbon dioxide of the pneumometra is cleared by the smoke evacuator. The smoke-containing gas is aspirated via the working channel of the hysteroscope and reinsufflated via the laser probe. The problem for hysteroscopic smoke evacuation was the relatively small volume of the uterine cavity, about 20–30 ml, coupled to the thick myometrium, requiring a high intrauterine pressure for sufficient distension. The smoke evacuator circuit therefore requires a pressure-controlled gas circulation system. While performing hysteroscopic surgery, collapse of the pneumometra should be avoided as this leads to both loss of vision and bleeding. Bleeding and probable mucous production, even in very small amounts, makes continuing hysteroscopic surgery more difficult.

Ringer's lactate is used for uterine distension and irrigation in less than 3% of cases by the authors. Generally a higher laser output of 60–80 W is required under these circumstances (Donnez et al 1990). As the fluid mixes with blood and mucus, a continuous-flow system is also preferable, the advantage being that there is no smoke to hinder the view.

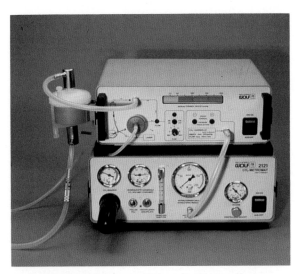

Fig. 13.15 The Metromat: Carbon dioxide insufflation machine for carbon dioxide hysteroscopy — on top of the Metromat is the new carbon dioxide cleaner (Wolf Knittlingen, Germany).

Laser target

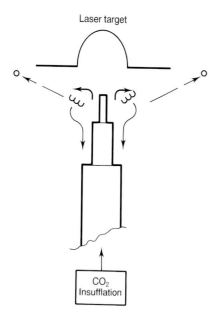

Fig. 13.17 The Teflon-coated probe is used for carbon dioxide gas insufflation. At the same time the smoke-containing carbon dioxide is aspirated via the working channel of the hysteroscope. The view remains clear.

TECHNIQUE

Submucous fibroids are a common finding in women complaining of menorrhagia or abnormal uterine bleeding (DeCherney & Polan 1983, Deutschmann & Lueken 1984, Desquesne 1987). Hysterography or curettage are old-fashioned techniques with high failure rates (Valle & Sciarra 1974, Wamsteker 1977, Hepp 1978). There are several studies showing that polyps and submucous fibroids are frequently undetected by curettage alone (Wamsteker 1984, Parent et al 1985, Donnez & Nisolle 1989). As discussed earlier, hysteroscopy introduces a very precise diagnostic technique (Valle 1981) and, nowadays, enables transcervical treatment of these diseases, avoiding classical management of myomectomy and, especially, hysterectomy. Pre-operative diagnosis, as well as postoperative follow-up, is today ideally performed by high-resolution vaginal ultrasound.

Preoperative therapy

Having confirmed the presence of submucous myoma, preoperative treatment may be required, depending on the size of the myoma. Myomata 2 cm in diameter or more should be treated by Gonadotrophin-releasing hormone (GnRH) agonists. After treatment, especially with larger myomata, shrinkage by an average of 38% occurs (Healy et al 1984, Donnez et al 1989,1990). In addition to the shrinkage, the myometrium and the covering endometrium are rendered less vascular, making surgery much easier.

Non-touch technique

In the early days of treatment of myomata, the authors used a non-contact technique. With pedunculated myomata, the pedicle close to the uterine wall was vaporized shot by shot (Fig. 13.18). By this technique there were long working gaps due to smoke production. After having vaporized the whole pedicle the shrunken myoma was removed with the biopsy forceps. By this technique, vessels are sealed and there is no bleeding (Fig. 13.19). With the additional coagulating effect, intramural parts of the myoma are simultaneously coagulated.

Intramural myomata are completely vaporized at high laser power. The smoke evacuator gives good cooling of the laser probe, otherwise the tip of the probe can be renewed intraoperatively if needed. With larger myomata this non-contact technique is, however, very time-consuming, although there is no bleeding.

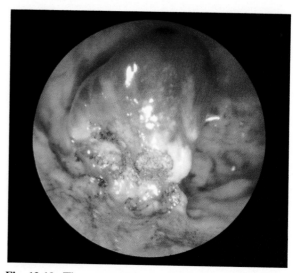

Fig. 13.18 The craters of the first Nd:YAG laser shots at the base of a submucous myoma.

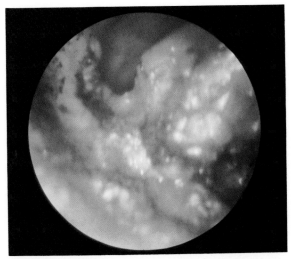

Fig. 13.19 The whole anterior part of the base of the myoma is vaporized, the posterior part is coagulated. There is no bleeding.

Touch technique

Having gained experience with the use of the Nd:YAG laser probes, the authors changed to a contact technique. The tip of the fibre was slightly pressed against the surface of the myomata and the myoma vaporized. Additional intramural parts were coagulated using a non-contact technique. The whole procedure is much faster, and there is almost no bleeding.

Combination of contact and non-contact techniques

Nowadays, with pedunculated myoma the authors cut the pedicle using the bare fibre technique. Before the pedicle is cut, and particularly if there has been no preoperative hormonal treatment, the pedicle can first be coagulated using the non-contact technique to seal the vessels, although the strong coagulating effect of the Nd:YAG laser, especially when using a gaseous distension medium, means there is virtually no bleeding (Figs. 13.20 and 13.21).

With intramural myoma, the intramural portion is also cut in contact with the bare fibre, starting at the lowest point of the myoma. As there is often slight bleeding the operation should be started at the lowest point. Using this bare fibre cutting technique, the intramural part of the

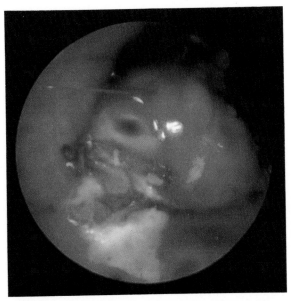

Fig. 13.20 Bare fibre cutting. The anterior part of this large submucous myoma is transversally cut.

myoma is cut at the level of the adjacent endometrial wall or a little below, whereby intramural remnants are simultaneously coagulated. If the largest part of the myoma is located intramurally, according to Donnez et al (1990) an additional

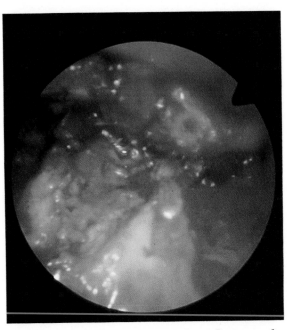

Fig. 13.21 The pedicle of the myoma is cut. Remnants of the pedicle at 12 o'clock are simultaneously coagulated.

coagulation is performed by inserting the Nd:YAG laser probe a few millimetres into the remnants of the myoma. In these patients, post-operative GnRH treatment is essential, such as two or three injections of goserelin (Zoladex) within 4–8 weeks (Donnez et al 1989). The bare fibre cutting technique has been shown to be the fastest way to cut myomata, or parts of myomata. There is only a small amount of smoke production with this technique, and bleeding is minimal.

With fibroids which are lateral or at the anterior or posterior wall, the base of the myoma is easily reached by the fibre (Fig. 13.20). At the fundus or near-fundal position the pedicle is hidden by the myoma itself. In these situations the fibre is placed behind the myoma and, under light pressure by the Teflon coating, the relatively stiff laser probe cuts the pedicle directly at the wall.

Smaller myomata (Fig. 13.22) are just coagulated in contact or non-contact mode. The high laser output guarantees coagulation of the whole myoma, especially the intramural part. The larger ones are cut. If the myoma is situated partly intramurally (Fig. 13.23) and the base cannot be seen, the authors split the myoma directly with the bare fibre, and both parts of the myoma are cut independently (Fig. 13.24). Ideal for Nd:YAG laser treatment is the larger myoma arising from the anterior wall. With a transverse cut the whole pedicle is cut close to the wall and the whole myoma is completely removed (Figs. 13.20 and 13.21). Larger-sized myomata often cannot be removed, but there are no problems associated with leaving the tissue in situ (Donnez et al 1990), as the tissue vanishes without symptoms, as confirmed by a second hysteroscopy or vaginal ultrasound follow-up.

Using carbon dioxide hysteroscopy the Nd:YAG laser output is between 30 and 40 W, while a liquid distension media power output of 80 W is required (Goldrath et al 1981, Donnez 1989). An additional advantage of using carbon dioxide hysteroscopy is that the major part of the laser energy is applied directly at the site of exposure when using either the touch or non-touch technique. Having a liquid medium, the point of maximal laser concentration is found below the surface secondary to the cooling effect of the liquid (see Fig. 7.15).

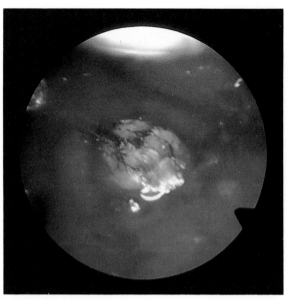

Fig. 13.22 A small intramural myoma which is coagulated. The diameter of this myoma is about 4 mm. The strong coagulating effect of the Nd:YAG laser guarantees complete coagulation of the whole intramural part.

Larger-sized intramural myomata very often require a second hysteroscopic treatment. During the first treatment as much mass of the myoma as possible should be removed. By performing intramural coagulation as many deeper

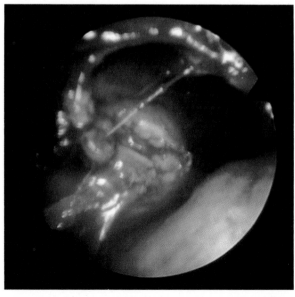

Fig. 13.23 A myoma of the left side wall, where the pedicle is hidden. The myoma is split into two parts.

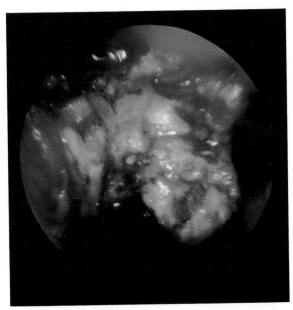

Fig. 13.24 The Nd:YAG laser probe is placed between the side wall and part of the split myoma. Parts of the myoma are vaporized by the Nd:YAG laser one after the other.

vessels of the myoma as possible are sealed. Postoperative GnRH therapy leads to shrinkage of the myoma while the vessels are diminishing. At the follow-up hysteroscopy, 6–8 weeks later, the myoma will have vanished while the remnants protrude into the cavity, and if needed can be separated easily by the Nd:YAG laser (Donnez et al 1990). As opposed to laparoscopic myoma preparation, tissue can be left in situ without problems.

If at the second hysteroscopy, blood and blood coagulum is found around the myomata, the walls being partly covered, Nd:YAG laser application is almost impossible. In these cases it is possible to flush the uterine cavity with physiological saline or other fluid medium (the authors use Ringer's lactate solution) until the blood clots spill out via the cervix. Using the same liquid, the myomectomy can be completed as described earlier using a maximum power output of 40 W.

ANAESTHESIA AND RECOVERY

All these procedures are performed in the authors department on an out-patient basis under general anaesthesia. This has been shown to be very agreeable for the patients. The authors consider that, especially in the postoperative period, the patients have less pain and feel better. After hysteroscopic treatment, patients normally leave the department after 2–4 hours. Only following prolonged operations did a very few patients need 12 hours of hospitalization. There have been no complications due to anaesthesia.

COMPLICATIONS

In the immediate postoperative period, cramping pains may be experienced. After endometrial ablation, where the entire cavity is treated, nearly half of the patients have this cramping whereas, following treatment of myomata, very few patients complain of cramping. Analgesics such as metamizole (Novalgin), pentazocine (Fortral) or naloxone hydrochloride (Valoron) are very effective for severe cramps. The day after the operation all patients are free of pain. In the authors' series, there were no operative complications during surgery. Postoperatively, there is only a slight discharge lasting for a few days which the patients did not find unacceptable.

In 1988 the authors had one severe postperative complication. Following vaporization of a large fibroid on the posterior wall using the touch technique, the operation itself was performed without difficulty. 4 days after surgery, severe bleeding started. In contrast, the authors have not seen postoperative haemorrhage associated with endometrial ablation. This may be due to the high power densities achieved during Nd:YAG laser surgery performed with carbon dioxide distension, resulting in a deeper than usual tissue coagulating effect.

Considering these results, the authors think that this technique is superior, as there are almost no complications (no intraoperative complication and only one postoperative bleeding in more than 4 years).

CONCLUSION

Nd:YAG laser treatment using carbon dioxide hysteroscopy is the safest method in modern hysteroscopic surgery. Restrictions for the use of carbon dioxide (special insufflation apparatus, no extra carbon dioxide gas tank) must be considered. Depending on the size and localization of the pedicle of the myoma, there are advantages to using either the resectoscope or the Nd:YAG laser. In general the use of the resectoscope might be easier initially. Apart from the use of unipolar current, the authors consider the main disadvantage of this technique to be that, at the moment, there exists no distension medium which is non-conductive.

There have been two main factors of importance to progress in treatment of myomata in the last few years:

1. The introduction of the Nd:YAG laser to hysteroscopic surgery and, more importantly, how to employ modern Nd:YAG laser technology, especially the use of quartz glass probes

2. The importance of preoperative hormonal treatment with GnRH agonists and their postoperative use for intramural myomata in combination with follow-up hysteroscopy.

Nd:YAG laser treatment needs some experience and requires knowledge of the techniques, but it is the one with the lowest complication rate. Although the success rate of both laser and resectoscope techniques are the same, this is the most important point to consider.

REFERENCES

Buchwald W 1965 Die Verwendung schnell resorbierbarer Gase bei diagnostischen Gasinsufflationen. Kritische Stellungnahme zum Problem der Gasembolie. 103: 187–200

Decherney A, Polan M L 1983 Hysteroscopic management of intrauterine lesions and intractable uterine bleeding. Obstetrics and Gynecology 61: 392–397

Dequesne J 1987 Hysteroscopic treatment of uterine bleeding with the Nd:YAG laser. Lasers in Medical Science 2: 73

Dequesne J 1989 Focal treatment of uterine bleeding and infertility with Nd: YAG laser and flexible hysteroscope. Journal of Gynecologic Surgery 5: 177

Deutschmann C, Lueken R P, Lindemann H J 1984 Hysteroscopic findings in postmenopausal bleeding. In: Siegler A M, Lindemann H J (eds) Hysteroscopy principles and practice. J B Lippincott, Philadelphia, p 132–134

Donnez J, 1989 Instrumentation. In: Donnez J (ed) Laser operative laparoscopy and hysteroscopy. Nauwelaerts Printing, Leuven, p 207–221

Donnez J, Nisolle M 1989 Laser hysteroscopy in uterine bleeding. Endometrial ablation and polypectomy In: Donnez J (ed) Laser operative laparoscopy and hysteroscopy. Nauwelaerts Printing, Leuven, p 277

Donnez J, Schrurs B, Gillerot S, Sandow J, Clerckx F 1989 Treatment of uterine fibroids with implants of gonadotropin-releasing hormone agonist: assessment by hysterography. Fertility and Sterility 51: 947

Donnez J, Gillerot S, Bourgonjon D, Clercks F, Nisolle M 1990 Neodymium: YAG laser hysteroscopy in large submucous fibroids. Fertility and Sterility 54: 999–1003

Gallinat A 1978 Metromat — a new insufflation apparatus for hysteroscopy. Endoscopy 3: 234

Gallinat A 1983 The Effect of carbon dioxide during hysteroscopy In: v d Pas H, v Herendael B, v Lith D, Keith L (eds) Hysteroscopy. MTP Press, Boston

Gallinat A 1984 Carbon Dioxide Hysteroscopy. Principles and Physiology In: Siegler A M, Lindemann H (eds) Hysteroscopy principles and practice. J B Lippincott, Philadelphia

Gallinat A, Leuken R P, Möller C P 1989 The use of the Nd: YAG laser in gynecological endoscopy. Laser Brief 14

Getzen J H, Speiggle W 1963 Anaphylatic reaction to dextran. A case report. Archives of Internal Medicine 112: 168–170

Goldrath M H, Fuller T A, Segal S 1981 Laser photovaporization of endometrium for the treatment of menorrhagia. American Journal of Obstetrics and Gynecology 104: 14–19

Healy D L, Fraser H M, Lawson S L 1984 Shrinkage of a uterine fibroid after subcutaneous infusion of a LH-RH agonist. British Medical Journal 209: 267

Hepp H 1978 Diagnostics in hysteroscopy. Endoscopy 10: 232

Hoeffken W, Junghans R, Zykla W 1957 Die Grundlagen der Pneumodiographie des rechten Herzens mit Kohlendioxyd (Basic principles of CO_2 - pneumoradiography of the right heart). Fortschritte auf dem Gebiete der Röntgenstrahlen 86: 292–301

Hulf J A, Corall I M, Knights K M et al 1979 Blood carbon dioxide tension changes during hysteroscopy. Fertility and Sterility 32: 193

Knudtson M L, Taylor P I 1976 Überempfindlichkeitsreaktion auf dextran 70 (Hyskon) während einer Hysteroskopie. Geburtshilfe und Frauenheilkunde 36: 263–264

Lindemann H J 1972 The use of CO_2 in the uterine cavity for hysteroscopy. International Journal of Fertility 17: 221–224

Lindemann H-J, Gallinat A 1976 Physikalische und physiologische Grundlagen der CO_2 - Hysteroskopie. Geburtshilfe Frauenheilkunde 36: 729–737

Lindemann H-J, Mohr J, Gallinat A, Buros M 1976 Der Einfluss von CO_2 - Gas während der Hysteroskopie. Geburtshilfe und Frauenheilkunde 36: 153–162

Lindemann H-J, Gallinat A, Lueken R P, Mohr J 1980 Atlas der hysteroskopie. Gustav Fischer Stuttgart

Mikulicz-Radecki, F von, Freund A 1928 Ein neues Hysteroskop und seine praktische Anwendung in der Gynäkologie. Zeitschrift für Geburtshilfe und Gynekologie 92: 13

Neuwirth R S 1978 A new technique for an additional experience with hysteroscope resection of submucous fibroids. American Journal of Obstetrics and Gynecology 131: 91–94

Neuwirth R S 1983 Hysteroscopic management of symptomatic submucous fibroids. American Journal of Obstetrics and Gynecology 62: 509

Neuwirth R S 1984 Hysteroscopic resection of submucous fibroids. In: Siegler A M, Lindemann H J (eds) Hysteroscopy principles and practice. J B Lippincott, Philadelphia, p 135–137

Neuwirth R S, Amin H K 1976 Excision of submucous fibroids with hysteroscopic control. American Journal of Obstetrics and Gynecology 126: 95–99

Parent B, Guedj H, Barbot J, Nodarian P 1985 Hysteroscopie panoramique, Maloine Paris

Rubin I C 1925 Uterine endoscopy, endometroscopy with the aid of uterine insufflation. American Journal of Obstetrics and Gynecology 10: 313

Rubin I C 1947 Uterotubal insufflation. C V Mosby, Philadelphia

Schroeder C 1934 Über den Ausbau und die Leistungen der Hysteroskopie. Archiv für Gynekologie 156: 407

Siegler A M 1975 A comparison of gas and liquid for hysteroscopy. Journal of Reproductive Medicine 15: 73

Valle R F 1981 Hysteroscopic evaluation of patients with abnormal uterine bleeding. Surgery, Gynecology and Obstetrics 153: 521

Valle R F, Sciarra J J 1974 Diagnostic and operative hysteroscopy. Minnesota Medicine 57: 892

Wamsteker K 1977 Hysteroscopie. Thesis, Women's Clinic of the University Hospital, Leiden

Wamsteker K 1983 Hysteroscopic surgery. In: van der Pas H, van Herendael B, van Lith D, Keith L (eds) Hysteroscopy. MTP Press, Boston, p 165–173

Wamsteker K 1984 Hysteroscopy in the management of abnormal uterine bleeding in 199 patients. In: Siegler A M, Lindemann H J (eds) Hysteroscopy principles and practice. J B Lippincott, Philadelphia, p 128–131

14. Pathology

M. Colafranceschi   J. Crow

INTRODUCTION

The technique of uterine curettage is so familiar to both gynaecologists and histopathologists that its use and limitations as a diagnostic and therapeutic procedure are well established and understood. The introduction of hysteroscopy, together with the associated possibilities of directed endometrial biopsy and of therapeutic endometrial resection or ablation, necessitates a consideration of the pathological effects of these various procedures, and a reconsideration of the common pathological conditions of the uterus which may be diagnosed and which may or may not be suitable for treatment by these techniques.

EFFECTS OF CURETTAGE

Since the basal layer of the endometrium is not normally removed by curettage, regeneration is usually rapid, as it is after normal menstruation. The subsequent menstrual flow has been found to occur at the expected time in 82.6% of women with regular cycles if the curettage was performed early in the cycle (Jorgensen & Enevoldsen 1963). Regeneration is slower if curettage is performed during the secretory phase (McLennan 1969, Johannisson et al 1981) and is sometimes delayed, with the endometrium appearing thin or partly denuded and showing minimal secretory changes (Cove 1981). Residual secretory areas may be out of phase with regenerated areas (Dallenbach-Hellweg 1981) and benign regenerative atypia of the epithelium may be found in the glands (Gompel & Silverberg 1985). Such atypia, particularly if in association with adenomyotic foci,

should not be mistaken for residual carcinoma in a subsequent hysterectomy specimen.

If curettage has been particularly zealous and denuded areas of uterine wall come into contact with one another, intrauterine adhesions (synechiae) can develop. This is more common in the case of postpartum curettage (Sugimoto 1978, Hamou 1991a) and it may be that inflammatory changes predispose to this development (Polishuk & Sadovsky 1975). Post-traumatic obstructive hypomenorrhoea or amenorrhoea, which is accompanied by infertility, is known as Asherman's syndrome (Asherman 1948, Carmichael 1970, Dallenbach-Hellweg 1981) and the histopathological changes seen in this include endometrial atrophy and fibrosis with adhesions across the cavity (Foix et al 1966). Adenomyosis is said to be a commonly associated condition (Gompel & Silverberg 1985).

EFFECTS OF ENDOMETRIAL RESECTION AND LASER ABLATION

In contrast to curettage, endometrial resection includes most of the basal layer of endometrium and some underlying myometrium (Figure 14.1). Regeneration of endometrium in this situation is therefore only possible from isolated residual endometrial pockets or from the isthmus, and healing is more likely to take place by a non-specific process of organization and fibrous scarring. It is therefore possible that the formation of adhesions across the cavity will prove to be more common after this procedure than after classical curettage. Very few observations have been reported on the histological appearances of the uterus following loop resection or laser ablation

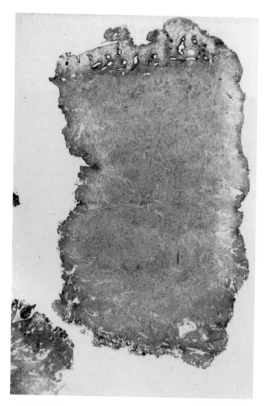

Fig. 14.1   Tissue fragment removed by transcervical endometrial resection showing endometrium and a considerable thickness of underlying myometrium.

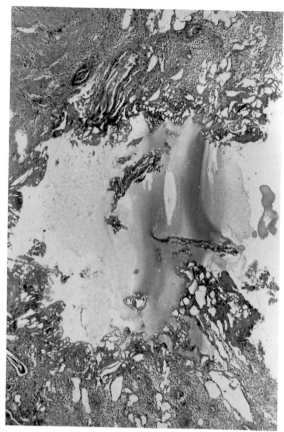

Fig. 14.2   Tissue damage as caused by laser or cutting loop of a resectoscope. The central cavity is caused by vaporization. Small surrounding cavities are produced by boiling due to direct thermal injury and further peripheral damage is due to heat conduction.

because it is only possible to examine this in patients who require hysterectomy at a later date, usually for recurrent symptoms.

The effects of laser vaporization have been reported in relation to the cervix (Colafranceschi et al 1988) and the effects in the uterine corpus are likely to be similar because the mechanisms of laser damage are the same in all living tissues. Water in tissue exposed to laser energy instantly boils and the heating of anhydrous molecules causes rapid vaporization when the energy density of the laser radiation is sufficiently high. Innumerable very small cavities are produced in the superficial layer, due to tissue disruption by flash boiling (Figure 14.2). This causes crusty carbonized debris to be removed and contributes to the vaporizing or cutting effect. Carbonization should not occur to a significant degree in correctly lasered tissue, unless the power density is so low that coagulating effects predominate. The superficial

layer of vaporization with minimal carbonization merges with an underlying dense and homogeneous layer of coagulative necrosis, devoid of microcavities, caused by an absorption of laser energy insufficient to cause vaporization. The depth of this layer is relatively constant (50–100 μm) and is not dependent on power density or exposure time. Thermal conduction causes a variable thickness of coagulative necrosis beneath this. Heat transfer through the tissue is also unrelated to power density but it is directly related to exposure time. Too low a power density (caused by low wattage or a defocused spot of laser beam) will result in a longer exposure time to reach vaporization and this will increase thermal conduction beyond the vaporized area. A slower elevation of tissue temperature also causes an increase in carbonization.

Since the correct use of the laser for a vaporising effect requires a high power density, laser endometrial ablation does not provide any tissue for histology. If such ablation techniques are to be used, it is important to obtain a representative preoperative endometrial sample for histology by either classical curettage or directed biopsies, in order to exclude atypical hyperplasia or carcinoma, which are unsuitable for treatment by endometrial ablation.

Endometrial resection performed with the heated cutting loop of the resectoscope causes similar thermal injury effects to those of laser vaporization but, because these are lesser in degree, the resected fragments are generally well enough preserved to provide material for histopathological study (Figure 14.3). Occasionally the areas of heat artefact are so extensive that

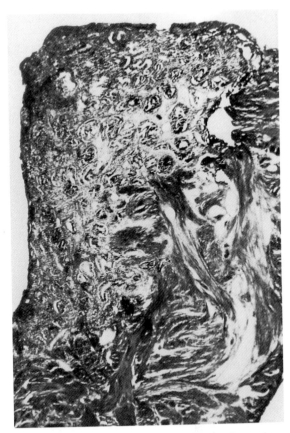

Fig. 14.4 Resected endometrial fragment showing such severe heat artefact that it is unsuitable for diagnostic histopathology.

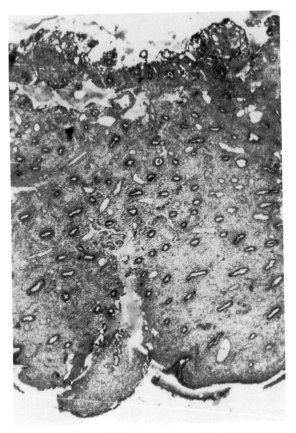

Fig. 14.3 Endometrial fragment removed by resectoscope showing thermal injury at the lower edge but quite adequate preservation to enable histopathological assessment of the endometrium to take place.

reliable histological assessment cannot be made (Figure 14.4). Endometrial resection includes the removal of up to 5 mm in depth of underlying myometrium (Hamou 1991b). Coagulation necrosis due to heat conduction is extensive in the superficial portion of the remaining myometrium and may also affect foci of superficial adenomyosis. Vessels may be dilated, or thrombosed with eosinophilic fibrinonecrotic walls (Figure 14.5) and complete obliteration of the lumen. Some preserved endometrial areas are usually found close to the tubal ostia (Figure 14.6) and these together with the spared isthmic epithelium represent sources from which epithelial regeneration may occur.

An exudative inflammatory reaction develops around the necrotic areas and is initially composed of neutrophils, macrophages, lymphocytes and plasma cells. After a few days, the

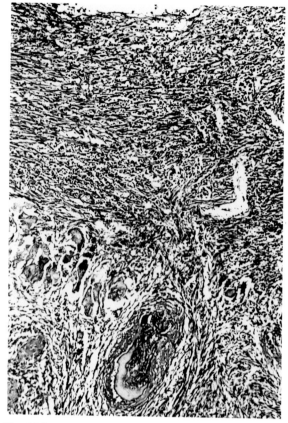

Fig. 14.5 2 weeks after endometrial resection there is a heavy inflammatory cell infiltrate in the uterine wall and extensive vascular occlusion (which may help to reduce postoperative haemorrhage).

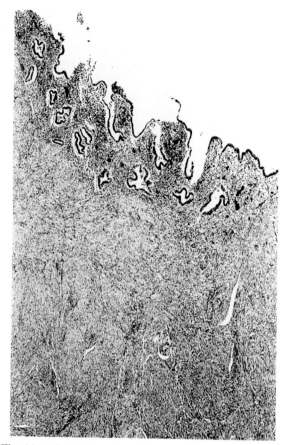

Fig. 14.6 Residual endometrium at cornu following endometrial resection.

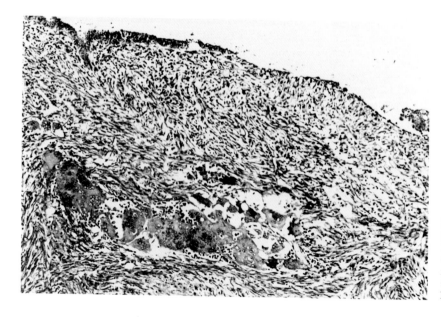

Fig. 14.7 Numerous foreign body-type giant cells are present and are lined up parallel to the endometrial surface. Such a reaction may be followed by sloughing of the overlying tissue and healing by fibrosis.

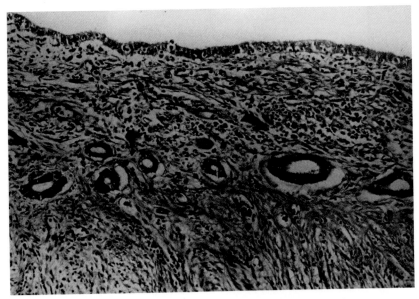

Fig. 14.8 Thin regenerated endometrium following resection.

inflammation becomes more severe and a marked giant cell granulomatous reaction develops (Figure 14.7). Foreign body giant cells can be very numerous and may show cytoplasmic inclusions. Although generally scattered in distribution, they can occasionally be arranged in palisades parallel to the uterine cavity, as though to demarcate necrotic areas which would subsequently slough.

Some regeneration of endometrium may be seen but this usually has an atrophic appearance with few glands and only a thin layer of stroma (Figure 14.8). In some cases, healing occurs by fibrosis and causes adhesions across the endometrial cavity (Figure 14.9). More rarely, a functional endometrium may be regenerated, probably from islands of endometrium which escaped the original thermal injury. If the original endometrium was hyperplastic and the patient continues to be hyperoestrogenic, it is possible for hyperplastic changes to recur.

ENDOMETRIAL SAMPLING

In the past, curettage has been the main source of endometrium for diagnostic purposes in patients presenting with abnormal uterine bleeding, and endometrial biopsy has been mainly reserved for the investigation of women with infertility or postmenopausal bleeding. Curettage may give a misleading sense of security based on the belief that the whole endometrial cavity has been sampled, although not more than 65–80% of endometrial mucosa is curetted (Stock and Kanbour 1975).

Hysteroscopy has changed the attitude of gynaecologists towards endometrial sampling, because with this technique directed biopsy can be performed under visual control. Although the biopsies obtained are small (often less than 1 mm^2) (Figure 14.10), in theory the visual control should ensure that they are a representative endometrial sample and the combination of hysteroscopic assessment and directed biopsy should enable diagnoses of hyperplasia or malignancy to be made and appropriate treatment instituted. Problems may arise, however, if there are microscopic foci of atypia which cannot be recognized on hysteroscopic examination and are therefore not biopsied and examined histologically; since it is theoretically possible for such foci to recur after ablation and possibly progress to malignancy. This possibility is lessened if multiple biopsies are taken from different areas of the endo-

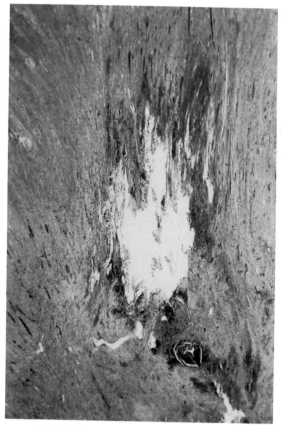

Fig. 14.9   Post-resection hysterectomy shows endometrial cavity partially obliterated by fibrous adhesions.

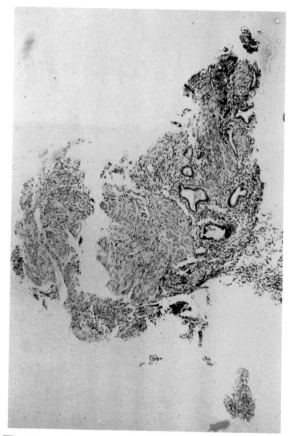

Fig. 14.10   Endometrial biopsy sample showing atrophic endometrium and underlying myometrium. The specimen is small and, to ensure adequate and representative sampling, multiple biopsies may need to be taken.

metrium, and taking multiple samples facilitates histological interpretation in general.

There is also an advantage in performing hysteroscopy immediately before an endometrial sampling technique such as Vabra, Novak or Pipelle, because this allows better orientation of the endometrial cavity and of the sample.

UTERINE PATHOLOGY

Adenomyosis

Adenomyosis is defined as the presence of endometrial tissue within the myometrium, beyond its 'normal' limits (Figure 14.11). It is a common condition, being detected in about 15–20% of uteri (Tiltman 1980). However, since the endomyometrial border is normally quite irregular and the depth of myometrial penetration in adenomyosis is variable, the incidence of the condition

also varies according to the exact diagnostic criteria being followed. A distance of more than one (Gompel & Silverberg 1985) or one-half low-power field (Zaloudek & Norris 1987) between the adenomyotic focus and the lower border of the endometrium has been assumed as a prerequisite for the diagnosis of adenomyosis. Other pathologists relate the depth of penetration of the endometrial tissue to the thickness of the myometrium and express this value as a proportion.

Macroscopically, adenomyosis appears as pink or greyish soft areas within whorled tissue that resembles a rather indistinct intramural leiomyoma. The uterine body may be enlarged if adenomyosis is severe and deep, due to hypertrophy of the myometrial smooth muscle bundles around the adenomyotic foci (Anderson 1991a). If par-

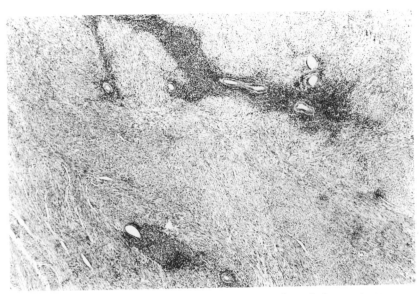

Fig. 14.11   Foci of adenomyosis deep within the myometrium of a hysterectomy specimen. Glands and stroma resemble the stratum basalis of the normal endometrium.

ticularly circumscribed and exaggerated, the lesion may be called an adenomyoma. There is an association with uterine leiomyomas in over 50% of patients (Weed et al 1966). Although adenomyosis is also sometimes (15%) associated with endometriosis externa (Weed et al 1966), these two disorders are probably unrelated and the term 'endometriosis interna' sometimes used to designate adenomyosis, should be discarded (Clement 1987). Cystic dilatation of adenomyotic glands and haemorrhage in the adenomyotic foci are uncommon histological findings, since the ectopic tissue retains the properties of the basal layer of the endometrium and is generally non-functional. However, stromal decidualization during pregnancy (Sandberg & Cohn 1962) or slight secretory changes may occasionally occur. Generally, adenomyosis is easily recognized as benign because the glands are separated by the characteristic stroma and do not show atypical features. However, when an endometrial carcinoma is also present, problems can arise in distinguishing between infiltrating adenocarcinomatous foci and adenomyotic glands.

Adenomyosis rarely undergoes malignant transformation (Colman & Rosenthal 1959, Winkelman & Robinson 1966, Hernandez &

Woodruff 1980) but multifocal atypical changes of the adenomyotic glands may be observed in uteri resected for atypical hyperplasia or endometrial carcinoma, suggesting a field change due to the influence of an oncogenic agent on all endometrial tissue.

It is possible that the presence of adenomyotic foci is one reason for recurrence of symptoms such as pain or abnormal bleeding following endometrial ablation or resection (Figure 14.12). Pathologists are therefore frequently asked to comment on the presence or absence of adenomyosis in hysteroscopically resected fragments of tissue. It should be understood that this a difficult or impossible assessment to make because the resected 'chippings' undergo twisting and distortion when they are fixed in formalin and endometrium which was originally on one surface of the myometrium may appear in histological sections on both sides and even within the myometrium, depending on the plane of section (Figure 14.13). This effect, combined with the irregularity of the endo-myometrial junction, means that to see endometrium apparently surrounded by myometrium cannot be taken as diagnostic of adenomyosis in this type of specimen. It is also not always possible to tell whether an individual fragment has come

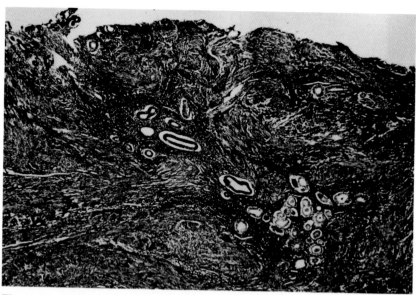

Fig. 14.12   Residual focus of adenomyosis following endometrial resection. This may be a cause of continued or recurrent symptoms postoperatively.

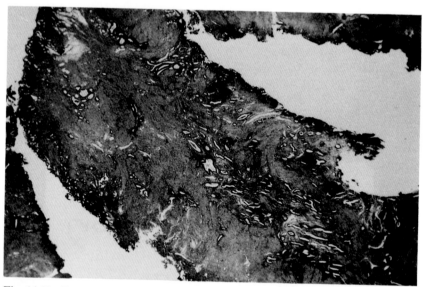

Fig. 14.13   Resected fragment of endometrium and myometrium. A combination of twisting during fixation, random plane of sectioning and an irregular endometrial–myometrial junction gives rise to an appearance falsely suggestive of adenomyosis.

from a superficial or a deep area and hence no assessment can be made of how far an endometrial area is from the endo–myometrial junction. One way around this problem is for the gynaecologist to take samples of the myometrium as a separate specimen after the completion of the resection procedure, which can then be assessed by the histopathologist for the presence or absence of any endometrial tissue. The presence of endometrial tissue within these deep myometrial fragments is suggestive of adenomyosis.

Endometrial hyperplasia

Hyperplasia is defined as 'an increase in the number of cells in an organ or tissue which may then have increased volume' (Robbins et al 1984). Endometrial hyperplasia is characterized by a variable increase of glands and stroma and includes a whole spectrum of changes ranging from a slightly disordered proliferative pattern at one end, up to appearances difficult to distinguish from adenocarcinoma at the other extreme. Some of these changes produce a prominent and irregular hysteroscopic appearance to the endometrial cavity, but in other cases the changes may be focal and unaccompanied by recognizable hysteroscopic changes.

There are numerous classifications of endometrial hyperplasia in the literature which attempt to define the variable morphology and there is much confusion because the same terms may be used with different meanings (Colafranceschi et al 1983). It must be stressed that, whatever nomenclature is chosen, there should be mutual understanding of the interpretation between the histopathologist and the gynaecologist so that appropriate treatment is always adopted irrespective of the pathological classification used. It is reasonably well established that hyperplasia displaying severe architectural and cytological atypia carries a significant risk of developing into invasive carcinoma (Kurman et al 1985). The most important aspect of classifying endometrial hyperplasia is to try and distinguish these from simple hyperplasia, often associated with anovular cycles, which is not thought to carry a significant risk of malignancy.

The modern classification owes much to the work of Welch & Scully (1977), who referred to the concepts of architectural and cytological atypia. This has been modified by the International Society of Gynaecological Pathologists to include three types: simple, complex and atypical hyperplasia. In the UK however, the terms 'simple' and 'cystic' hyperplasia are considered to be synonymous and the changes may be graded as mild, moderate or severe. Atypical hyperplasia is subclassified according to the presence and severity of architectural atypia and/or cytological

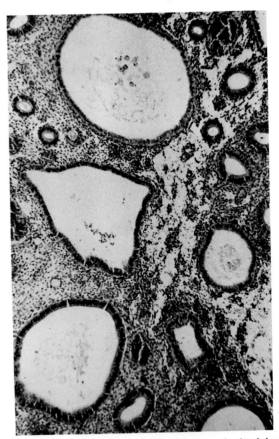

Fig. 14.14   Typical appearance of simple or cystic glandular hyperplasia. The dilated glands are the most prominent feature and, although there may be some multilayering of epithelial cells, the proportion of glands to stroma is not significantly increased.

atypia (Anderson 1991b), and the term 'complex' is not commonly used.

Histological examination is needed in order to make a diagnosis of endometrial hyperplasia. Endometrial cytology may help to identify the possibility of hyperplasia or neoplasia in asymptomatic women but patients with positive endometrial cytology or with symptoms require further investigation. Atypical hyperplasia cannot reliably be distinguished from well-differentiated endometrial carcinoma by either cytology or hysteroscopy and can often be difficult even by histology in small tissue samples.

'Simple' hyperplasia shows an exaggerated proliferative pattern characterized by lengthening and irregularity of the gland lumen, with focal dilatations. The epithelium is pseudostratified, with numerous mitoses, ciliated cells and regular oval nuclei with diffuse chromatin and small nucleoli. In the UK this is referred to as a 'disordered proliferative pattern'. In cystic glandular hyperplasia, the epithelium of the cystic glands may appear pseudostratified, cuboidal or flat, according to the degree of hormonal activity or due to pressure atrophy because of secretions into the gland lumen (Figure 14.14). Ciliated or eosinophilic metaplasia may be present.

'Complex' hyperplasia shows a more prominent architectural disturbance (in the UK this would be called hyperplasia with architectural atypia). The glands are crowded in an irregular fashion and dilated with infolding and budding of the epithelial lining (Figure 14.15). The gland epithelium is pseudostratified or stratified with frequent mitoses and easily recognizable nucleoli.

Atypical hyperplasia usually shows both architectural abnormality and various degrees of cytological atypia (Figure 14.16). There is loss of cell polarity, decrease or absence of ciliated cells, increased nuclear pleomorphism, prominent nucleoli, clumping or irregular distribution of chromatin and irregular thickness of the nuclear membrane.

Endometrial hyperplasia is associated with oestrogenic stimulation. Simple or cystic glandular hyperplasia is frequent around the time of the menarche and the menopause when anovular cycles are common. Long-term exposure to unopposed oestrogens for hormone replacement therapy is associated with development of a variety of appearances including atypical hyperplasia and carcinoma (Cramer 1980). It is generally considered that oestrogen-dependent hyperplastic

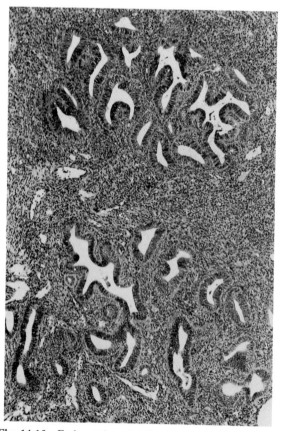

Fig. 14.15 Endometrium showing (complex) hyperplasia with architectural atypia. The glands show focal crowding and irregular shapes with infolding and budding.

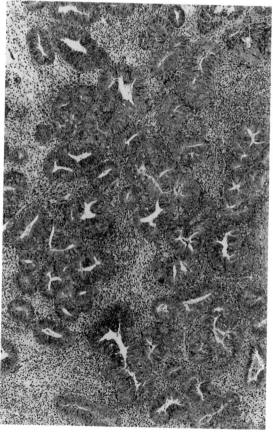

Fig. 14.16 Atypical hyperplasia of endometrium. There is crowding and architectural abnormality of the glands together with cytological atypia of the epithelium.

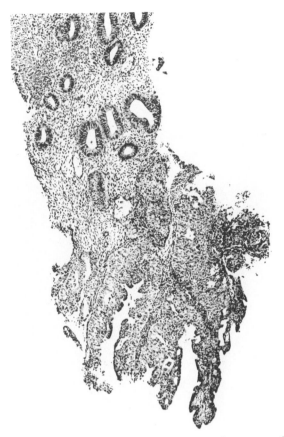

Fig. 14.17 Biopsy of endometrial polyp showing an area of architectural atypia adjacent to an area of more normal endometrium.

patterns progress in a stepwise fashion through atypical hyperplasia to invasive carcinoma but the data available at present do not allow the estimate of progression or regression in an individual patient nor of the likely time course of the changes, although it is probable that the more severe the architectural and cytological atypia, the higher the likelihood of progression (Kurman et al 1985, Ferenczy & Gelfand 1989).

As a practical guideline, patients with biopsies or curettings showing features of atypical hyperplasia are not suitable for treatment by endometrial resection or ablation. Hysterectomy is needed for full histological assessment of malignant potential. On the other hand, patients with histologically confirmed simple or cystic glandular hyperplasia are suitable for treatment by endometrial ablative techniques, bearing in mind the potential for recurrence if residual endo-

metrium is left behind and unopposed oestrogen activity continues.

Endometrial polyps

Some hyperplastic endometria have a polypoid architecture but, in addition, solitary polyps occurring on a background of normal endometrium are quite a common finding. Sometimes these are hormonally responsive with a glandular and stromal architecture similar to that of the surrounding endometrium. More often they have a rather fibrous stroma with a leash of thick-walled vessels at the base and glands which are less hormonally reactive than the surrounding endometrium and often show cystic dilatation. The pathogenesis of such local overgrowth of tissue is not understood. Possibly they result from local variation in hormone responsiveness, producing an increased bulk which, once it becomes manifest as a protrusion, is exaggerated by the muscular activity of the myometrium (Anderson 1991c). Atypical areas of epithelium (Figure 14.17) or even carcinoma can develop in a polyp so, when these lesions are identified at hysteroscopy, it is advisable to resect and submit them for histological examination rather than ablate them in situ.

Small submucous leiomyomas can also present as polypoid protuberances into the endometrial cavity.

Endometrial carcinoma

If curettage or hysteroscopic biopsy reveals histological features of endometrial carcinoma, the case is not suitable for treatment by endometrial resection or ablation. The problem of differentiating between atypical hyperplasia and adenocarcinoma in biopsy or curettage specimens has been exhaustively examined in the literature, but without achieving any solution other than identifying as invasive carcinoma a lesion in which the histologic features of stromal invasion are present (Tavassoli & Kraus 1978, Hendrickson & Kempson 1980, Robertson 1981, Fox & Buckley 1982, Kurman & Norris 1982, 1986, King et al 1984). Malignant invasion of stroma is confirmed by the sclerosing periglandular reaction (Figure

14.18) more effectively than by cytological or architectural atypia. However, if a hyperplastic lesion is associated with endometrial atrophy in late menopause, where the stroma has become fibrotic, this diagnostic criterion may not be applicable and in any case may be very difficult to apply in small biopsies. Back-to-back crowding of glands without intervening stroma, intraluminal cellular bridges, cribriform or papillary patterns, cellular anarchy and necrosis with neutrophil polymorphs are features suggestive of adeno-carcinoma (Fox & Buckley 1982) but, in order to avoid possible undertreatment of malignancy in this difficult diagnostic area, it is better to treat both atypical hyperplasia and adenocarcinoma by hysterectomy so that full pathological assessment can be made.

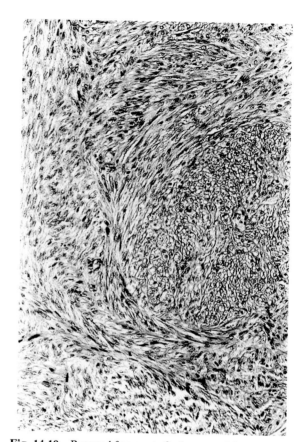

Fig. 14.19   Resected fragment of submucous leiomyoma.

Leiomyomas

Piecemeal resection of submucous leiomyomas can also be carried out via the hysteroscope. Although leiomyomatous tissue may be easily recognized by the operator due to its different colour and texture compared with the adjacent myometrium, it can be surprisingly difficult to differentiate leiomyomatous tissue from myo-metrium in the tissue 'chippings' submitted for histopathological examination (Figures 14.19 & 14.20). The smooth muscle cells of the benign tumours are actually very similar to those of the normal myometrium both histologically and ultrastructurally (Crow 1992) and leiomyomas are recognized in hysterectomy specimens large-ly by their overall architecture, which is difficult to discern when removal is performed in a piecemeal fashion. Assessment of possible smooth muscle malignancy can, however, be

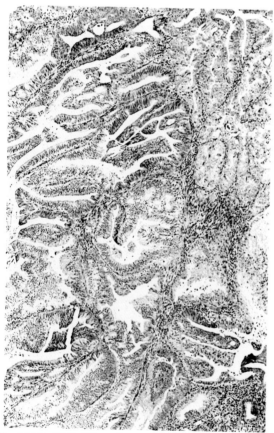

Fig. 14.18   Well-differentiated adenocarcinoma showing epithelial bridges and a sclerosing periglandular reaction. These are two of the features which help to differentiate between carcinoma and atypical hyperplasia.

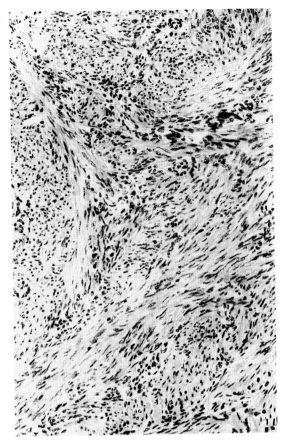

Fig. 14.20 Superficial cellular myometrium in a resected fragment showing a pattern of interlacing bundles of smooth muscle which may be difficult to distinguish from fragments of leiomyoma.

made in the usual way by the number of mitoses per high power field and the presence or absence of pleomorphism (Kempson & Hendrickson 1987) even though peripheral invasion may not be assessable in fragmented specimens.

REFERENCES

Anderson M C 1991a Adenomyosis. In: Anderson M C (ed) Female reproductive system. Symmers W St C (gen ed) Systemic pathology, 3rd edn, vol 6. Churchill Livingstone, Edinburgh, p 234–236

Anderson M C 1991b Endometrial hyperplasia. In: Anderson M C (ed) Female reproductive system. Symmers W St C (gen ed) Systemic pathology, 3rd edn, vol 6. Churchill Livingstone, Edinburgh, p 171–184

Anderson M C 1991c Functional and inflammatory disorders of the endometrium. In: Anderson M C (ed) Female reproductive system. Symmers W St C (gen ed) Systemic pathology 3rd edn, vol 6. Churchill Livingstone, Edinburgh p 147–170

Asherman J G 1948 Amenorrhoea traumatica (atretica).

Journal of Obstetrics and Gynaecology of the British Empire 55: 23–30

Carmichael D E 1970 Asherman's syndrome. Obstetrics and Gynecology 36: 922–928

Clement P B 1987 Endometriosis, lesions of the secondary Mullerian system, and pelvic mesothelial proliferations. In: Kurman R J (ed) Blaustein's pathology of the female genital tract, 3rd edn. Springer-Verlag, New York, p 517–559

Colafranceschi M, Taddei G L, Mencaglia L, Scarselli G 1983 La istopatologia delle lesioni precancerose dell'endometrio. Oncologia Ginecologica 2: 15–27

Colafranceschi M, Taddei G L Santucci M, Tinacci G, Longo L, Mencaglia L 1988 Laser radiation effects on the uterine cervix examined through light microscopy and scanning electron microscopy. Laser 1: 13–16

Colman H I, Rosenthal A H 1959 Carcinoma developing in areas of adenomyosis. Obstetrics and Gynecology 14: 342–348

Cove H 1981 Postcurettage endometrium. In: Surgical pathology of the endometrium, 1st edn. J B Lippincott, Philadelphia, p 46

Cramer D W 1980 Epidemiology of endometrial cancer. In: Koss L G (ed) Recent advances in endometrial neoplasia (27th Annual Scientific Meeting of the American Society of Cytology). Acta Cytologica 24: 478–482

Crow J 1992 Uterine fibroids: histological features. In: Shaw R W (ed) Uterine fibroids-time for a review. Carnforth Parthenon Carnforth, Lancs. (in press)

Dallenbach-Hellweg G 1981 Iatrogenic changes of the endometrium. In: Histopathology of the endometrium, 3rd edn. Springer-Verlag, Berlin, p 255–256

Ferenczy A, Gelfand M M 1989 The biologic significance of cytologic atypia in progestogen-treated endometrial hyperplasia. American Journal of Obstetrics and Gynecology 160: 126–131

Foix A, Bruno R O, Davison T, Lema B 1966 The pathology of postcurettage intrauterine adhesions. American Journal of Obstetrics and Gynecology 96: 1027–1033

Fox H, Buckley C M 1982 The endometrial hyperplasias and their relationship to endometrial neoplasia. Histopathology 6: 493–510

Gompel C, Silverberg S G 1985 The corpus uteri. In: Pathology in gynecology and obstetrics, 3rd edn. J B Lippincott, Philadelphia, p 149–277

Hamou J E 1991a Uterine adhesions. In: Hysteroscopy and microcolpohysteroscopy. Text and Atlas, 1st edn. Appleton & Lange, Norwalk, p 139–154

Hamou J E 1991b Partial endometrial ablation. In: Hysteroscopy and microcolpohysteroscopy. Text and Atlas, 1st edn. Appleton & Lange, Norwalk, p 186–199

Hendrickson M R, Kempson R L 1980 The differential diagnosis of endometrial adenocarcinoma. Some viewpoints concerning a common diagnostic problem. Pathology 12: 35–61

Hernandez E, Woodruff J D 1980 Endometrial adenocarcinoma arising in adenomyosis. American Journal of Obstetrics and Gynecology 138: 827–832

Kempson R L, Hendrickson M R 1987 Pure mesenchymal neoplasms of the uterine corpus. In: Fox H (ed) Haines and Taylor Obstetrical and Gynaecological Pathology, 3rd edn. Churchill Livingstone, Edinburgh, p 411–456

Johannisson E, Fournier K, Riotton G 1981 Regeneration of the human endometrium and presence of inflammatory cells following diagnostic curettage. Acta Obstetrica et Gynecologica Scandinavica 60: 451–457

Jorgensen V, Enevoldsen B 1963 The occurrence of the first menstruation after curettage. Acta Obstetrica et Gynecologica Scandinavica 42 (suppl 6)

King A, Seraj I M, Wagner R J 1984 Stromal invasion in endometrial carcinoma. American Journal of Obstetrics and Gynecology 149: 10–14

Kurman R J, Norris H J 1982 Evaluation of criteria for distinguishing atypical hyperplasia from well-differentiated carcinoma. Cancer 49: 2547–2559

Kurman R J, Norris H J 1986 Endometrium. In: Henson D, Albores Saavedra J (eds) The pathology of incipient neoplasia. W B Saunders, Philadelphia, p 265

Kurman R J, Kaminski P F, Norris H J 1985 The behaviour of endometrial hyperplasia. A long-term study of 'untreated' hyperplasia in 170 patients. Cancer 56: 403–418

McLennan C 1969 Endometrial regeneration after curettage. American Journal of Obstetrics and Gynecology 104: 185–190

Polishuk W, Sadovsky E 1975 A syndrome of recurrent intrauterine adhesions. American Journal of Obstetrics and Gynecology 123: 151–158

Robbins S L, Cotran R S, Kumar V 1984 Pathologic basis of disease, 3rd edn. W B Saunders, Philadelphia, p 32

Robertson W B 1981 The endometrium In: Crawford S T (ed) Postgraduate pathology series, 1st edn. Butterworths, London, p 20–21

Sandberg E C, Cohn F 1962 Adenomyosis in the gravid uterus at term. American Journal of Obstetrics and Gynecology 84: 1457–1465

Stock R J, Kanbour A 1975 Prehysterectomy curettage. Obstetrics and Gynecology 45: 537–541

Sugimoto O 1978 Diagnostic and therapeutic hysteroscopy for traumatic intrauterine adhesions. American Journal of Obstetrics and Gynecology 131: 539–547

Tavassoli F A, Kraus F T 1978 Endometrial lesions in uteri resected for atypical endometrial hyperplasia. American Journal of Clinical Pathology 70: 770–779

Tiltman A J 1980 Adenomatoid tumours of the uterus. Histopathology 4: 437–443

Weed J C, Geary W L, Holland J B 1966 Adenomyosis of the uterus. Clinical Obstetrics and Gynecology 69: 794–799

Welch W R, Scully R E 1977 Precancerous lesions of the endometrium. Human Pathology 8: 503–512

Winkelman J, Robinson R 1966 Adenocarcinoma of endometrium involving adenomyosis. Cancer 19: 901–908

Zaloudek C, Norris H J 1987 Mesenchymal tumors of the uterus. In: Kurman R J (ed) Blaustein's pathology of the female genital tract, 3rd edn. Springer-Verlag, New York, p 401–402

15. Epidemiology

K. McPherson

INTRODUCTION

This chapter will cover the epidemiological aspects of transcervical endometrial ablation. Essentially, this includes the distribution and the aetiology of the condition(s) for which ablation might be appropriate treatment, the evaluation of the efficacy and safety of ablation and the epidemiology of the treatment which ablation might replace and hence the prospective epidemiology of endometrial ablation itself.

All of these issues are surrounded by a certain amount of uncertainty and controversy. Hysterectomy is a gynaecological procedure which has been performed for increasingly liberal indications and with considerably varying populations, based on standardized rates between countries and indeed between neighbouring hospital areas. The agreement of appropriate surgical indications is clearly difficult. Hence, the definitive measurement of the incidence or prevalence of any relevant gynaecological conditions is, outside special medical surveys, in this instance, extremely problematic.

However, endometrial ablation will be carried out predominantly for functional disorders of menstruation, usually menorrhagia and submucous fibroids. In the absence of objective studies of the quantity of blood loss, the diagnosis of excessive menstrual loss is in part real and in part impressionistic (Chinbira et al 1980). This fact, combined with differences in a woman's propensity to seek advice in the first place, explains in part the enormous epidemiological uncertainty.

CAUSES OF MENORRHAGIA

The possible pathological causes of menorrhagia are well known (Rees 1987). Since, for example, uterine fibroids are a common cause the designation of unexplained menorrhagia is generally only possible after a physical examination. Thus, because epidemiological studies require large numbers of cases, the aetiology of unexplained menorrhagia has been hardly studied and the comparison of incidence rates by age, social class, time and geography not reliably performed. Polyps and endocrine disorders can cause menorrhagia as well as certain bleeding disorders, as can, of course, the intrauterine contraceptive device.

CAUSES OF HYSTERECTOMY

Until recently the dominant surgical treatment for menorrhagia has been abdominal or vaginal hysterectomy. Much interest has concentrated over the last several decades on the age-standardized rate of this operation. Unlike the incidence of unexplained menorrhagia, hysterectomy is an easily defined and hence a well-measured event and thus is amenable to epidemiological study. People have been interested in studying the use of hysterectomy among different populations for a long time. The original interest lay in the observed differences in the rate of this operation between communities, and the inability to explain these differences by known differences in disease rates. However, the true incidence of diseases for which hysterectomy is an appropriate treatment is difficult to measure reliably and therefore the extent to which rates of the operation are determined by relevant morbidity among populations difficult to ascertain. Much evidence of various kinds is used to address the question and the general conclusion that hysterectomy rates are determined by factors other than morbidity much more than they are by morbidity itself remains very persuasive.

Firstly, the operation rate varies around sixfold between developed countries (McPherson 1989) (and, of course, by much more between the developed and developing world), and those countries with high rates tend to be countries with high rates of intervention for conditions which are known not to vary a great deal. For example, the rate in the USA is around 560 per 100 000 of the population, while in England and Wales it is around 250 and in Japan it is around 90 per 100 000 (Table 15.1).

Secondly, the variation in the incidence of well-measured medical conditions between countries is only exceptionally of this kind of magnitude and then there is usually a well-understood set of reasons. The incidence of breast cancer between Europe and Japan does, for instance, vary by about a factor of six, but much of this difference can be explained by differences in the prevalence of known risk factors. The incidence of breast cancer between European countries and North America is much less variable than the incidence of hysterectomy between these countries.

However, by far the most persuasive evidence concerning the relative independence of hysterectomy rates from the incidence of appropriate conditions comes from the study of hysterectomy between neighbouring small areas. Traditionally, hospital service areas or catchment populations provide opportunities for comparing the practice style of the consultants and the primary care physicians and the referral process for these hospitals. Such work indicates a systematic variation between such areas within countries of around three- or fourfold. Of course, such differences in the true incidence of relevant conditions (such as menorrhagia) between relatively homogenous populations is less plausible. An example recently published by Teo (1990) from Scottish data is shown in Table 15.2. He compared the rate of hysterectomy for particular indications between the Western health boards and the Eastern health boards.

Of course there are opportunities for coding artefacts to distort these data in Table 15.2 a little and hence the interpretation, but assiduous study of hysterectomy rates for all causes between small areas in many countries shows the same magnitude of variation. McPherson et al (1982) found very comparable differences for the very different mean levels among small areas in New England, USA, the districts of the West Midlands, UK, and the counties of Norway (Fig. 15.1).

These differences were judged to be determined as much by clinical uncertainties surrounding the correct indications and possibly differences in access or the supply of appropriate

Table 15.1 Hysterectomy rates in developed countries per 100 000 of the population (1980s)

Country	Rate
Australia	405
Canada	479
Denmark	255
Ireland	123
Japan	90
Netherlands	381
New Zealand	431
Norway	130
Sweden	145
UK	250
USA	557

Source: McPherson (1989).

Table 15.2 Hysterectomy rates (per annum) by selected diagnostic category in Scotland 1980–1984. Rate per 100 000 of the female population

	Eastern health board	Western health board	Significance of difference (P)
Menstrual disorder	81.6	65.4	<0.0001
Fibroids	46.9	40.9	0.0001
Genital prolapse	25.6	14.4	0.0001
Malignant neoplasm	20.9	14.2	0.0001
Benign neoplasm	3.5	1.9	0.0001
Pelvic inflammatory disease	2.7	3.5	0.01
Carcinoma in situ	2.2	6.2	0.0001

From Teo (1990).

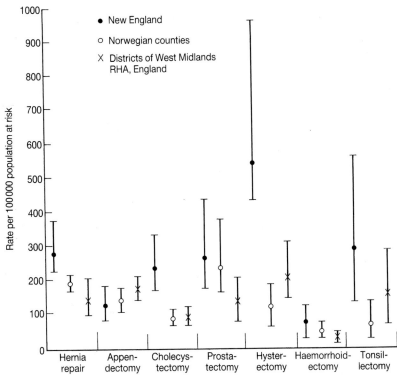

Fig. 15.1 Mean and range of age and sex-standardized rates for common surgical procedures in New England, USA, Norway and the West Midlands, UK. (Reproduced from McPherson et al (1982) by kind permission of the Massachusetts Medical Society.)

facilities as by local variations in morbidity incidence. Coulter and McPherson (1986) in trying to investigate the possible effect of women's preferences investigated hysterectomy rates in a variety of settings. They performed a survey of 3000 randomly selected women from general practice to investigate any social class or occupational differences in the prevalence of hysterectomy. There was no difference in the rate of hysterectomy standardized by age and parity between social class at all. Women with an older terminal educational age tended to have had fewer hysterectomies, and nurses of common occupational groups the highest rate. This was similar to a finding of Bunker and Brown (1974) in the West Coast of America in the 1970s showing wives of doctors having a much higher rate of hysterectomy than wives of other professionals.

Also using data from a large cohort study of different methods of contraception, Coulter et al (1988) found a threefold difference in the age-standardized rate of hysterectomy for uterine bleeding between users of different family planning clinics. The highest standardized rate was 4.82 per 1000 women years among this cohort of women aged in their 40s, while the lowest was 1.48. In a detailed examination of these data (Vessey et al 1992) a highly significant gradient in hysterectomy rates, standardized for age and parity, was found for menstrual problems by social class of husbands. Lower social class women had a higher rate — 2.72 among women whose husbands were manual workers and 2.12 per 1000 women years among wives of non-manual workers. This might explain to some extent the finding above that women with a lower terminal educational age had a higher hysterectomy rate.

Of course these variations in rates might also to some degree be determined by the propensity of general practitioners to refer patients with menstrual problems for a consultant opinion. Coulter et al (1988) noted a sevenfold difference in the referral rate for hysterectomies between general practitioners, but this was inevitably based on small numbers. The referral rate for disorders of menstruation was much more variable, ranging astonishingly from less than ten per 10 000 female patients per annum to more than 100 per 10 000.

This work tends to emphasize that hysterectomy remains a fairly controversial procedure which is favoured to varying degrees by different professionals for different reasons. In part this is because the properly controlled prospective studies comparing the benefits of competing treatments have not been done. This is a lesson for the widespread implementation of medical or surgical procedures which seem highly beneficial but in fact for a large proportion of patients represent treatments of highly marginal cost effectiveness (Bunker et al 1977).

In terms of the implementation of transcervical endometrial ablation there is another particular problem in its evaluation illustrated by recent research on transurethral resection of the prostate (TURP) for benign hypertrophy of the prostate (BPH). Comparing TURP with watchful waiting again suggests that for some patients the choice is very finely balanced (Wennberg et al 1988). Prostatectomy, just like hysterectomy, shows striking variations in its rate both between small areas and between countries. This suggests the possibility that the use of a policy of watchful waiting is more common in those areas with low prostatectomy rates.

Discussion with urologists and a systematic review of the literature has revealed important and unsettled uncertainties concerning the indications for prostatectomy. Clinicians are faced with two options among men with symptoms of BPH: to operate during the 'early course' of development, and so prevent any deterioration of the condition, operating when the patient is relatively young; or, alternatively, delay the operation and reduce the risk and inconvenience of surgery, but also accept a possible deterioration of symptoms, and hence the prospect of non-elective surgery at a later time.

Using evidence from the literature and from longitudinal studies it was possible to assess the life expectancy associated with prostatectomy versus watchful waiting. For men with uncomplicated BPH, the average life expectancy is somewhat lower when prostatectomy is chosen instead of watchful waiting (Barry et al 1988). When adjustment was made for quality of life, however, the operation increased the average expectation of quality-adjusted life months. Hence the choice depends on the particular preferences of patients: some may prefer the risks of the operation, including risks of incontinence and impotence as well as death, in order to gain a likely relief of symptoms, whilst others may not wish to take the risk and prefer to put up with the symptoms.

In parallel with this work, other choices regarding prostatectomy have been investigated: wide variations have existed in the type of operation performed — TURP or open surgery. In the USA, readmission and death rates can be calculated from Medicare data for the majority of men undergoing prostatectomy, in order to compare outcomes for the two procedures (Fowler et al 1988, Wennberg et al 1988). These data indicated a higher long-term mortality among men receiving TURP compared to the open operation (Roos et al 1989). Such a hypothesis generated from observational data can, in principle, only be tested using randomized studies. However, practice patterns and incomplete contemporary knowledge make such randomized comparisons seem unethical (Anonymous 1989a, Baum 1989).

In order to proceed scientifically, longitudinal and independent databases in Oxford, Denmark and Manitoba were analysed to investigate the same hypotheses and in each the same excess mortality was found for TURP (Roos et al 1989). That is, a 50% excess mortality in the 8 years following surgery. Clearly, the decision to use the transurethral approach could be made more safely for small prostrate glands and perhaps for patients with more co-morbidity. Such selection could lead to higher subsequent mortality itself, independent of the effect of the particular operation.

However, examination of the Manitoba data with adjustment for important information on previous medical history and anaesthesiologists' risk categories made no difference to the apparent mortality excess. Moreover, comparing men with benign hypertrophy only and similar men admitted for TURP and open surgery compared to men admitted for other elective surgery continued to confirm the excess. Further work analysing case records in Manitoba in greater detail and making more fine statistical adjustments failed to eliminate the excess (Malenka et al 1990). Indeed, work in Denmark (Andersen et al 1990) with detailed case mix adjustment also failed to eliminate the excess.

As a consequence the American Urological Association (Anonymous 1989b) has decided to mount a randomized study of treatment for BPH in which men with large glands will be randomly allocated between TURP and open prostatectomy. This has yet to actually happen because the finance and details have not been finally agreed, but the need is now well understood. Indeed, assessment of transcervical endometrial ablation, which uses similar technology, will as a consequence be difficult to introduce without rigorous experimental evaluation (Magos et al 1989).

Further cross-sectional follow-up studies of patients undergoing prostatectomy in the USA, UK and Denmark provide insights into the level of symptoms present preoperatively and the changes attributable to the operation (Fowler et al 1988, Black et al 1992). It is fascinating to observe that the average prostate size is larger in the UK, and the prevalence of serious symptoms much higher preoperatively than in the USA. The average level of symptoms and complication postoperatively is, however, much the same in the two countries. The standardized rate of prostatectomy is around twice as high in the USA, where presumably the indications for surgery are more liberal.

CONCLUSION

Clearly, with an operation for which the indications are not tightly defined, and for which the individual preferences of patients might be important, the outcomes associated with all levels and extents of symptoms require assessment. While the short-term outcomes may be well understood, it still remains that a lack of proper evaluation in the early experience of transurethral resection for benign prostatic hypertrophy is responsible now for great uncertainty concerning long-term and serious side-effects. Such results were not expected at the time. The analogy to endometrial ablation is obvious.

REFERENCES

Andersen T F, Bronnum-Hansen H, Seyr T, Roepstorff C 1990 Elevated mortality following transurethral resection of the prostate for benign hypertrophy! But why? Medical Care 28: 10

Anonymous 1989a TU or not TU. Lancet i 1361–1362

Anonymous 1989b Databases for health care outcomes. Lancet ii: 195–196

Barry M J, Mulley A G, Fowler F J, Wennberg J E 1988 Watchful waiting versus immediate transurethral resection for symptomatic prostatism: the importance of patients preferences. Journal of the American Medical Association 259: 3010–3017

Baum M 1989 Treatment of benign prostatic hyperplasia. British Medical Journal 299: 979–980

Black N, McPherson K, Doll H 1992 A comparison of symptom level among US and British patients receiving surgery for BPH. Unpublished

Bunker J P, Brown B W 1974 The physician as an informed consumer of surgical services. New England Journal of Medicine 290: 1051–1055

Bunker J, McPherson K, Henneman P 1977 Elective hysterectomy. In: Bunker J, Barnes B, Mosteller F (eds) Cost, risks, and benefits of surgery. Oxford University Press, New York.

Chinbira T, Anderson A, Turnbull A 1980 Relationship between measured blood loss and the patients subjective assessment of loss, duration of bleeding, number of sanitary towels, uterine weight and endometrial surface area. British Journal of Obstetrics and Gynaecology 87: 603–609

Coulter A, McPherson K 1986 The hysterectomy debate. Quarterly Journal of Social Affairs 4: 379–396

Coulter A, McPherson K, Vessey M 1988 Do women undergo too many or too few hysterectomies. Social Science and Medicine 27(9): 987–994

Fowler F J, Wennberg J E, Timothy R P et al 1988 Symptom status and the quality of life following prostatectomy. Journal of the American Medical Association 259: 3018–3022

McPherson K 1989 International differences in medical practices. Health Care Financing Review, Annual Supplement

McPherson K, Wennberg J, Hovind O, Clifford P 1982 Small area variations in the use of common surgical procedures: an International comparison of New England, England and Norway. New England Journal of Medicine 307: 1310–1314

Magos A L, Baumann R, Turnbull A C 1989 Transcervical resection of the endometrium in women with menorrhagia. British Medical Journal 293: 1209–1212

Malenka D J, Roos N, Fisher E et al 1990 Further study of the increased mortality following transurethral prostatectomy: a chart based analysis. Journal of Urology 144: 224–220

Rees M 1987 Menorrhagia. British Medical Journal 294: 759–762

Roos N P, Wennberg J E, Malenka D J et al 1989 Mortality and reoperation after open and transurethral resection of the prostate for benign prostatic hyperplasia. New England Journal of Medicine 1120–1124

Teo P 1990 Hysterectomy a change of trend or a change of heart, In: Roberts H (Ed) Women's health counts. Routledge, London

Vessey M, Villard L, McPherson K, Coulter A, Yeates D 1992 The epidemiology of hysterectomy: findings in a large cohort study. British Journal of Obstetrics and Gynaecology (in press)

Wennberg J, Mulley A Henley et al 1988 An assessment of prostatectomy for benign urinary tract obstruction. Geographic variations and the evaluation of medical care outcomes. Journal of the American Medical Association 259: 3027–3030

16. Blood loss studies

A. L. Magos   J. H. Phipps   T. Smith   B. V. Lewis

PART 1
ENDOMETRIAL RESECTION
A. L. Magos

INTRODUCTION

It is well recognized that there can be a considerable discrepancy between a woman's perception of the volume of her menstrual loss and her measured blood loss (Chimbira et al 1980). Currently, the gold standard method for such an objective assessment is the alkaline haematin method (Hallberg & Nillson 1964) and, using this technique, genuine menorrhagia can be defined as a menstrual blood loss of greater than 80 ml/cycle (Hallberg et al 1966). By this criterion, the mean menstrual blood loss for an unselected population of women is 35–40ml per cycle and, conversely, only 40% or so of those who complain of excessive menstruation are in fact truly menorrhagic with measured losses above the threshold of 80 ml/cycle (Haynes et al 1977; Fraser et al 1984).

The unreliability of subjective self-reports of menstrual bleeding has meant that, in drug studies at least, the objective measurement of menstrual blood loss is essential to prove the efficacy of any treatment (Rees 1987). Surprisingly perhaps, no such studies have yet been carried out with respect to endometrial ablation, despite the fact that this form of therapy has been available for over a decade. While such reluctance is understandable as many women either become amenorrhoeic or reduce to minor degrees of spotting following surgery, a considerable number do continue to menstruate, and it remains to be proven in what proportion of such cases are the periods truly 'normal', that is, associated with menstrual blood loss within the normal range as defined above.

Data are now available concerning this aspect of treatment for endometrial resection and radio frequency-induced thermal ablation. First, the menstrual effects of total and partial endometrial resection as assessed by the alkaline haematin method will be described in women with symptomatic menorrhagia.

PATIENTS

The author studied 52 women with a mean age of 42.4 years (standard deviation 4.6 years) before and after endometrial resection who agreed to provide serial samples (sanitary towels, tampons and blood samples) for objective blood loss measurements. They all complained of excessive menstruation and were offered this form of surgery as an alternative to hysterectomy. 46 (85%) underwent total and eight (15%) underwent partial endometrial resection, that is, either the entire uterine cavity was treated down to the endocervical canal as described in Chapter 9, or a 1 cm rim of endometrium was left around the isthmic part of the uterus. Simultaneous hysteroscopic myomectomy was performed in 15 (27.8%) cases. Two patients required repeat surgery within 1 year of their initial procedure, one after total and the other after partial resection, and so were assessed after both treatments.

METHODS

Menstrual blood loss was assessed using the standard alkaline haematin method as described by Hallberg & Nilsson (1964). Measurements were made during at least one untreated cycle prior to surgery (mean 1.4 cycles per patient, range 1–4 cycles), and continued at intervals after surgery for up to 1 year (mean 4.3 cycles per patient, range 1–12 cycles). For comparative purposes, the postoperative results were averaged over 2 monthly time periods.

RESULTS

The mean menstrual blood loss prior to surgery for the 52 women was 159.3 ml/cycle, ranging from as little as 13 to 922 ml/cycle. Women with fibroids were considerably more menorrhagic (mean 248.6 ml/cycle, range 13–454 ml) than those with a normal uterus (mean 126.7 ml/cycle, range 13–454 ml). Overall, 33 (61.1%) of the patients were found to have genuine menorrhagia before surgery.

Surgery was followed by a reduction in menstrual blood loss measurements in all but one case, irrespective of whether surgery involved total or partial resection or additional myomectomy (Fig. 16.1). Of the group who underwent total endometrial resection ± myomectomy, 15 (34.1%) became amenorrhoeic and the mean menstrual blood loss during the follow-up period was 17.7 ml/cycle (range 0–135 ml), a reduction compared to pretreatment of 90.2%. Even if the patients who stopped menstruating are excluded

from the calculation, the mean menstrual loss of those still bleeding after surgery averaged only 26.2 ml/cycle (range 0.3–135 ml), an overall improvement of 82.4%. The therapeutic effect of surgery was usually immediate, and there was only a slight tendency for any further menstrual improvement. The presence of fibroids and thus the need for hysteroscopic myomectomy appeared to have minimal influence on the outcome of surgery.

Instead, the most important determinant of success was the extent of surgery, women undergoing partial endometrial resection having a less dramatic improvement; for the eight women in this group, menstrual blood loss reduced to a mean of 38.3 ml/cycle (range 17–85 ml), an improvement of 66.3%. However, the small number of this subgroup makes it difficult to interpret these results.

Objectively, proven menorrhagia persisted in a total of six women, four (9.1%) after total and two (25%) after partial resection; however, three of these patients only provided one menstrual collection after their surgery. Two of the menorrhagic patients underwent repeat surgery, and their menstrual blood loss results are shown in Figure 16.2. One initially underwent partial resection with myomectomy, and although her blood loss reduced from 922 ml/cycle preoperatively to 214 ml/cycle at 8 months, she was still menorrhagic. She then underwent total resection, blood loss measurements showing a further improvement to a mean of 83.8 ml/cycle

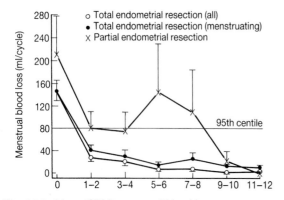

Fig. 16.1 Mean (SEM) menstrual blood loss measurements before and after total and partial endometrial resection. Results for total resection expressed for the group as a whole and the subgroup who were still menstruating following surgery.

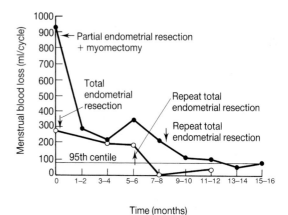

Time (months)

Fig. 16.2 Menstrual blood loss measurements for the two patients who required repeat hysteroscopic surgery.

over the subsequent 8 months (range 108–54 ml). The second patient had a total resection as her initial procedure, but after 4 months her menstrual blood loss only improved to 199 ml/cycle from a preoperative assessment of 274 ml/cycle. Surgery was repeated after 6 months, and the two measurements she had made during the next 8 months averaged 21.5 ml/cycle (range 5–38 ml).

DISCUSSION

These results confirm to a large part the reports of the author's patients that endometrial resection, particularly when the entire uterine cavity is treated, is followed by considerable improvement in the amount of bleeding, with normalization of menstrual loss in the majority of patients. Endometrial resection appears superior to those medical treatments which are both well tolerated and can be used in the long term (e.g. prostaglandin synthetase inhibitors, combined contraceptive pill), a 50% improvement with these agents being typical in contrast to over 90% following total endometrial resection (Magos 1990). The author's data also show that this form of hysteroscopic surgery is successful not only in cases of 'functional' menorrhagia but also when the uterine cavity is distorted by fibroids, an important consideration bearing in mind the prevalence of submucous fibroids in such women. Transcervical resection of the endometrium appears to be more effective than medical treatments for menorrhagia but less traumatic than hysterectomy.

ACKNOWLEDGEMENTS

I am grateful for the technical assistance of Margaret C. P. Rees, Parke Davis Lecturer in the Nuffield Department of Obstetrics and Gynaecology, John Radcliffe Hospital, Maternity Department, Oxford, for performing the menstrual blood loss assays in her laboratory.

REFERENCES

Chimbira T H, Anderson A B M, Turnbull A C 1980 Relationship between measured menstrual blood loss and patient's subjective assessment of loss, duration of bleeding, number of sanitary towels used, uterine weight and endometrial surface area. British Journal of Obstetrics and Gynaecology 87: 603–609

Fraser I S, McCarron G, Markham R 1984 A preliminary study of factors influencing perception of menstrual blood loss volume. American Journal of Obstetrics and Gynecology 149: 788–793

Hallberg L, Nilsson L 1964 Determination of menstrual blood loss. Scandinavian Journal of Clinical and Laboratory Investigation 16: 244–248

Hallberg L, Hogdahl A-M, Nilsson L, Rybo G 1966 Menstrual blood loss — a population study. Acta Obstetrica et Gynecologica Scandinavica 45: 320–351

Haynes P J, Hodgson H, Anderson A B M, Turnbull A C 1977. Measurement of menstrual blood loss in patients complaining of menorrhagia. British Journal of Obstetrics and Gynaecology 76: 763–768

Magos A L 1990 Management of menorrhagia. British Medical Journal 300: 1537–1538.

Rees M 1987 Clinical algorithms. Menorrhagia. British Medical Journal i: 759–762

PART 2
MEASUREMENT OF MENSTRUAL BLOOD LOSS BY WHOLE-BODY COUNTING

J. H. Phipps   T. Smith   B. V. Lewis

INTRODUCTION

It is usually accepted that a menstrual blood loss of up to 80 ml/cycle is normal. Chamberlain (1981) defines normal menstrual blood loss as 25–75 ml, and abnormal loss as 125 ml or more. The simplest methods of measuring blood loss use either chemical or radioisotopic analysis of blood on collected sanitary pads. Whole-body counting provides an alternative method of estimating blood loss which avoids some of the potential errors inherent in pad-saving techniques because the calculation is based on differences between whole-body retentions and therefore does not depend on the measurement of radioactivity lost from the body. In this technique, a known quantity of radioactive iron (iron-59, ^{59}Fe) is given intravenously and allowed to bind to newly formed erythrocytes. With high incorporation of tracer into circulating erythrocytes, iron loss from the body is almost entirely due to blood loss, and a measured fall in ^{59}Fe retention over a given time period (after allowing for radioactive decay) reflects the amount of blood loss during the same period. If the patient's blood volume and/or ^{59}Fe concentration are known, the fall in retention can be equated to the proportion of the total blood volume that is lost. This technique has been used for almost 30 years to measure blood loss, mainly gastrointestinal, using a variety of types of whole-body counters (Warner 1973). Price et al (1964) used such a technique to quantify menstrual blood loss in six patients with convincing histories of menorrhagia which revealed blood losses of 110–550 ml/cycle. Similarly Holt et al (1967) reported a blood loss of 870 ml measured during a single 'menorrhagic' menstrual cycle, and Flach and Deckart (1977) measured losses ranging from 142 to 1237 ml (mean 353 ml) in 11 women with menorrhagia compared to 74–144 ml (mean 105 ml) in six women reporting normal menstruation.

Although the technique involves the injection of radioactive isotopes and is more time-consuming compared to pad-saving techniques, it was decided that whole-body counting should be used to objectively demonstrate the effects of radio frequency endometrial ablation (RaFEA) because of its greater accuracy. Patients are also saved the task of saving used sanitary pads.

METHOD

Blood losses were measured in a group of 19 patients (age range 35–51 years) who attended the gynaecology clinic complaining of heavy menstrual bleeding, and who agreed to take part in the trial. In 15 patients, repeat studies were performed 4 weeks after treatment. Informed consent was obtained from all the participants and approval for the investigation was given by the district ethical committee.

After an initial measurement in the whole-body counter to obtain a background reading, each patient was given intravenously 37 kBq (1 µCi) ^{59}Fe ferric citrate via an antecubital vein and then remeasured in the whole-body counter. Sterile ^{59}Fe citrate was diluted with isotonic saline and filtered before injection. A period of 9–14 days then elapsed to allow equilibration of ^{59}Fe uptake into circulating erythrocytes, after which a further whole-body measurement was made and a blood sample was taken for estimation of the level of radioactivity. The initial

injection and equilibrium measurements were arranged to occur respectively shortly after the end of a menstrual period and before the onset of the subsequent period. The equilibrium measurement was taken as the starting point for a measurement period extending over two menstrual cycles, after which further measurements of whole-body and blood radioactivity were made. The blood samples were measured in an automatic counter.

Whole-body counting was performed in a 15 cm thick steel cubicle with a multidetector system (Smith et al 1979). Counts were obtained in the energy range 0.99–1.42 MeV to include both photopeaks of the ^{59}Fe gamma ray spectrum. Whole-body counting time was 400 seconds, ensuring that errors due to counting statistics were less than 1%. On all counting occasions, care was taken to reproduce the position of the patient as accurately as possible to limit potential errors due to variations in counting geometry. Whole-body and blood radioactivity measurements were corrected for radioactive decay of ^{59}Fe, and blood loss was calculated from the equation

$$\text{Blood loss (ml)} = \frac{2\,(\text{WB1} - \text{WB2})}{\text{B1} + \text{B2}}$$

where WB1 and WB2 are the whole body retentions (percentage of administered ^{59}Fe) at the start and end of the observation period, respectively, and B1 and B2 are the measured concentrations of ^{59}Fe in blood samples (percentage of administered ^{59}Fe per millilitre) withdrawn at the same times. For patients who were examined after treatment, an initial whole-body count was performed and a blood sample taken, to allow correction for residual ^{59}Fe from the first injection. A second injection of 37 kBq of ^{59}Fe was then given and the same measurement procedure was repeated for two consecutive menstrual cycles or, where amenorrhoea was achieved, for a time period similar to that for the pretreatment measurement. A 4 week interval between treatment and the second measurement was allowed, to minimize errors arising from blood loss due to post-treatment sanguineous vaginal discharge. A diagram illustrating the protocol for the procedures is shown in Fig. 16.3.

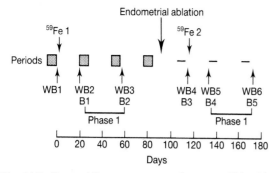

Fig. 16.3 Protocol for measurement of menstrual blood loss before and after endometrial ablation.

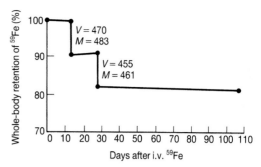

Fig. 16.4 Comparison of volumes of blood removed (V) with estimations by whole-body counting (M) in a polycythaemic patient.

RESULTS

Repeated whole-body measurements, requiring repositioning of the patient, gave a mean paired difference of only 0.66% (standard deviation 0.48%, $n = 18$) of the mean whole-body count rate, showing that the geometry error can be minimized by careful positioning. If 1% of errors are ascribed to counting geometry, sample pipetting and weighing, the standard error of the blood loss technique is estimated to be approximately 70 ml, and errors due to blood sample preparation and counting are not significant in relation to the error involved in serial whole-body counting.

When the technique was compared directly in a polycythaemic patient undergoing serial venesections, excellent agreement was obtained; volumes of 470 and 455 ml were removed (measured by weighing and calculated using blood density) and estimated by whole-body counting to be 483 and 461 ml, respectively (Fig. 16.4).

Pretreatment blood losses were very variable (Fig. 16.5) with a range from 97 to 1330 ml and a mean value of 561 ml. After RaFEA, the mean blood loss in 15 patients was 104 ml with a range of 0–266 ml (Fig. 16.6). The mean reduction in blood loss over the two cycles after treatment was 389 ml (SEM 79 ml, $p = < 0.001$), i.e. a mean reduction of 195 ml/cycle.

At follow-up of 15 patients 6–12 months after treatment, seven were amenorrhoeic and seven had experienced a reduction in menstrual blood loss to acceptable levels. One patient was unhappy with her result and elected to undergo hysterectomy.

DISCUSSION

Many attempts have been made in the past to measure menstrual blood loss objectively in women complaining of heavy bleeding, almost universally with the conclusion that less than half are losing more than a 'normal' amount. The majority of such studies have involved patients saving used sanitary pads for elution by alkaline extraction of haemoglobin (Haynes et al 1977, Chimbera et al 1980). However, different sanitary materials may not only retain different amounts of blood at saturation point (Grimes 1979), but possess different affinities for blood, resulting in variable extraction efficiency during haemoglobin elution. Improvements in technique may overcome this, however (van Eijkeren et al 1986, Vasilenko et al 1988). A further inaccuracy may result due to micturition during menstruation. Corstens et al (1989) measured sanitary pad and urine radioactivity after labelling the blood with ^{59}Fe. They calculated that an average of 25% (range 1–69%) of menstrual blood was lost

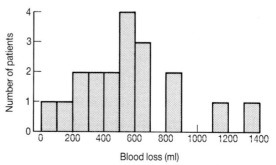

Fig. 16.5 Distribution of menstrual blood loss over two cycles in preoperative group ($n = 19$).

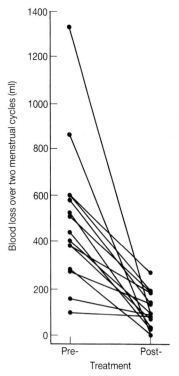

Fig. 16.6 Effect of radio frequency endometrial ablation on measured menstrual blood loss.

during micturition and therefore not observed on pads. In addition, despite careful instruction, some blood may conceivably be lost at the time of pad change, especially if clots have formed within the vagina.

The accuracy of whole-body counting techniques has varied according to the type of instrument used and the complexity of the chosen method. In the simplest case, total incorporation of administered ^{59}Fe into circulating erythrocytes has been assumed, and observed fractional decreases in body retention equated directly to the same fractions of total blood volume, the latter usually estimated empirically from body parameters (Holt et al 1967). When red cell labelling is increasingly less than 100%, this method can involve significant errors. A more accurate technique involves the periodic assessment of ^{59}Fe concentration in blood, which can be used with the observed whole-body retention deficit, to yield a value of blood loss that is independent of the patient's blood volume or a knowledge of the red cell ^{59}Fe incorporation value

(Werner et al 1972). Assessment of the accuracy of the whole-body counting technique has traditionally been performed with polycythaemic patients requiring venesections. The estimated blood loss following venesection has been compared with the known volume removed. Accuracy depends largely on the type of the whole-body counter and, in general, the standard error obtained for venesections of 500 ml or more has been reported to be of the order of ± 50 ml (Werner et al 1972). Holt et al (1967) concluded that their technique was sensitive enough to detect blood loss of 100–300 ml but, to increase the accuracy of estimating losses in menorrhagia, retention changes over several menstrual cycles should be measured. On theoretical grounds the accuracy of the authors' technique is in accord with that claimed by other workers using similar types of whole-body counter and suggests a standard error of 70 ml of blood. In confirmation, the authors have obtained satisfactory results on a polycythaemic patient measured during two sequential venesections and, in view of the similar assessments that have appeared in the literature, the authors did not feel justified in subjecting more polycythaemic patients to this procedure. The authors' method was adapted to quantify blood loss during two menstrual cycles to provide more reliable estimates, even though the patients in this study were expected to be having heavier than normal menstrual blood loss.

CONCLUSION

The multidetector whole-body counter method of quantifying menstrual blood loss has been shown to be satisfactory for patients with menorrhagia, when observed during two consecutive menstrual cycles. Contrary to current gynaecological theory, the authors found that most of their patients complaining of menorrhagia (17/19) were losing amounts of blood greater than the accepted normal rate of 80 ml/ cycle. The observed range was 97–1330 ml over two cycles with a mean of 561 ml ($n = 19$) (i.e. a mean loss of 281 ml/cycle). All 15 patients treated by RaFEA had reduced levels of blood loss post-treatment. The mean blood loss over two cycles after RaFEA was 104 ml ($n = 15$) and individual losses were reduced by 14–100% (mean 71.1%, $p = < 0.001$).

Although the technique has the advantages of greater accuracy and not having to save used pads, there are certain drawbacks. The necessary equipment is expensive and only available in a very few centres. Moreover, it is invasive and requires that the patient is exposed to radioactivity, although the dose is minute. Despite this, the need for an accurate assessment of the efficacy of these new ablative techniques perhaps justifies the use of whole-body counting.

REFERENCES

Chamberlain G 1981 Dysfunctional uterine bleeding, Clinical Obstetrics and Gynecology 8: 93–101

Chimbera T H, Anderson A B M, Turnbull A C 1980 Relation between measured menstrual blood loss and patients' subjective assessment of loss duration of bleeding, number of sanitary towels used, uterine weight and endometrial surface area. British Journal of Obstetrics and Gynaecology 87: 603–609

Corstens F, van den Brock W, Buijs W, Rolland R 1989 Measurement of blood content in sanitary wear underscores menstrual blood loss, 36th Annual Meeting of The Society Of Nuclear Medicine, St Louis (Poster 1109)

Flach von W, Deckart H 1977 Quantitative Bestrimmung des Menstruellen Blutverlustes mit dem Klinischen Ganzkorperzahler, Zentralblatt für Gynakologie 99: 679–683

Grimes D A 1979 Estimating vaginal blood loss, Journal of Reproductive Medicine 22: 190–193

Haynes P J, Hodgson H, Anderson A B M, Turnbull A C 1977 Measurement of menstrual blood loss in patients complaining of menorrhagia, British Journal of Obstetrics and Gynaecology 84: 763–768

Holt J M, Mayet F G H, Warner G T, Callender S T 1967 Measurement of blood loss by means of a whole body counter, British Medical Journal 4: 86–88

Price D C, Forsyth E M, Cohn S H, Cronkite E P 1964 The study of menstrual and other blood loss, and consequent iron deficiency, by ^{59}Fe whole body counting, Canadian Medical Association Journal 90: 51–54

Smith T, Hesp R, Mackenzie J 1979 Total body potassium calibrations for normal and obese subjects in two types of body counter, Physics in Medicine and Biology 24: 171–175

van Eijkeren M A, Scholten P C, Christiaens G C M L, Alsbach G P J, Haspels A A 1986 The alkaline haematin method for measuring menstrual blood loss — a modification and its clinical use in menorrhagia, European Journal of Obstetrics, Gynecology, and Reproductive Biology 22: 345–351

Vasilenko P, Kraicer P F, Kaplan R, de Masi A, Freed N 1988 A new and simple method of measurement of menstrual blood loss, Journal of Reproductive Medicine 33: 293–297

Warner G T 1973 The use of total body counters for the study of iron metabolism and iron loss, Postgraduate Medical Journal 49: 477–486

Werner E, Kaltwasser J P, Becker H 1972 Quantitative Bestimmung von Blutverlusken mit dem Ganzkorperzahler, Klinische Wochenschrift 50: 543–547

17. Future prospects

Adam L. Magos, B. Victor Lewis

. . . For I dipt into the future,
far as human eye could see,
Saw the Vision of the world,
and all the wonder that would be . . .
                              Alfred, Lord Tennyson

There can be little doubt in the mind of anyone who has read even a few of the chapters in this book that the surgical management of abnormal uterine bleeding is undergoing a major revolution. Hysterectomy is no longer the logical choice for those who have failed with medical treatment and, instead, an ever-growing selection of less invasive and disfiguring procedures is becoming available. All these new alternatives share similar advantages compared with hysterectomy, namely, faster surgery, shorter hospitalisation and quicker recovery, and fewer operative and post-operative complications. They also all suffer from the same disadvantages, the chief of these being that none of the currently available techniques can guarantee total amenorrhoea, and we do not yet know the long-term consequences of these interventions. For many women, the benefits still outweigh the drawbacks, and the pendulum is swinging away from hysterectomy.

The ablation techniques described in this book are, however, only the beginnings of a new chapter in gynaecological therapy for menorrhagia. Although often termed 'minimally invasive', all the methods currently practised are associated with potentially serious operative risks as well as the shortcomings already noted, and the ideal approach to endometrial ablation has still to be found.

What could the future hold? Clues to further developments can be found in some of the chapters in this book. Laser ablation, currently performed using Nd:YAG laser energy applied via a narrow 0.6 mm fibre, could obviously be improved if the tip size were increased, thereby allowing for faster and more efficient surgery. The use of other laser sources, possibly combined with tissue sensitisers to target the endometrium and to protect the myometrium, is another approach which may produce better menstrual results, particularly in women with adenomyosis.

Hysteroscopic electrosurgery will also be improved. Current instrumentation is identical to the equipment used by urologists for prostatic surgery. As the uterine cavity is quite unlike the bladder in volume, compliance and shape, even the modern continuous-flow resectoscope is not the ideal instrument for intrauterine surgery. The rounded cutting loops mean that ridges are left between resected furrows possibly containing residual endometrium; the small size of the outflow perforations mean that the resected debris is not aspirated from the cavity as it is cut but remains to gradually obstruct the view and can only be extracted by first removing the resectoscope. A gynaecological resectoscope which overcomes these shortcomings would have great advantages, not only during endometrial resection, but also with hysteroscopic myomectomy.

Hysteroscopic techniques, whether using laser energy or electrosurgery, involve uterine distension, usually with a fluid medium. Although fluid overload is easily prevented by ceasing surgery before there is any risk to the patient, better

211

control of intrauterine pressure and particularly automated monitoring of the volume of fluid absorbed would considerably enhance surgical safety. The pumps currently available only partially address these aspects of surgery and, as with hysteroscopes themselves, technical advances are to be expected.

Conceptually as well as technically simpler are those approaches to endometrial destruction which are performed blindly and merely involve the placement of a probe or agent within the uterine cavity. This is how endometrial ablation started in the 1960s, and it may be that we will go full circle by the start of the next century. Radiofrequency thermal ablation is one such technique which is already available, but restricted to the treatment of dysfunctional bleeding. Other approaches suitable for women with enlarged fibroid uteri would be the next logical development in this area.

Of course, the ultimate 'minimally invasive' solution to menorrhagia would be one that is non-invasive. For instance, antibodies specifically active against endometrium would be the easiest, and theoretically the most effective, solution to the eternal problem of menorrhagia. The surgeon gynaecologist would become a physician, and lasers, electrosurgical generators and the like would be moved from the operating theatre to the museum as items of medical history. This day may not be too far away, as advances in molecular biology influence more and more aspects of medical practice.

Now, however, we have at our disposal the techniques described in this book. Their use is becoming increasingly widespread as medical thinking accepts that hysterectomy may be the ultimate, but not the only, surgical solution to abnormal menstruation. In the immediate future, the most important future prospect must be the safe and appropriate application of these procedures by trained personnel. The tales and rumours which pervade the gynaecological community suggest that this may not always have been the case. If nothing more, this book will hopefully play a part in improving our understanding and use of this exciting treatment, endometrial ablation.

Index